CLINICAL LABORATORY SCIENCE

Education & Management

M. Ann Wallace, MS, MT(ASCP), CLS
Assistant Professor
Clinical Laboratory Science/Medical Technology
Wayne State University
College of Pharmacy and Allied Health Professions
Detroit, Michigan

Deanna D. Klosinski, PhD, MT(ASCP), DLM
Assistant Professor
Division of Medical Education
Department of Family Medicine
School of Medicine
and
Adjunct Assistant Professor
College of Pharmacy and Allied Health Professions
Wayne State University
Detroit, Michigan

Department of Clinical Pathology
William Beaumont Hospital
Royal Oak, Michigan

CLINICAL LABORATORY SCIENCE
Education & Management

W.B. SAUNDERS COMPANY
A Division of Harcourt Brace & Company
Philadelphia London Toronto Montreal Sydney Tokyo

W.B. SAUNDERS COMPANY
A Division of Harcourt Brace & Company

The Curtis Center
Independence Square West
Philadelphia, Pennsylvania 19106

Library of Congress Cataloging-in-Publication Data

Clinical laboratory science education and management / M. Ann Wallace, Deanna D. Klosinski.

p. cm.

ISBN 0–7216–4543–7

1. Medical laboratory technology—Study and teaching. 2. Pathological laboratories—Management. I. Klosinski, Deanna D. II. Title.

RB37.5.W35 1998 616.07′068—dc21

DNLM/DLC 96-49581

CLINICAL LABORATORY SCIENCE AND MANAGEMENT ISBN 0–7216–4543–7

Printed in the United States of America.

Last digit is the print number: 9 8 7 6 5 4 3 2 1

"To all of my students, who have helped me become a better teacher."

M. Ann Wallace

"To my family, colleagues, co-workers, students, and other learners who challenge me to live by the principles I espouse."

Deanna D. Klosinski

Preface

Clinical Laboratory Science Education and Management presents the basic tenets of both education and management for practical applications in the field of laboratory medicine. This book resulted from our observation, over the several years we co-taught this course, of the lack of textbooks appropriate for individuals exposed to teaching and supervising, perhaps for the first time. Out of necessity, we began to develop extensive handouts, notes, and exercises to convey essential principles and help students to build relevant skills. A primary objective for writing this text stemmed from our commitment to provide cohesive teaching materials. We were challenged to grow from where we were as accomplished teachers in classroom settings to authors sharing our combined experiences in this textbook. We believe learning is best accomplished through interaction; therefore, we designed activities to engage readers, as adult learners, to be involved in their learning. We identified and collected the components of the processes and arranged their presentation in an orderly and consecutive manner.

This text provides an assortment of introductory materials for several groups of readers. The first group is made up of students in academic and clinical laboratory science programs at the undergraduate and graduate levels: clinical laboratory science/medical technology, cytotechnology, histotechnology, molecular biology, pathology assistant, and other medical, allied health, and bioscience disciplines. Another group of readers is the practicing laboratorians and scientists and other health caregivers who have been designated to take on or have advanced to clinical teaching and supervision responsibilities. This text will enable them to gain confidence through planned practice. It would assist individuals who are actively teaching and/or supervising but who have not received formal instruction in educational and managerial principles and processes. The information and activities presented in this text would be of benefit for teaching and supervising training in other health care disciplines.

Components of both education and managerial processes are presented, discussed, and applied by incorporating a variety of activities and review questions in each chapter. The activities represent real-life situations involving learning/teaching, supervising, and managing. Many of the activities have been developed following the small group learning model and are adaptable to individual effort. This format allows for each reader to assume leadership (of the group) and engage in opportunities to experience listening, translating, compromising, and summarizing the group's reactions and conclusions. The wide scope of readers will find the comprehensive list of topics covered in both disciplines pertinent in meeting their current and future needs as educators and managers.

The Education chapters are sequentially arranged and start with remote preparation, the formation of objectives, and the investigation of the hierarchical domains to culminate with correctly correlating the level of domain to each specific objective. The variety of teaching methodologies, testing, and the correction of tests follows. The evaluation of both readers (as students or laboratorians) and teachers is discussed. The teacher receives attention within these topics in several chapters. The roles, which have grown in number and in depth, are explored, as are the attributes that fall under the headings of technical, teaching, and personal qualities. The last education chapter summarizes the contributions that governmental and professional organizations and agencies have made and continue to make for clinical laboratory science education.

The topics presented in the management chapters, 11 through 20, address the broad range of knowledge and skills that would be used by anyone who is in leadership, supervisory, or managerial roles. Selected information is presented in each chapter to give readers different and relevant experiences applicable for the variety of work settings in health care.

Using the organized and logical approach that adheres to traditional management theories, the sequence of the topics in management is similar to the sequence of the topics in education. Planning should precede all work in order to fulfill the desired outcomes. Organizing, directing, controlling, and coordinating functions consume many hours that managers devote in order to fulfill their responsibilities. Evaluating the processes, the people, and the products or services completes this cycle.

External factors that influence managerial activity are presented in other chapters. Two major forces are regulations and finance. These topics are quite comprehensive for supervisors and managers in the workplace. For readers of this text, information and activities were chosen that most likely represent what the beginning supervisor would be expected to do.

Several additional miscellaneous topics are introduced with the encouragement to readers to seek more information on the basis of their interest and needs. These topics, which are outcomes management, marketing, empowerment, and customer relations, are no less important in the workplace but may not be in much demand initially of a new supervisor.

We hope that this book will fulfill the needs of readers. Some may seek training and opportunities to teach, lead, and supervise. For others who are experiencing challenges as teachers or supervisors, we believe they will find practical applications from the text and activities.

Both educating and managing are dynamic processes. Educators and managers are not born, they are taught and trained to blend the objective processes of each science with the facets of their minds and the expression of their personalities. Those who have innate abilities and talents for educating and managing will enjoy these disciplines as art.

M. Ann Wallace, MS, MT(ASCP), CLS
Deanna D. Klosinski, PhD, MT(ASCP), DLM

Acknowledgments

We would like to thank Daniel C. Smigell, education sales representative, and Selma Kaszczuk, Senior Acquisitions Editor at W.B. Saunders Company, who believed in the idea and need proposed by M. Ann Wallace for a combined book in education and management. We thank Rachael Kelly, Assistant Developmental Editor, for the attention and time she gave to us. We also want to acknowledge Edna Dick, Copy Editor, Jeff Gunning, Production Manager, and Karen O'Keefe, Designer, who contributed to the beautiful presentation of the book and text through their transcribing, editing, and designing. Matt Andrews and Sharon Iwanczuk, the artists who contributed the cartoons throughout the book, are appreciated for their talents in "translating" our words into characters and mini-scenes. Acknowledgment is well deserved for the special mentors, Martha Winstead, Bettina G. Martin, Thomas F. Dutcher, and Daniel H. Farkas, and the many professional colleagues of Deanna Klosinski for their tolerance of her ideas and convictions that principles can be valued in the workplace. Several co-workers at William Beaumont Hospital, Royal Oak, Michigan, likewise contributed to the thoughts written by Deanna Klosinski in their collaboration on laboratory manuals and policies: Joyce M. King, Frederick L. Kiechle, Joan C. Mattson, Noelle Procopio, Nancy F. Ramirez, JoAnn Logue-O'Malley, and Sandra L. Collins.

Further acknowledgment by M. Ann Wallace is extended to Cris Ford of the CLS/MT Department at Wayne State University for her continual support during the writing of the education segment, and to Deanna Klosinski for joining her in this great venture.

Contents

Education

There has always existed a need in clinical laboratory science to instruct students in the Educational Process, the science of teaching, and all it encompasses. The recognition and understanding of the various learning patterns is also essential and critical.

Reorganization in the hospital setting is witnessing the destruction of traditional department structures together with the advent of multiskilled personnel who are providing better patient care. As a result, clinical laboratory scientists are finding themselves in positions as instructors not only for the laboratory staff but also for those in other departmental specialties.

This has been recognized by all educators in the health care field with the result that emphasis in training is being placed on providing activities that will develop not only better communication skills (listening, discussing, compromising) but will also provide a generation of clinical laboratory scientists who have been trained to teach.

Enough! Turn the page and let's get started!

The Education Process: Getting Ready

OBJECTIVES

Upon completion of this chapter, the reader should be able to:

- Outline a plan of work in preparation for teaching a course. By priority, list the necessary steps to be taken while organizing the strategy.
- Identify the components of the Educational Process. Define and explain the significance of each.
- Define "effective teaching" from your own experiences and observations of the various instructors you have had throughout your education and through reading.
- Write a short paper within your group on what you think the philosophy of teachers in Clinical Laboratory Science should reflect.

KEY WORDS

educational process
effective teaching
instructional preparation

Introduction

Why is it always so difficult to start anything? We say to ourselves, "Where do I begin"? Also, as you prepare to teach, you may remember outstanding teachers and recall how everything just seemed to be in place, how the hour lecture flowed so smoothly. After serious consideration, you will realize that there are so many facets of teaching of which you are not even aware, that the question "Just where **do** I start?" will arise again and again. With every activity you have ever tackled in your life, your approach was systematic. You defined your objectives in pursuing the project and organized all the aspects and details that would sooner or later demand your attention.

Getting Started

In preparing to teach in the Clinical Laboratory Science (CLS) program, you would do likewise. Whether you plan to teach in the clinical or academic setting, remote preparation does not differ significantly; only the scope of the teaching load will vary. Some suggestions on how you approach the teaching assignment might help to get you started:

1. In the university, ask your chairperson for a written description of your assignment; look to see what it specifically encompasses, including scheduled contact hours and free time. In the clinical setting, meet with your department head and ask for the department syllabus that accompanies the area to which you have been assigned. Read the syllabus carefully to identify specifically those areas for which you will be held responsible.

2. If you have been assigned to teach an established course, ask to see previous course outlines. These should be found in the department self-study manual. These outlines will present various organizational plans of lecture and laboratory material. This can be done in the clinical laboratory also. These outlines provide the distinct advantage of allowing you to visualize another

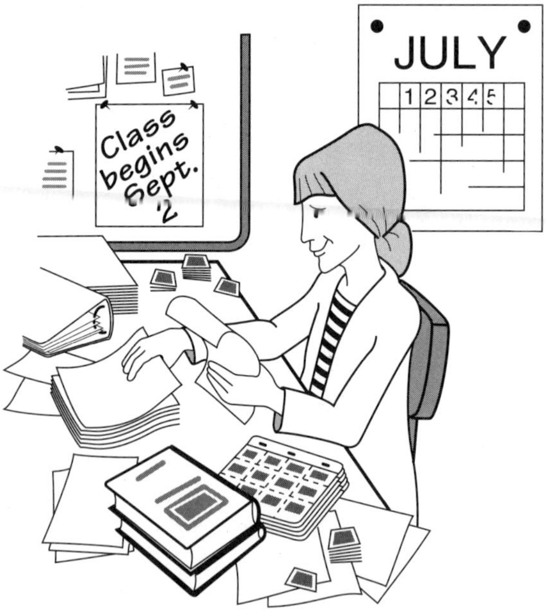

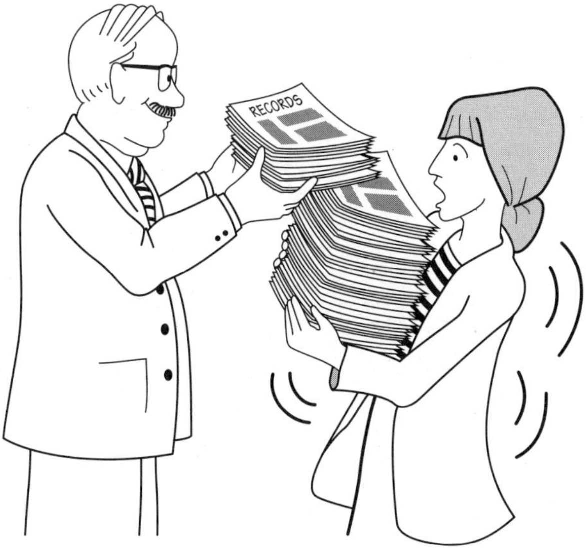

teacher's systematic planning and recognize the sequential presentation of material and the accompanying planned laboratory exercises. It surpasses the other alternative: starting from scratch.

3. Review the textbook that had been adopted as the official text for the students. Study its organization, presentation of material, charts, and photographs. Check the publication date; books become outdated very quickly, especially in the sciences. Investigate other texts on the market. Publishers' sales representatives are eager to provide *free* examination copies, hoping that you will adopt their book as your text.

4. Investigate the file cabinets in your office. Look for a class syllabus the previous teacher used to see which aspects of the discipline were emphasized.

5. Ask for the average number of students who are admitted annually. In addition, get a feel for the diversity of the class. In the clinical laboratory, it is most likely that you will have two students rotating through your department at the same time. Planning for this number presents no problems.

6. Check the laboratory equipment and the reagents you will be using. Find out if the instructor provided a laboratory manual to be used by the students or the back part of a text that contains laboratory procedures.

7. Ask to see the forms used by students in evaluating instructors. This will tell you what the students expect of you. The clinical laboratories provide lengthier forms for evaluation of instructors. This will provide a helpful check-off list of activities dealing with teaching, student/teacher relationships, and methodology.

This type of remote preparation is helpful because you begin to engage in planning, whether you realize it or not. You are *data gathering;* as you gather, you automatically make judgments regarding what you have found: "This is good"; "No, I can't use this"; "What terrific notes!" "This teacher has saved me a lot of time in planning, at least for the first year." "What a terrific reference library this instructor has collected!"

You have accomplished the following:

- You got your feet wet, and it wasn't too traumatic. We are all good data collectors.
- You established the overview of the course in the university department/ in the clinical setting, for which you will be responsible.

- You have a good idea of which texts are available for adoption.
- You have a concise knowledge of what to emphasize in your course.
- You know what laboratory equipment is running, which pieces of equipment need to be "fixed" before classes start, and which reagents need to be ordered.
- You can breathe a little bit easier! You feel you have things under control.
- And further, upon investigation, you have found an excellent collection of educational books in the departmental library, many of which have teaching tips for teachers at all levels of experience.

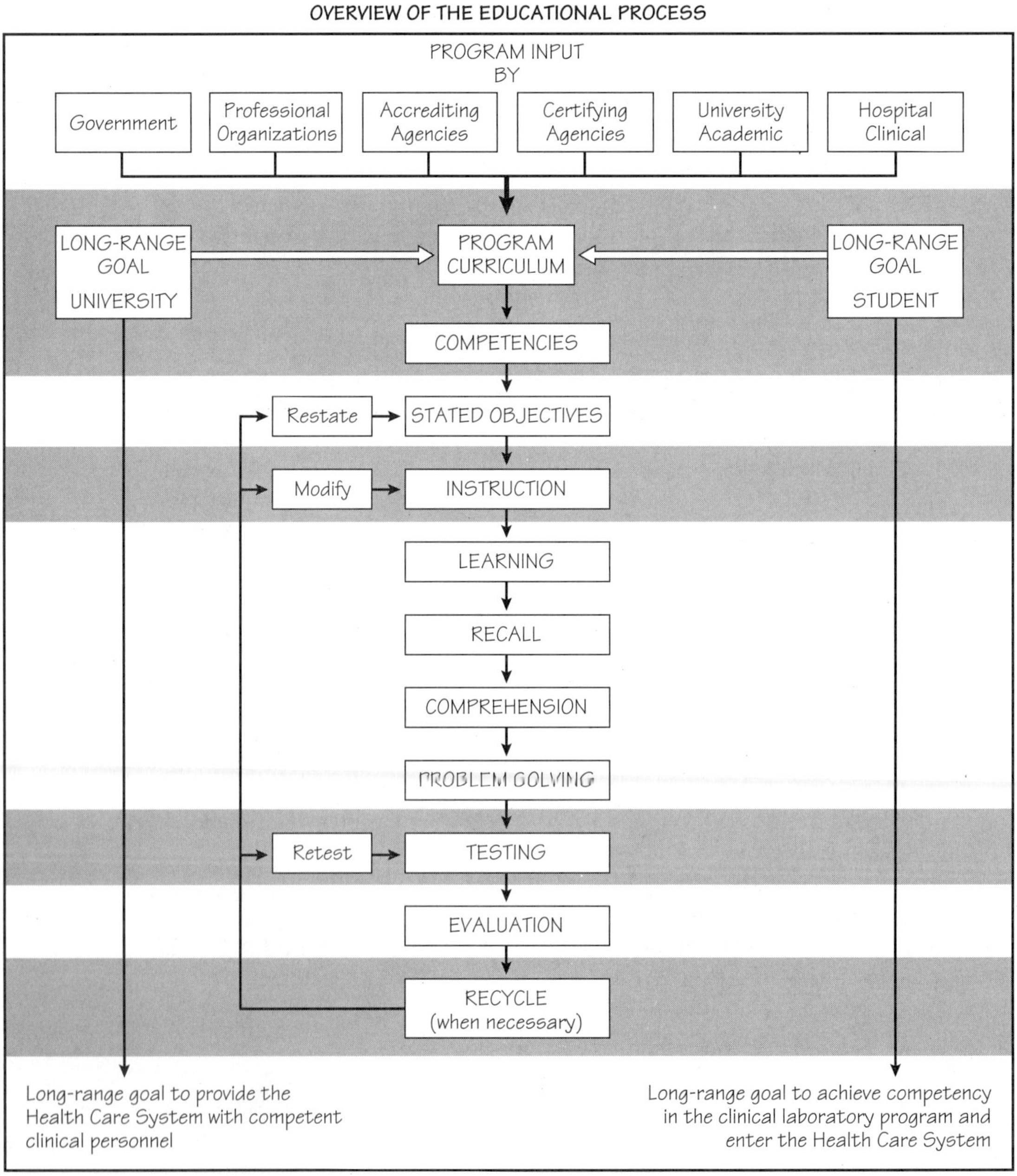

Figure 1–1 Overview of the Educational Process.

The Educational Process (See Fig. 1–1)

Once all the preparatory organization has been initiated, you will become aware of the "Educational Process" as applied to CLS and the other professions. For every profession and business, there is an organizational chart that defines and clarifies the process that must be followed in order to efficiently and profitably achieve the objectives of the organization. Applying this principle to the profession of education has resulted in the construction of a directional educational flow chart that guides the instructor to recognize the sequential steps in the process of teaching/learning. This flow chart is found in most educational texts. Although they might differ in minor aspects, they all depict the basics of the "Educational Process" in essentially the same manner. However expressed, the process must include the following essentials:

- *Competencies* defined and incorporated into the "Essentials" by the professional organizations and agencies that comprise and specify the body of knowledge and skills that must be mastered by students attending accredited CLS programs
- Trained faculty teaching in accredited educational programs that represent both university academic and departmental clinical rotation segments
- Stated objectives established by the educators in translating and stating the *competencies* into behavioral, observable directives
- Instruction that provides for the acquisition and mastery of specific knowledge and development of high-level psychomotor skills
- Development and use of testing mechanisms that measure the degree of learning by the students
- Evaluation tools that indicate to what degree the competencies have been mastered
- Formation of a professional attitude that identifies with the moral and ethical practice of laboratory medicine
- A mechanism whereby the retention of learners with different styles of learning is activated. (Some mechanisms are having the student use a tutor, establishing group learning sessions, and meeting with students individually.)

After a clinical laboratory scientist enters the educational aspect of the

COMPONENTS OF THE EDUCATIONAL PROCESS	
1. PROGRAM CURRICULUM	5. TESTING PROGRAM
2. COMPETENCIES	6. EVALUATION
3. STATED OBJECTIVES	7. REPETITION OF THE CYCLE when necessary
4. INSTRUCTION	

profession, there are several "first steps" to be taken. The newly appointed instructor and the newly appointed graduated CLS student in the clinic must (1) examine the educational process and identify that section of basic knowledge and skills for which they will be responsible and (2) become cognizant of the science of teaching and the educational resources available for them to become effective teachers. Step 1 has been carried out. Now you devote your time and efforts on how to become "effective teachers." The following charts should provide guidance to clinical instructors.

GUIDELINES FOR CLINICAL INSTRUCTION

I. Preparatory: Prior to Arrival of Students

A. Establish overall goal and objectives.

1. Review the Competencies and Stated Objectives for the specific rotation.
2. Develop a pretest to assess knowledge and skills of the students.
3. Construct a plan of work based on daily activities for the number of weeks spent in that rotation.
4. Clearly list the responsibilities of students during rotation.
5. Develop a form through which students can express their personal expectations from this rotation.

II. Implementation of Program

A. Establish rapport with the new students.

1. Administer the pretest; establish academic and laboratory needs for each student.
2. Establish a dialogue, and communicate with each student; clearly state the behavioral objectives and relate to entry-level abilities.
3. Ensure that the learner clearly understands the professional expectations of performance.

B. Provide a structured schedule of activities.

1. Relate the activities to the goals and stated objectives.
2. Include a variety of experiences through which students can achieve the objectives.
3. Schedule "free time" to be used by students in activities that reinforce the objectives.
4. Provide for "group learning experiences."
5. Remain available for consultation.

C. Develop reliable testing and evaluation tools.

1. Use questions that have been tested for wording and objectivity.
2. Provide immediate feedback.

Chart continued on opposite page

GUIDELINES FOR CLINICAL INSTRUCTION *(Continued)*

3. Review all test items with students.
4. Evaluate performance against objectives.
5. Reteach and retest when necessary.
6. Reevaluate performance together with the student.

D. Terminate learning.

CLINICAL EXPERIENCE EVALUATION

Atmosphere

Relaxed, conducive to learning
Help of personnel other than the instructor
Availability of space for student to work and study
Availability of supplies and equipment

Comments:

Material

Quality of specimens
Quality of abnormal specimens for students

Comments:

Rotation Coordinator

Interest in student
Patience with student
Time available for student when needed
Ability to impart knowledge of material
Periodic constructive appraisal of student progress
Keeps student informed of teaching schedule
Keeps student on schedule
Informs student of any schedule changes

Comments:

Instructor

Interest in student
Patience with student
Develops learning objectives based on job expectations
- Informs student of objectives
- Creates an atmosphere in which student expresses ideas and asks questions

Chart continued on following page

CLINICAL EXPERIENCE EVALUATION *(Continued)*

Ability to impart knowledge of material
Ability to answer questions
Interest in material taught
Demonstrations well organized
Time available for students
Sets a good example for students

Comments:

---

1. a. For this rotation, indicate the approximate time (in %) spent (should add up to 100%):
   _____ Performing technical procedures with direct or indirect supervision
   _____ Performing technical procedures without supervision
   _____ Studying during *assigned* study periods with no specific activity assigned
   _____ Other (please explain)

   b. If specific activity was not assigned, how did you spend your time?

---

2. a. Indicate the types of instruction used during the supervised training time:
   _____ demonstrations
   _____ lectures and/or discussions
   _____ reading manuals
   _____ A/V aids
   _____ study questions
   _____ case-study discussions
   _____ other (please identify)

   b. Which methods did you find most helpful?
   c. Was the material presented at a rate that permitted you to comprehend and absorb details?

---

3. Did you find the theoretical information offered in discussions:
   a. relatively easy
   b. moderately in-depth
   c. difficult but challenging
   d. none of the above (please comment)

---

4. Did you find the theoretical information offered in *reference* material:
   a. insufficient
   b. sufficient but relatively easy
   c. organized and moderately in-depth or difficult
   d. organized, concise, and challenging
   e. none of the above (please comment)

---

5. Were you provided with a schedule of topics to be covered and the necessary reference material?
   a. always
   b. sometimes
   c. usually
   d. rarely

Chart continued on opposite page

CLINICAL EXPERIENCE EVALUATION *(Continued)*
6. How well did the examinations correlate with and cover the subject matter? a. inadequately b. sometimes adequately c. adequately d. very adequately
7. Were you informed of your progress after completing each task? a. always b. usually c. sometimes d. rarely
8. Would you like to work in this area? Comment.

Signs of Effective Teaching

Every year toward the end of the final semester in academia, and in the hospital toward the end of clinical training rotation, awards are given to those individuals chosen as "Outstanding Teachers of the Year." In the academic setting, a special assembly of the university faculty is held at which these honors are awarded. As each teacher's name is announced, he/she is escorted to the stage, and a short narrative is delivered on the reasons that this teacher is being honored, including such academic achievements, as publications, patents, discoveries, and presentations. Accompanying the list of these personal achievements is a testimony, submitted by students, as to how they were intellectually stimulated by that teacher to achieve and accomplish recognition for their own academic work.

In the hospital setting, the criteria for the awards are established by the senior CLS students. This includes the personal involvement the teacher has established with the students, the specific methodology of teaching used to

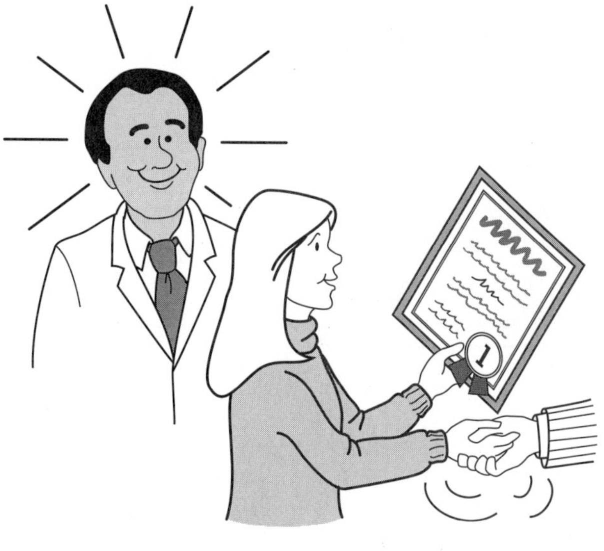

cover the required material, and the special attention they received from the teacher that helped them to learn. Thus, the first aspect of "Effective Teaching" involves the student. The criteria used by students in identifying an exceptional teacher reveal that it was neither their personal knowledge nor accomplishments but rather *how* the teacher perceived and treated the students, the respect the teachers demonstrated during instruction, and the *type* of instruction that led students to want to learn and achieve independently. Barbara G. Davis, in her book *Tools for Teaching* states the following:

> Research on students' academic success and intellectual development and on theories of learning and cognitive development, has demonstrated the effectiveness of modes of instruction that emphasize *active learning* and collaborative activities that *engage* students in intellectual activity.[1]

The implication is that the instructor knows and understands the students in his or her class; works at knowing what they already know; interacts with them by providing activities and assignments in which they can learn independently, thus building onto their already acquired base of knowledge and skills. To this end, Davis encourages instructors to concentrate their efforts on four main considerations:

1. Organize and vary the methodology of teaching in such a way that the material can be understood by all the students
2. Create an environment conducive to learning,
3. Encourage students to learn on their own, to become autonomous, and
4. Evaluate yourself periodically to see that the learning process by the students is continual. This reflects the consistency of your effective teaching.

It's obvious! One of the keys to successful teaching is to know the subject matter so well, so completely, that in the hands of the teacher, it can be manipulated and presented in one manner, and again, if necessary, in a

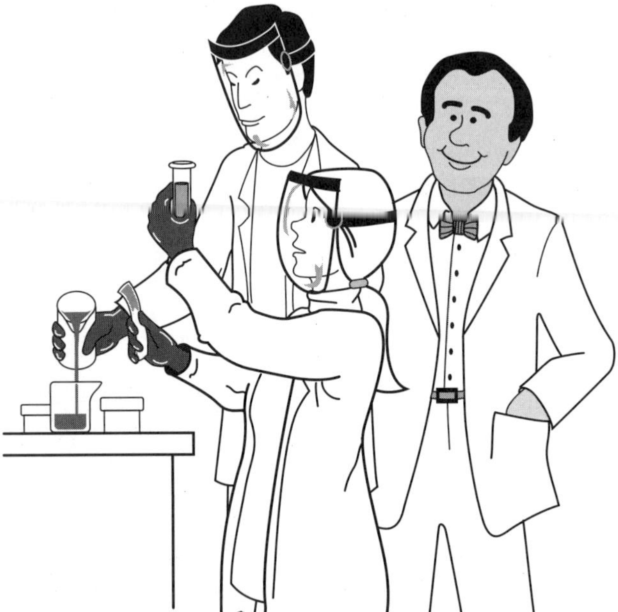

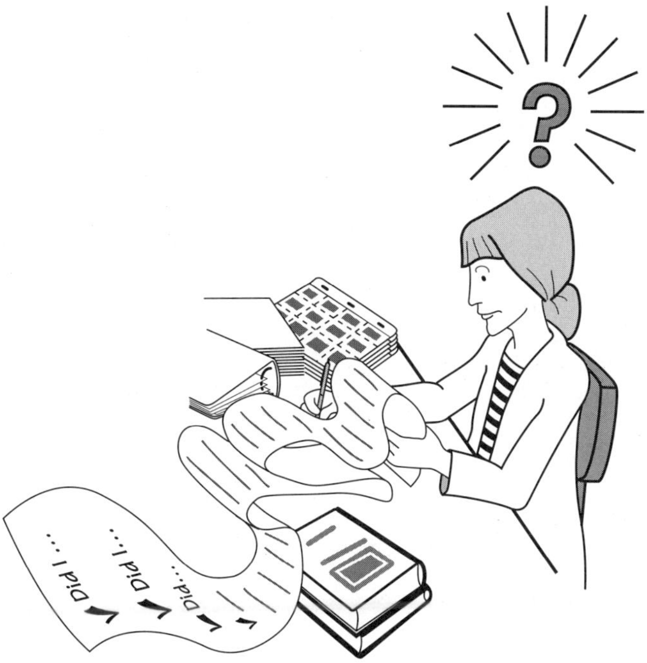

completely different format, perhaps a story, or through the use of an analogy and for one purpose alone: *to reach all students.*

Did you notice the verbs used by Dr. Davis? "Organize, create, encourage, evaluate." These are very active verbs: activities that should challenge the teacher in planning her lecture/activities. Lowman, in describing what "masterful teaching" is, describes three different situations: an awe-inspiring scholar lecturing from a stage of an amphitheater to a spellbound audience leaning forward, eager to catch every word that is spoken. A second scene depicts a warm person, seated at a table with a group of students, facilitating a discussion and encouraging critical thinking. The third describes a group of students in the professor's study, drinking beer with students in close proximity, able to observe how the teacher thinks and how he has committed his life to the development and expression of ideas and the achievement of knowledge through discussion. Lowman identifies these examples in which effective teaching can take place and identifies the types of skills necessary for superior teaching to take place: The instructor must demonstrate the ability to deliver clear, intellectually exciting lectures, and he or she must possess interpersonal skills. He states, "To become an excellent instructor, one must be outstanding in one of these sets of skills and at least competent in the other."[2]

Lowman emphasizes that the student is indeed No. 1 and that effective teachers must develop and master a style, a means of communication, that is consistent with their personae: one that is authentic and one in which both instructor and students feel comfortable. What works so well for one instructor can fail for another.

Weimer adds:

> . . . that the component of effective instruction can be acquired. Some of the difficulty derives from the fact that characteristics of good teaching are highly abstract. They are not concrete entities that one goes out and acquires. However, the characteristics manifest themselves as behaviors. Enthusiastic instructors *do*

> certain things that convey their interest and energy. We can identify what those behaviors are: they move about, look intently at students, and vary their tone of voice, for example.[3]

Adding to the ingredients that characterize *effective teaching,* Weimer has added the expressions of teachers that are so personal and unique to each, that the same motion and facial expression could not be duplicated or mimicked by another in an attempt to convey the same message. Hanna and McGill state the following:

> Four sets of competencies described in various ways by researchers seem to stand out when teachers, identified as excellent at the community college level, describe how they behave in various situations. According to Baker, Boggs, and Putnam (1983), these effective teachers displayed the following:
>
> - A student-centered orientation
> - A value for the learning process
> - A need to influence individual behavior, and
> - A belief that they possessed the power to produce a desired effect in the learner[4]

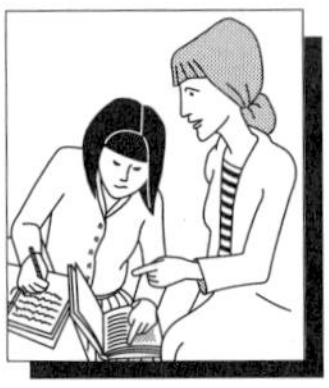

Activity 1

From the references above (and any other sources or experiences), compose a definition or a description of "Effective Teaching."

By priority, list the characteristics in that order (Group Activity).

Definition:

Characteristics:

Activity 2

Research the literature for publications dealing further with *Effective Teaching.* Summarize and write a critique of your article. Make an outline of your critique. Include the *reference, journal name, title of article, date, and author name(s).*

RESOURCES AVAILABLE FOR TEACHER FORMATION

The formation of the teacher is our next consideration. The definition of a teacher is one who *causes* someone to know a subject, to *cause* an individual *to know how; to cause students to think for themselves.* The types of activities and resources available to assist the instructors in developing the art of teaching are many.

On the Job

When a CLS program advertises for an individual with specific expertise in a discipline to teach in the educational program, the advertisement never includes any requirement for indication of instructional background. *It is only when the candidate is hired that his or her instruction in the Educational Process begins.* Newly hired teachers are made aware of the "competencies" and the correct stating of the behavioral objectives for their courses. In some departments, new faculty members are assigned mentors—senior faculty members—to assist them in becoming proficient instructors. In some universities, very informal interdepartmental meetings are held (all voluntary) during lunch time to discuss ways of becoming effective teachers.

Observation

Instructors known and recognized as outstanding teachers are more than willing to be observed by those learning to teach. Give attention to the following:

- The presentation of the objectives for the lecture
- The format of the handouts and the syllabus
- The methodology of instruction
- The ability to generate student discussion
- The caliber of discussion that provokes intellectual stimulation
- The activity of the students
- The instructor–student rapport
- The ease displayed by the instructor in fielding questions
- The energy level and excitement that pervades the classroom

Then apply and adapt those factors to your own style and expression.

Educational References

A visit to the Education section of the university and the departmental libraries in the hospital will yield numerous journals and books related to instruction. Every aspect of the Educational Process continues to be studied, re-

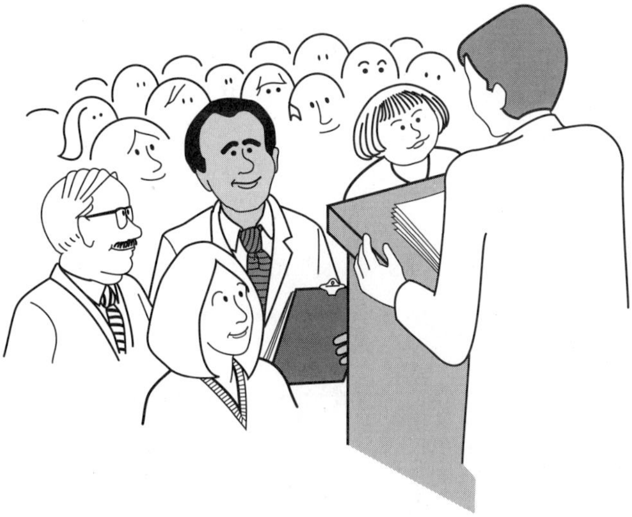

viewed, and improved. Excellent texts published solely to share "Teaching Tips" are very accessible. (See Suggested Reading section.)

Local Seminars, Conventions, Continuing Education in the Professional Journal

The rising concern of educating students for their roles in the clinical laboratory, which includes the science of teaching, has resulted in including programs dealing with instruction, especially "Problem-Solving" and the "small group" method of learning, at the various professional meetings. The presenters are teachers who have used the methods of instruction in their own teaching and provide, by simulation, a class of students experiencing (consisting of the teachers), with direction, the dynamics of the "small group" approach.

Student Evaluation

Both the university and the clinical programs require students to evaluate each instructor at the end of each course. The students are asked to comment on the course and the instructor. When analyzing the questions contained on the evaluation questionnaire, the questions reflect the information contained on the "Syllabus" instructors give to students the first day of class. These questions are directed to the organization of the class, the communication given to students regarding lecture schedule, exam schedule, and so forth. What is helpful to new teachers is to review the evaluation form to see what factors the university considers important enough to include in a university-wide teacher evaluation form.

Examples of questions referring to the evaluation of the instructor include the following:

- At the beginning of the course, the overall class plan was clearly presented.
- The class plan was followed reasonably well.
- At the beginning of the course, my responsibilities as a student were made clear.
- All things considered, the instructor was available to me.
- The grading procedures were explained at the start of the class.
- The material presented in the class and in assignments was fairly represented on examinations.

And dealing with the Affective Domain:

- The instructor *treated* all students, including me, fairly, and with respect.
- The instructor *provided* prompt feedback on my performance on assigned activities.
- Overall the instructor *did* a good job of teaching this course.

Basically, students are honest and tell it as it is. An instructor, on reading their comments, has to realize their responses reflect how *they* see him/her, not how the *instructor* sees himself/herself. These evaluations provide good reading matter for self-reflection. Many changes in an instructional course have taken place because of substantial comments made by students through these evaluations. It is the practice of the university that there always be anonymity.

The evaluation forms used in the clinical program give equally good feedback to the *novice student teacher.* Similar feedback provided by the new students finishing a rotation through the departments covers similar factors in their evaluations. These include the method of teaching, the manner in which it was taught, the provision of meaningful activities, the establishment of a good instructor/student relationship, and an expressed concern by the teacher for the students' achievement and success.

Administrators of CLS Programs

Administrators of CLS programs accept the responsibility to try and provide for the individuals teaching and training students in their programs, a means by which they can learn to become effective teachers. A certain amount of the budget is usually targeted for such purposes. Teachers: keep an eye open to programs you think will be of assistance to you.

Self-Evaluation for Self-Improvement by the Instructor

No matter the number of years an instructor has been teaching the same course—whether one, few, or many—it is good, wholesome, and wise to conduct a self-evaluation on one's own teaching just about the time the students perform theirs. Examples of questions instructors could consider regarding their performance are as follows:

- Why did I choose to be a teacher?
- What is my philosophy on teaching?
- Have I been aware of the expression *effective teacher?* Can I identify with it?
- Have I made an effort to improve my teaching? If the answer is yes, specifically what action have I taken?

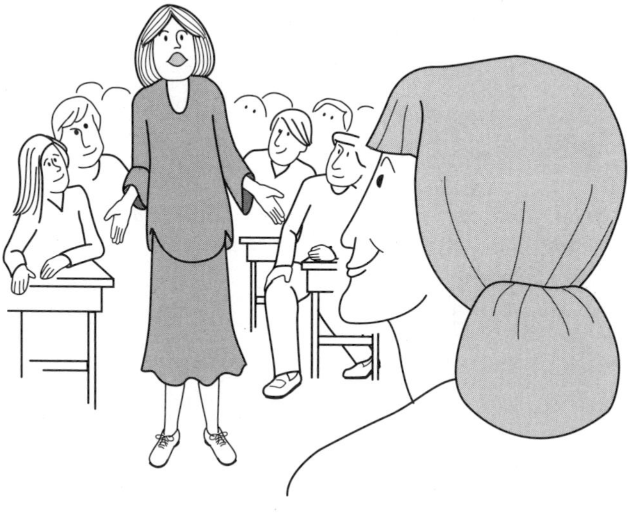

- On what basis do I choose a text for the discipline I teach?
- What criteria do I use when I change my test? How often have I done this?
- How often do I review my handouts in order to update the information?
- Have I improved the kodachromes I used in my lectures? (If applicable.)
- Do I relate feature stories released by the news media dealing with the topic I teach in order to emphasize a relevancy of the condition, the disease state?
- Have I tried to eliminate unnecessary material from my lecture? (Such material tends to confuse students in discerning what is and what is not essential information.)
- Have I improved the language of my stated objectives?
- Do I refer to the stated objectives when I teach and test?
- Have I recently reviewed the competencies set forth by the professional organizations and agencies to see if they are stressed in the stated objectives?
- Do I discuss what I teach with others in the field to see what insights they have on both teaching and teaching methods?

Efforts to Improve Teacher/Student Relationships

- Do I treat students as adults? Do I show them respect?
- *How* do I show it? How often do I show it?
- Have I tried to improve my relationship with students by trying to understand their situations outside the lecture room and how their life away from the classroom affects their academic studies?
- Do I communicate to the students that it is important to me that they *must understand* what is taught?
- Do I encourage them to come for help? Let me reword this: *Do I invite them to come for help?*
- Do I act as a friend to the students? Do I show interest in helping them succeed?

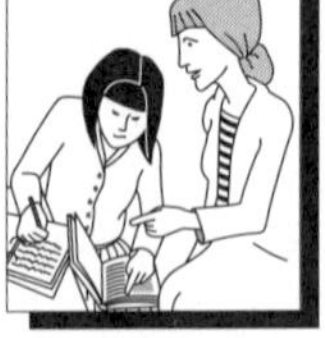

Activity 3:

Within your group, discuss and summarize those factors important to the group members that deal with instructor behavior in the classroom. List the items by priority (group chosen).

Summary

The 80s and early 90s have been extraordinary decades with respect to the influx of instructional and educational programs through new texts and other publications for those instructors involved in CLS teaching. The availability of "teaching tips" that apply to all facets of CLS instruction—both in the academic and clinical aspects of the program—assist all instructors in achieving the goal of becoming effective teachers.

The recognition that feedback from students in portraying ourselves as they see and experience us should be recognized as essential in helping us to see ourselves as they see us. Attention should be given to how your students relate to you. Treat them as your best friends. Respect and honor their minds and their persons. Let them feel this and rest secure in it.

Review Questions

1. List in order the eight components that comprise the Educational Process.
2. In retrospect, can you relate to or recognize the Educational Process as described in this chapter? In what classes can you associate its planning to that which best follows and reflects the process?
3. Describe, in your own words, an Effective Teacher.

See p. 405 for answers.

References

1. Davis BG. Tools for Teaching. San Francisco, Jossey-Bass Publishers, 1993, Preface pp xiii–xxiii.
2. Lowman J. Mastering the Techniques of Teaching. San Francisco, Jossey-Bass Publishers, 1984, pp 1–22.
3. Weimer M. It's a Myth: Good Teachers are Born, Not Made. *In* Weimer M, Neff R, eds. Teaching College. Madison, Wisc, Magna Publications, 1990, pp 15–16.
4. Hanna SJ, McGill LT. Nurturing Environment and Effective Teaching. *In* Weimer M, Neff R, eds. Teaching College. Madison, Wisc, Magna Publications, 1990, pp 17–20.

Suggested Reading

1. Baker G, Boggs G, Putnam S. Ideal Environment Nurtures Excellence. Community and Junior College Journal Oct. 1983.
2. Neff R, Weimer M, eds. Classroom Communication: Collected Reading for Effective Discussion and Questioning. Madison, Wisc, Magna Publications, 1989.
3. Davis BG. Tools for Teaching. San Francisco, Jossey-Bass Publishers, 1993.
4. Eble KE. The Craft of Teaching. 2nd ed. San Francisco, Jossey-Bass Publishers, 1990.
5. Reiguth CM, Erlbaum L, eds. Hillsdale, NJ, Association Publishers, 1983.
6. Johnson GR. First Steps to Excellence in College Teaching. 2nd ed. Madison, Wisc, Magna Publications, 1990.
7. Michels E. Enhancing the Scholarly Base: The Role of Faculty in Enhancing Scholarship. Commentary. Journal of Allied Health Winter 1989, 129–141.
8. One hundred forty-seven practical tips for teaching professors. The Teaching Professor. Madison, Wisc, Magna Publications, 1990.
9. Weimer M, Neff R, eds. Teaching College—Collected Readings for the New Instructor. Madison, Wisc, Magna Publications, 1990.
10. The Teaching Professor. All Issues. Madison, Wisc, Magna Publications.
11. Udolf R. The College Instructor's Guide to Teaching and Academia. Chicago, Nelson-Hall Publishers, 1976.

2

Roles of the Teacher: Multifunctional

OBJECTIVES

Upon completion of this chapter, the reader should be able to:

- Identify and *identify with* the roles of the teacher.
- Discuss each role as in depth as possible and construct a list of further attributes, areas of involvement, in which the instructor will become involved.
- List, by importance the essential qualities of the teacher.
- Enumerate the factors involved in immediate preparation for a lecture/laboratory session.
- List the advantages and limitations of the various types of audio/visual (AV) equipment; discuss several types of AV equipment and qualify how they would enhance specific types of instruction.

KEY WORDS

roles
skills
attributes

Introduction

In Chapter 1, the "remote preparation" of the teacher was discussed. All the activities undertaken fulfilled the task of introducing the teacher to considerations that had to be faced, preparations that had to be made, prior to entering the classroom. Constructing a check-off list would be of help until the actual time comes when all of these preparatory concerns should be in place.

This chapter deals with the individual instructor: what roles he/she has to be aware of in advance in order to not only assume these roles with ease and naturalness, but to blend and mold them to his/her *person.* Not an easy thing to do! It does not take students long to see through a facade when instructors are "acting" a role. Individuals entering the educational arena learn early in their teaching experience that it is a total commitment of their person and time. It is the "personality" (the totality of an individual's behavioral and emotional tendencies) that students observe, and communicate with, in order to learn *from.*

> A decisive fact in health education is that educational work relies heavily on the person of the educator; his/her personality is decisive as to whether the information and explanations given by him/her and the resulting motivation and exercising of new behavior patterns will ultimately produce a permanent change in the patients' (students') attitude.[1]

Activity 1

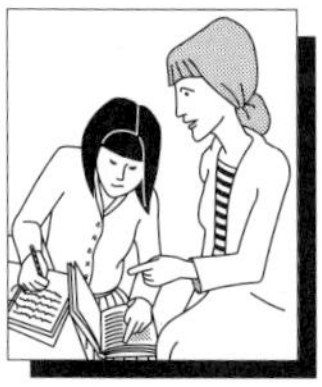

Read and reread the above quotation and discuss among your group. Identify the key message you believe the writer is making. How does it affect each of you? Do you relate to it? Summarize your comments.

Let's take a look at the various "roles" the instructors must identify with in their profession as a teacher.

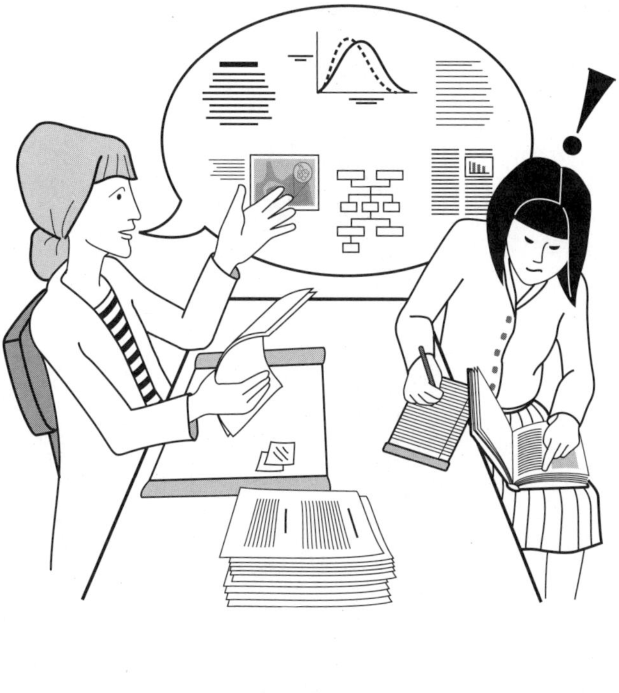

The "Roles" of the Teacher

(Clarification: The word *role* is defined by Webster as either a part played, or function. Its application in this section emphasizes the internalizing of the attributes by the instructor so much so that he/she is characterized by that function. The individual *becomes* the roles given below.)

THE EXPERT

An important functional aspect of an instructor is that he/she be *knowledgeable;* all else flows from this. It can be no other way. Knowledge of the subject is essential before an instructor can use his/her array of teaching techniques and engage personal attributes in the act of teaching. To remain knowledgeable implies constant updating and attendance at meetings and seminars. The information that becomes outdated the fastest is that which relates to the sciences: not only that which pertains to the body of knowledge but also the advancement in technology of instrumentation. The communication of new information—regardless of where in the world it comes from—is so efficient, that an information data base becomes obsolete in a short time. This mimics what is experienced in the production of automobiles. The '94 cars are sold in the Fall of '93, and in Spring of '94, the '95s are being displayed at the auto shows. Clones of all types of counters and analyzers purchased by clinical laboratories, once installed, become outdated by better engineering applied to new clones; they break the records of time, number of specimens analyzed, accuracy and reliability of performance, and they are available *now!*

How do you keep up with this pace of productivity in education? You do your best. Continual reading of journals and references pertaining to your subject is essential. And further, if possible, involvement in research in order to contribute original information in your area of *expertise* results in peer recognition and applause. Knowledge begets *credibility;* credibility begets

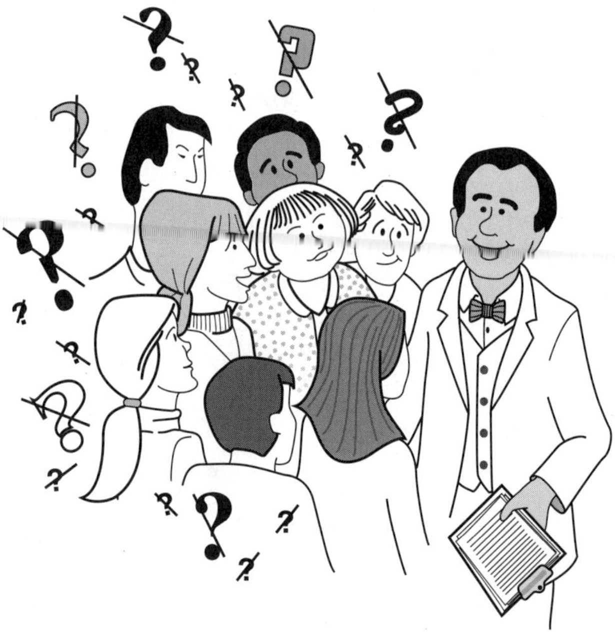

respect. And there are always occasions when a student will ask a question on a far-out angle of a subject, one of which you may not be sure. The only response is to state: "I'm not sure. Let me look it up and I'll get back to you as soon as I can." This honest answer gains respect, understanding, and acceptance by all.

Activity 2

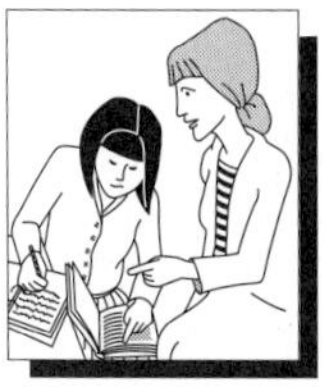

Discuss within your group the various attitudes you have experienced regarding the academic readiness of the various instructors you have had. Summarize your comments. All groups will read and discuss their summaries to the entire class at the end of the exercise.

THE AUTHORITY

The authority conferred on teachers by their immediate supervisor encompasses many activities and functions in which the teacher *serves* in the capacity of *the formal authority.*[2] All teachers have the authority to do the following:

- Establish guidelines, policies, rules, regulations that contribute to the structure of the course
- Develop course content with accompanying course description and course objectives
- Compose behavioral objectives to reflect competencies

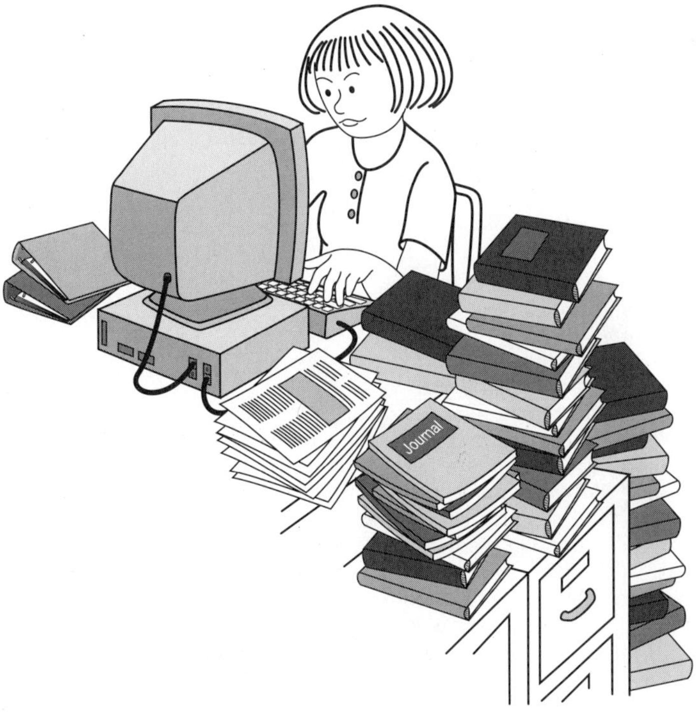

- Establish criteria for the grading system
- Construct quizzes and exams
- Assign grades
- Evaluate students regarding their performance
- Determine (and record) students' grades
- Control the classroom and laboratory in the interest of maintaining an environment in which the other students can learn[3]

Discussion

What is of essence to students regarding authority is *how* the instructor uses, abuses, and displays it. Each instructor who has been delegated authority in his/her class must be aware of the responsibility that accompanies that authority. It is no small task to be responsible for the learning process of a class of adult learners. This entails the unfolding of the educational process along with the personal involvement of assisting the achievement of each individual enrolled in the course. No small feat!

Instructors are respected by students who genuinely care about their progress and display this by showing encouragement, giving praise when deserved (and aloud), listening and responding to the questions and contributions students make.

Additional responsibility involves trying to motivate the students to want to learn and succeed in the class, not just to receive a good grade. McKeachie refers to this attitude as "extrinsic motivation": raising students' motives from "grade-based" to *learning for learning's sake.*

"Learning for learning's sake" is perhaps the highest motive one can have while studying. The son of one of the teachers in our department sent her the following composition. It has no designated author to acknowledge. The son mentioned that someone had tacked it onto a bulletin board at Michigan State University.

THE JOY OF TEACHING

Then Jesus took his disciples up to the mountain and gathering them around him, he taught them saying:
Blessed are the poor in spirit, for theirs is the kingdom of Heaven.
Blessed are the meek.
Blessed are they that mourn.
Blessed are the merciful.
Blessed are they that thirst for justice.
Blessed are you when persecuted.
Blessed are you when you suffer.
Be glad and rejoice for your reward is great in Heaven.
Then Simon Peter said, "Are we supposed to know this?"
And Andrew said, "Do we have to write this down?"
And James said, "Will we have a test on this?"
And Phillip said, "I don't have any paper."
And Bartholomew said, "Do we have to turn this in?"
And John said, "The other disciples didn't have to learn this."
And Matthew said, "May I go to the bathroom?"
Then one of the Pharisees who was present asked to see Jesus' lesson plan and inquired of Jesus, "Where is your anticipatory set and your objectives in the cognitive domain?"
And Jesus wept.

On giving a copy of this narrative to the students in my class, one approached me afterward and confessed, "I've used each one of those statements in one class or another. I can identify with this very easily."

Activity 3

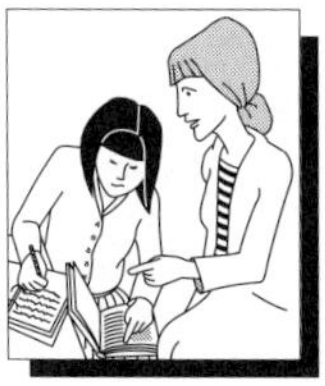

Within your group, discuss your experiences on how the various teachers you have had have exercised their authority: for example, for the good of the group, to maintain order, etc. Have you ever been affected by a teacher who abused authority? Summarize your comments.

FACILITATOR

To facilitate: to make easy.

The role of a facilitator involves presentation of subject matter in such a way as to make it clearly understood. If some students do not grasp the knowledge or skills taught at the same time as the majority of the class, the ability of the instructor to perceive, recognize, and identify a specific learning difficulty demonstrated by a student is essential, but it cannot stop there. The instructor must respond by providing exercises or activities to assist the student in learning. The difficulties in learning, whether caused by or related to an intellectual or psychological block, should be at least recognized by the instructor. If no improvement is realized following a review and additional explanation, the recommendation of special educational instruction for these students should be made. In these situations, the instructor, through identification of a learning disability, can direct placement of the student in an environment with a special education teacher who, through special techniques, can facilitate learning.

But for that population of students that gives evidence of different learning patterns, a different *rate* of learning (and this includes students with accelerated rates as well as those with different rates), the instructor must have a plan, including activities, reading, and projects, that will assist all types of students to achieve according to their ability. Experience has borne out that many students need to hear information expressed different ways. Some need to talk with the instructor alone and work out problems on a one-to-one basis. There are many solutions to problems.

Equally important is the ability of the teacher to exercise and raise the level of thinking of students in the cognitive domain. This is often achieved by presenting questions or comments for discussion during lecture/lab. The emphasis is placed on *exercising* the students' minds; the response might not result in "a right answer." That is not important; "the right answer" will eventually emerge. What *is important* is the opportunity provided for students to engage their minds in formulating a response indicative of a higher cognitive level.

Students should be aware of what the instructor is doing. When higher-level questions are asked based on given information, students often label these as "trick questions." The majority of students learn information and expect (and hope for) questions that involve regurgitation of facts. This type of learning provides a security blanket for those who do not engage in the higher forms of mental activity. These students are not prepared to use or apply the facts in situational problems. Conducting lectures and laboratory sessions as described above prepares the student to realize an all-important fact: "It does not matter how much you know if you can't apply your knowledge." Instructors' greatest challenge is to help students engage in the thinking process. How do we look at the process of *thinking?*

> Thinking constitutes the performance skills that we use in order to apply our intelligence to a knowledge-base, derived from the totality of our experience.
> Getting people to think is an on-going bout.
> Thinking eliminates another frame of mind . . .
> Thinking examines.
> Questions that have a *puzzle* quality about them get students to think.
> Thinking satisfies a curiosity.
> Thinking serves a purpose.
> Thinking always wonders *how.*
> Thinking is hard, but it can be fun.[4]

The Facilitator provides assistance in learning for:

- the general population of students
- the accelerated student
- the students with different learning rates
- the advancement to a higher cognitive level
- the students who need special education

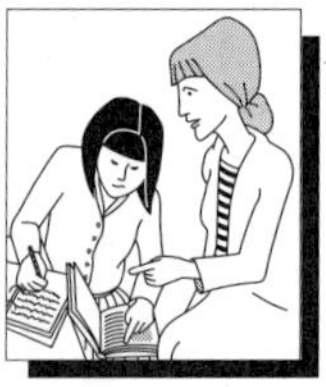

Activity 4

Within your group, relate experiences in *how* the various instructors you have had, have facilitated your learning. Summarize the comments. These will be shared with the class.

THE TEACHER AS A FRIEND

The very fact that teachers and students are human beings identifies an equality factor that establishes a commonality of qualities, attributes, and feelings that are perceived, communicated, interpreted, felt, and understood by both groups. Individuals born and raised in the United States share common language including "body language." The instructor expresses friendship toward a student with care, never crossing that "invisible line" between faculty and student. The instructor does not need to. The teacher, in how he/she conducts himself/herself while teaching and facilitating, establishes the "friend" aspect of his/her person.

Friendship is defined as "one showing kindly interest and good will." It is sufficient that the instructor communicates this to the students while on the job. "Friendship" is not dependent on social activities to demonstrate how an instructor feels about students. Familiarity expressed by identifying with the student and identifying with his/her interests or value system, which is foreign to your own, is taboo. The quickest way to lose respect from students is to engage in such practice; "familiarity breeds contempt."

Newly hired graduates assigned to bench teaching will realize that, in some cases, there is hardly an age difference between themselves and the new students. They must recognize that they represent an authority figure while engaged in instructing these students. It is the "power" that is invested in them by their superior that places them in a different social status.

The role of the instructor is made more complex by the influx of a diversified student body: each group reflecting its own value system, religious convictions, practices, and language. It has become essential for all instructors to become aware that words, expressions, and gestures translate differently to different groups. What perhaps is not meant as an intentional slur can be perceived, identified, and interpreted as one.

Activity 5

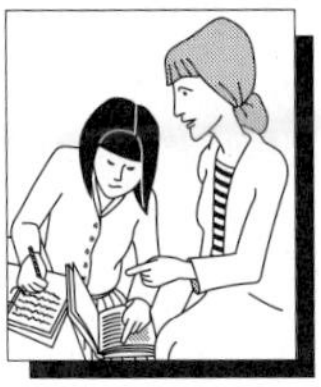

Within your group, relate an instance in which you felt the "friendship" aspect of a teacher and how it was demonstrated.

THE TEACHER AS A LEGAL DEFENDER

This role is seldom included along with the more obvious ones, yet it is the one that has us constantly on the alert. We must ensure that students do not fracture the structure of the course, disregard the policies, and flout authority. To compound the problem, some students influence others, multiplying the infractions committed. Disregard for authority is shown in a multitude of ways; we have all experienced them. The "legal defender" role of the teacher is a passive watchfulness that is activated once infractions are committed. Familiarity with regulations and policies and their explicit expression on all levels of university and hospital involvement that relate to the program is essential. It is important to be aware of their location in the proper manuals

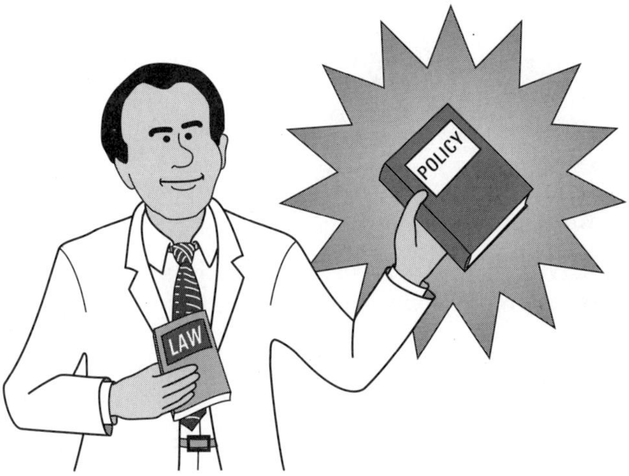

so that "specifics" regarding various policies can be referenced. (The subject will be discussed in Chapter 9.)

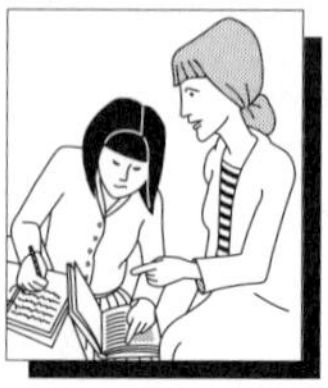

Activity 6

Within your group, discuss if you have ever witnessed a situation involving infraction of policies or regulations by a student and how it was handled.

The Essential Qualities versus Desirable Qualities

The literature is inundated with studies based on students' opinions and feelings regarding qualities of a good instructor. And so stated by such a student several years ago:

> Qualities which an instructor *MUST* possess are:
>
> thorough knowledge of subject matter, ability to convey information to the students, respect for students as fellow human beings, availability to the students, and fairness.

When a list of attributes (generated by students) was constructed and organized, the categories that seemed to encompass them all were *technical skills, teaching skills, and personal qualities.* The question that haunts the educator is: Are these essential or just desirable? The first and most important conclusion after studying the list of qualities and skills (Table 2–1) is that they are essential to a good teacher and they must become identified with the skill or attribute, so that, in time, the skill characterizes the individual. Exercising these skills, as we do different parts of our bodies, assists in their development.

When the fall semester began, the author asked the class to write what they hoped to achieve from the class during the semester and what they expected of the teacher. The results were not surprising. The total number responding was 25. The majority qualified their remarks. The results are shown in Table 2–2.

"To help change my aptitude for science" was an unexpected response. But the most important response was as follows: "Be fair, try to explain stuff without getting upset. At the end of the course, I would like to be proud of what I left this class with."

In placing them in the established categories and interpreting the findings it showed the following:

1. The majority of students recognized the importance of knowledge and having skills that represent entrance level skills necessary to perform in a clinical laboratory
2. An equal number listed concerns in teaching techniques
3. The majority of students not only listed but qualified the importance of the instructors' personal attributes and their expression when dealing with students individually and when in groups.

Table 2–1
SKILLS AND ATTRIBUTES OF TEACHERS

Technical Skills	Teaching Skills	Personal Attributes
Technical knowledge	Writing, speaking skills	Pleasant
Techical experience	Vocabulary	Respectful
Technical skills	Correct usage and grammar	Friendly
Expertise in both manual and automated instrumentation	Organization of topic	Enthusiastic
	Lecturing skills	Warm
	Mechanics of delivery	Honest
Electronic experience	Articulation, voice, volume	Understanding
	Clear	Fair
	Use of eye contact, gestures	Happy
	Ability to move about	In control
	Facial expressions	Patient
	Student involvement	Wise
	Ability to field questions, lead discussions, involve students, be aware of each student during lecture and lab, keep their attention	Tolerant
		Even-tempered
		Aware of limitations
		Well groomed
	Use of A/V equipment	Encouraging
	Test construction skills	Caring
	Development of front sheet with behavioral objectives	Flexible
		Ethical
	Conduct reviews	High moral fiber
		High value system
		Approachable
		Able to motivate
		Dedicated
		Available
		Open minded
		Reasonable
		Displays common sense
		Aware of student needs

There were no unrealistic "requests" from the class. Everything listed represented that which constitutes students' rights.

It is a good practice on the first day of class, after handing out the syllabus of *your* course (designating student responsibilities and *your* specific expectations of them), to have *them* express their expectations of *you,* their instructor. The responses provide excellent material for review and a reminder of one's performance before and while teaching.

INTERRELATIONSHIP OF ATTRIBUTES

Every business or profession that depends on the employee to "make a sale," concerns itself with the "whole person": the image that is projected. Emphasis is placed on the individual being qualified, articulate, personable, innovative, business-minded, organized, warm, and concerned. To be people-oriented in this context means to realize individual needs and to sell the best product that best fits their needs. Many workers are even sent to enroll in the Dale Carnegie course with the objective of enhancing their communication skills and self-image. And why is all this effort spent in developing the person? To make a better salesperson. To sell what? There should be no difference be-

Table 2–2
STUDENT EXPECTATIONS

Teacher Attribute	Number of Responses with Qualifying Statement
Knowledge	17 . . . I expect to come out of this class with a thorough understanding of basic hematology . . . so that I will be able to perform in a hematology lab without feeling lost or needing guidance . . . I expect to leave this class feeling confident regarding the material
Clear teaching	6 . . . to be taught in an intelligent and understanding manner
Will assist, review, answer questions	11
Fairness	7 . . . by *fair,* I mean that anything on the examinations will have been introduced in lecture or contained in the text. I do not expect any tricks or ambiguities on exams and quizzes . . . I expect you to be fair and unbiased in decision making
Understanding	4
Available	7
Patient	6
Organized	4

tween those preparing to teach and those already teaching. We are knowledgeable, and we should develop the ability to communicate clearly and effectively and with conviction (if we don't already possess it). And we do this for one purpose alone: to advertise that our products of *knowledge and skills* are of exceptional value, and we want to convince the customers (students) to recognize and desire them.

Teachers need to assess their strong and not-so-strong assets in regard to *technical and teaching skills, and personal attributes.* This assessment has to start with an awareness of seeing yourself in the most realistic light possible. Reviewing your reactions to incidences that take place while teaching affords a good review of how you have acted or reacted. It takes a lifetime of many situations, both good and bad, to form the teacher-person we would like to be. As the young child who was being corrected by his mother said, "Be patient with me, Mother; God isn't finished with me yet." Becoming an effective teacher does not happen overnight. As Weimer states in her article, "It is a myth to believe that good teachers are born, not made."[5] It takes a lifetime and great effort.

You the educator should realize you are not the only teacher in the educational life of a student. A student takes one or two courses from you; you are not the only driving force in his/her life. Sometimes we act as if students' formation and total education depends on our instruction. Rather, let us do a good job in the little time we have with them. This good job will depend on the integration of the various skills, attributes, and attitudes that contribute to good, effective teaching.

Teacher Responsibilities

Some helpful points to remember in the physical preparation prior to either the formal lecture in the university or the bench teaching in the hospital are as follows:

1. *Handouts:* Factors to check include clarity of copy; adequate, complete number of pages in correct sequence; clearly labeled diagrams or figures, with large print; correct spelling and grammar.
2. *Text:* When using a text, have page numbers handy when referring to specific material for which the students are responsible. This includes references to charts, graphs, photographs, or the text proper.
3. *Overheads:* Avoid overcrowding an overhead. A short message and a simple diagram is much more effective. Try to prepare the overheads before the instruction period.

   Affix a reference number to one of the corners to identify the placement of the overhead within the lecture. When writing or printing on a transparency while lecturing, monitor the screen to be sure your words are not off the screen. Print legibly. Check the spelling. When using overheads with small print, move the overhead projector further back in the lecture room so that the writing can be seen by all students. Determine this before class starts.
4. *Kodachromes:* Always conduct a "dry-run" to ensure correct sequence of slides and correct position of the slide in the slot. Lock the underplate of the carousel to prevent slides from falling out. Make out a reference sheet for the students with identification of the substance (cell, crystal, parasite) on the slide accompanied with a mini explanation. Develop a numbering system in which the number 1 slide in slot 1 is identified by number 1 explanation on the key for that specific carousel. This appears to be rather simplistic; never take for granted that what appears to be organized in your mind is recognized as such

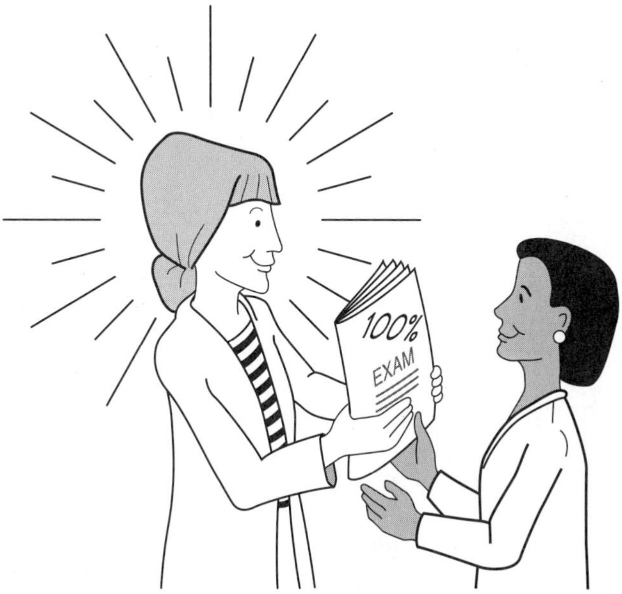

by the students. Run through the slides and commentary you have assembled and see if it runs smoothly and makes sense to you.

5. *Equipment:* Check out all equipment prior to the lecture: videos, monitors, 35-mm projectors, overheads, etc. All should be turned on to ensure working order. It is wise to be aware of the storage location of the various light bulbs specific to each piece of equipment. Become aware of "how" you replace light bulbs for each type of projector.

   When a bulb burns out during use, and you replace it with the backup, report it to the individual in charge of ordering supplies and equipment. It is helpful to take the small carton in which the bulb is packed that contains the correct catalog number and specific coding information to that person. Never leave a disfunctioning piece of equipment in a lecture room without having attended to its replacement. This will affect and inconvenience the next instructor who will use that lecture room and equipment.
6. *Microphone:* If the lecture room is large and equipped with a speaker, check the working order, and set the desired volume prior to class.
7. *Readiness of the Teaching Area* (The lecture room and the laboratory)
   a. *Preparation:* Never assume that chairs are in order in a lecture room (unless fixed to the floor). Go before the scheduled time to arrange the room in the order appropriate to your teaching. Check out the overall neatness, cleanliness of the floor, the condition of the blackboard (sometimes filled with writing from a previous lecture). Order and disorder affect the milieu the instructor attempts to create. Have chalk and eraser available on the chalk tray.
   b. *Window blinds:* Before lecture, prepare the blinds for the degree of darkness necessary for overheads/Kodachromes.
   c. *Windows/fan/air conditioner:* Provide adequate ventilation and coolness or warmth for the students.
   d. *Fire escape route:* Adjust rows of chairs as to provide wide aisles students can use in case of emergency. As students arrive, have

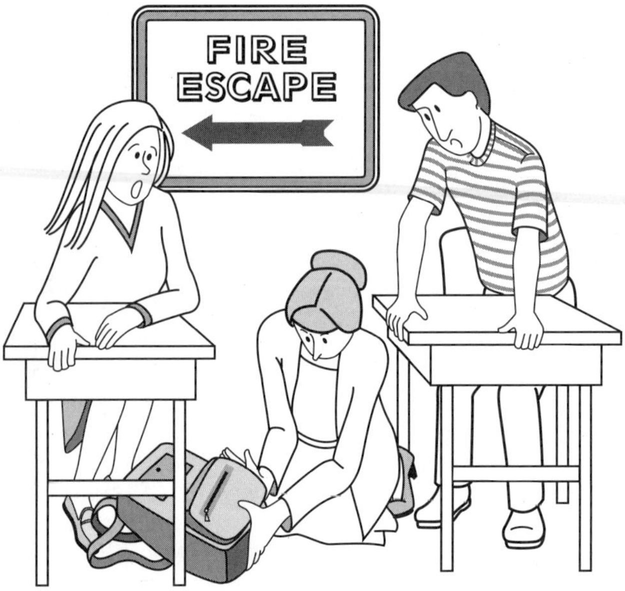

them place their book bags (and they are large) under the seats so as not to obstruct the aisles.

e. *Check out the light source in the ceiling.* If there are replacements needed, inform the correct person of the need.

f. *"Bench tech" area:* All of the above along with having cleaned table tops and decks with solution via procedure according to OSHA is essential.

Check equipment/reagents to be used in the procedures to be taught. Check the date of reagents for expiration. Have those solutions ready if they have to be made up in the laboratory. Check for nicks on pipettes, especially at the tips. Have masks, face shields, laboratory coats, and gloves available for the students you will instruct.

Have OSHA-approved materials nearby to neutralize chemical spills/possible organisms in blood spills. Know how to use these substances before the teaching session. Make this information available to the students. Know the OSHA symbols on the various receptacles and their location.

Summary

In the majority of cases, the remote preparation of a teacher involved in the educational aspect of the Clinical Laboratory Science Program takes place following the appointment to the department and prior to active instruction. Focus is placed on the availability of instructional programs that faculty can use to learn how to teach and how to become an effective teacher.

The various factors that contribute to the whole person of an effective teacher are enumerated, categorized, and described in this chapter. The various roles associated with the teacher that contribute to the overall make-up of the teacher were discussed and their importance emphasized. Instructors are encouraged to identify those areas that need to be developed or fine-tuned. Honest student evaluations yield valuable information that often shows how instructors come across when actively involved in teaching and in dealing with students outside the classroom on a more informal basis.

Immediate preparation by the instructor prior to lecturing or conducting a laboratory session provides numerous considerations that must be attended to before class starts. These include the instructor, instructional materials, equipment, reagents, and the lecture room.

Review Questions

1. What responsibility, as a result of the authority given instructors, must be exercised toward students?

2. List the three categories that encompass the essential attributes of an instructor. Place in the order of importance you believe to be essential.

3. At this point, express how you feel regarding the preparation of teachers for their jobs.

See p. 405 for answers.

References

1. Gottsching C. Limits of preventive health care and health education. Offentliche Gesundheitsweses 1990; 52(8-9):361–367.
2. McKeachie WJ. Teaching Tips: A Guidebook for the Beginning Teacher. 7th ed. Lexington, Mass, DC Heath Co, 1978, pp 68–82.
3. Eble KE. The Craft of Teaching. 2nd ed. San Francisco, Jossey-Bass Publishers, 1990, pp 197–213.
4. Weimer M, Neff RA, eds. It's a Myth: Good Teachers Are Born—Not Made in Teaching College. Madison, Wisc, Magna Publications, 1990, pp 15, 16.

Suggested Reading

1. Davis GD. Tools for Teaching. San Francisco, Jossey-Bass Publishers, 1993.
2. Gustafson KL, Tillman MH. Designing the General Strategies of Instructional Design: Principles and Applications. 2nd ed. Englewood Cliffs, NJ, Educational Technology Publications, 1991.
3. Hanna SJ, McGill LT. Nurturing Environment and Effective Teaching in Teaching College. Madison, Wisc, Magna Publications, 1990.
4. Johnson GR. First Steps to Excellence in College Teaching. 2nd ed. Madison, Wisc, Magna Publications, 1990.
5. Lowman J. Mastering the Technique of Teaching. San Francisco, Jossey-Bass Publishers, 1984.
6. Mager RF. Developing Aptitude Toward Learning. Belmont, Calif, Fearon, 1968.
7. Massachusetts Institute of Technology. You and Your Students. Washington, DC, American Society for Engineering Education, 1975.
8. Michels E. Commentary: Enhancing the scholarly base: The role of faculty in enhancing scholarship. Journal of Allied Health 1989, winter, pp 129–142.
9. Saunders RL, Saunders DS. Education in The Modern College by Chickering AW and Associates. San Francisco, Jossey-Bass Publishers, 1988, pp 500–511.
10. One hundred forty-seven practical tips for teaching professors. The Teaching Professor. Madison, Wisc, Magna Publications, 1990.
11. The Teaching Professor. All issues. Madison, Wisc, Magna Publications.

3

The Behavioral Objectives: Your Educational Map

OBJECTIVES

Upon completion of this chapter, the reader should be able to:

- Discuss competency-based education and its application to clinical laboratory science.
- Define and describe the *competencies*.
- Define and describe behavioral objectives and their relationship to the competencies.
- Identify, and give examples of the components that contribute to a behavioral objective.
- Convert covert verbs to overt verbs.
- Recognize and identify correctly-stated behavioral objectives.
- Write correctly stated behavioral objectives.
- Discuss the advantages of having accompanying behavioral objectives.

KEY WORDS

competency-based education
competencies
goals
behavioral objectives

Introduction

In Chapter 1, attention was given to the factors contributing to the instructor's preparation prior to teaching. Defining the boundaries of your course and researching possible texts to adopt enabled you to get a sense of what your course would entail. The structure of the educational process and its individual components were presented. Effective teaching was defined, and the various factors that contribute to *being effective* were introduced. In Chapter 2, focus was placed on the *person* of the teacher. Roles and essential attributes a teacher must develop to be effective were described. In both chapters, emphasis was placed on the *remote preparation* of the teacher, increasing awareness of what must be in place before instruction begins.

Chapter 3 introduces the mechanism of *competency-based education* (CLS) used in both academic and clinical instruction. Competencies target the essential information and skills required to function as a laboratorian in the clinical laboratory.

For clarification and differentiation: *Goals* are *broad, general* statements made by individuals, students, about what they hope to achieve following their instruction and how they will function in their jobs. *Objectives* are *specific* directives identifying the means by which they will achieve these goals during their instruction.

Competency-Based Education

What are these *competencies?* Where did they originate? Why are they important? The stated competencies of NAACLS (Accrediting Agency for Clinical Science), given in the *Essentials and Guidelines of Accredited Educational Programs at Baccalaureate Medical Technology Level (1996), The Competency Statements* of the American Society of Clinical Pathologists (ASCP) Board of Registry (1995), and the *Competence Assurance Documents, Statements of Competence* of the American Society of Clinical Laboratory Science (ASCLS) (early 1980s) are used by the educational programs as *fixed resource documents* for the development of all course work. Through a process known as *task analysis,* a study was conducted based on the observation of performance of clinical laboratory scientists while at work, with the purpose of identifying competencies involved in completing each laboratory procedure. Thus, the competencies listed by each of the three associations/agencies represent most accurately the total capabilities and knowledge that graduates must demonstrate in order to be hired by the clinical laboratory. This then constitutes *competency-based education* (CBE). The competencies originated from those associations/agencies just listed and are accepted as the criteria by which they (ASCP, National Certifying Agency [NCA]) grant certification to students who successfully graduate from an accredited program and pass their certifying examination.

Educationally then, CBE relates to certification granted by an external organization that recognizes students who have fulfilled all the requirements (the demonstration of having achieved the competencies) necessary to practice in the field. They have achieved this by having been graduated from an accredited program and having passed the certification examination. *Certification* relates to *competency. Practically,* it describes a person who has developed the ability to combine the realms of cognitive domain with the mastery

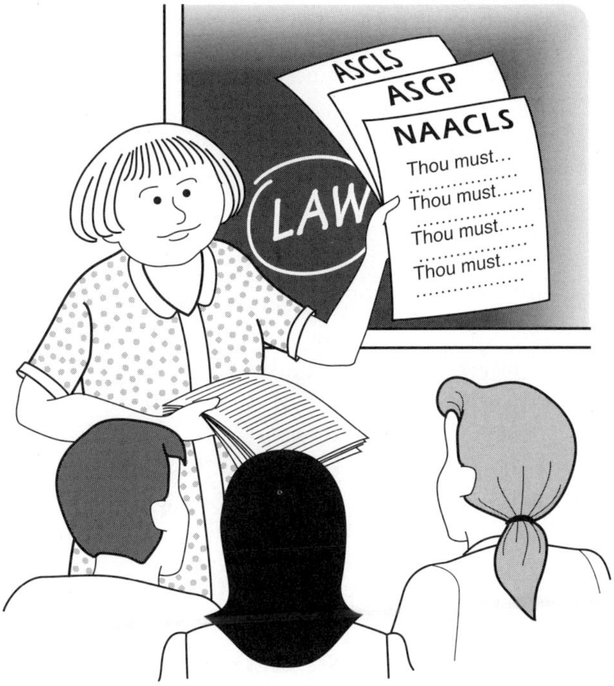

of technical skills in generating accurate and reliable results when performing laboratory procedures.

Advantages of CBE

The advantages of such a program are as follows: It defines a standardized-based performance . . . an end result that is *predetermined, fixed,* but the *means,* the variability of educational methodologies used in *achieving the end,* are multiple and diverse. This allows students with varied learning patterns to achieve the end in a reasonable time and by whatever means are available.

If the "fixed end" defines a procedure to be performed in a specific time limit, CBE allows students additional time to practice thus assisting them in meeting specified criteria. Educators can vary the style of teaching to one that would meet the needs of the students.

APPLICATION

CBE emphasizes mastering the skill (performance) that translates to generating accurate results of a test in a clinical setting. These results are used by doctors in diagnosing and treating patients. Doctors rely heavily on laboratory results to either confirm their diagnosis, assist them in establishing one, or define the degree of abnormality of a disease state with an established diagnosis.

CBE thus expresses the outcome of student performance. Some examples taken from the *Competency Statements* of *The American Society of Clinical Pathologists* (see Appendix 3–A) follow:

In regard to laboratory operations and the performance of laboratory tests involving Microbiology, Hematology, Chemistry, Body Fluids, Immunology, and Blood Bank at career entry, the Medical Technologist:

Applies
- Principles of basic laboratory procedures in order to perform tests
- Principles of special procedures related to testing

Selects . . .
Prepares . . .
Calculates . . . results from test data obtained from laboratory procedures
Correlates Laboratory Data . . .
Evaluates . . .[1]

Competencies are expressed in broad statements. They state that a recent graduate, when newly employed by a clinical laboratory, is required to demonstrate *entry-level* skills. The instructor needs to express these competencies in a language that defines, for the student, *the activity, the conditions of performance, and how accurate or in what range of acceptance the results must be . . . EXACTLY!* Students need specific directions that define and guide them to perform *competently.*

Behavioral, Measurable, Observable Objectives

Objectives are rooted in the competencies. Behavioral objectives are stated specific directives with a designated task, requiring special skills in order to be performed. Adherence to specific format provides for the development and acquisition of the competency. Objectives are sometimes described as behavioral, measurable, and observable: all terms expressing the essence of, the core, of stated objectives, that is, that the knowledge, the skill acquired by the student, be demonstrated by the student. Objectives, therefore, provide the mechanism by which competencies are stated, followed, acquired, tested, and evaluated.

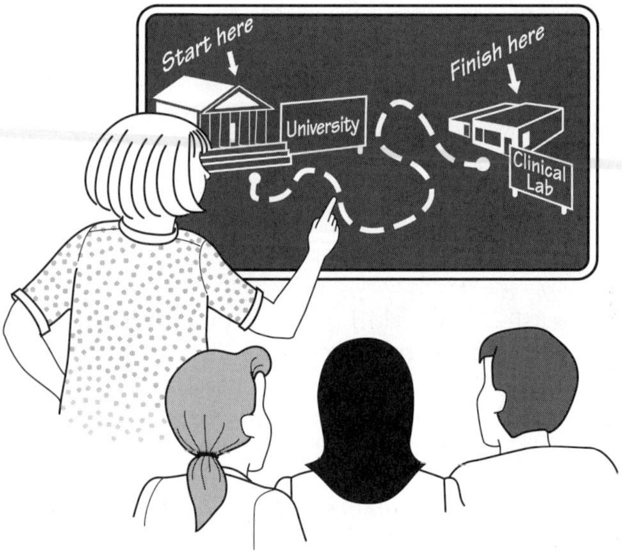

UTILIZATION OF BEHAVIORAL OBJECTIVES

Instructors construct behavioral objectives for their courses that identify the skills students should demonstrate at completion of instruction. These are found in the course syllabus and designated *course objectives.* In addition, each lecture and accompanying laboratory designates more concise objectives that identify specific competencies to be mastered during those sessions.

OBJECTIVES: BENEFIT TO THE STUDENT

These objectives, by design, are student-oriented. The implication is that students who take the course have in mind what they want to accomplish. They can see where the course, through its stated objectives, is going to take them and then decide if that is where they want to go. When the instructor composed and wrote the specific behavioral objective, he/she had one thing in mind: that the objective reflected the acquisition of one of the competencies and that it would contain clear directions that would enable the student to acquire it. The students have to trust the instructor in leading them to acquire those skills and knowledge necessary for being employed in a clinical laboratory. The instructor is really saying; "I know what you need to work in a lab; if you follow these instructions and are successful, you are on your way there." The variable functions/benefits of stated objectives for students found in the literature include the following:

- To assist students with the means to organize their own efforts toward accomplishment of those objectives.[2]
- Our teaching objectives must be to prepare men and women for a useful life.[3]
- The major reason for an objective is to facilitate clear communication between the student and the instructor.[4]
- Instruction is effective to the degree that it succeeds in changing students in desired directions and not in undesired directions. If it doesn't change anyone, it has no effect, no power.[2]
- It helps students begin a lifelong learning process; that is, we want to develop interest in future learning and provide a base of knowledge and skills that will facilitate future learning.[5]
- They are much more likely to meet expectations if these are clearly stated well in advance of expected performance.[6]
- Competence is essential to the possession of the objective; both because competence defines the individual's potential and because it is experienced as self-worth.[3]

A student could refer to the stated objectives of a course and say: "This is what is important. This is what I have to master." And he/she would be right.

What becomes obvious in the format of the required course work—with assigned reading, specific skills to acquire, and the degree of accuracy to be mastered—is the structure within the program, the exactness of performance demanded of all students. Structure and order beget discipline; discipline begets competence. Stated objectives give direction to achieving competence.

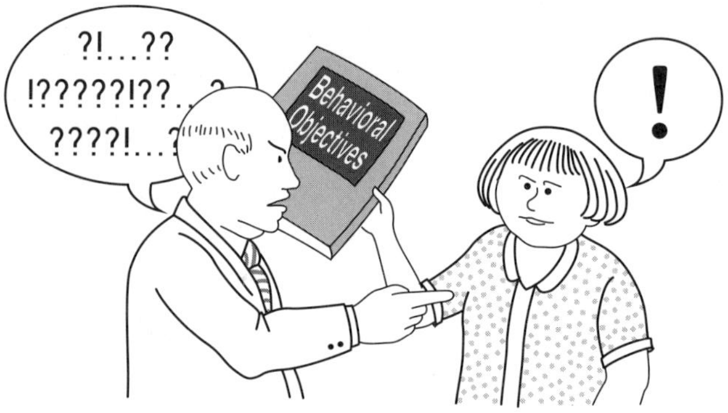

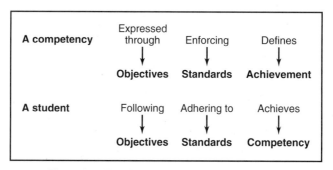

Being competent means being really good at something, and the students really know it.

OBJECTIVES: BENEFIT TO THE INSTRUCTOR

Instructors indirectly gain insight through experience as to how students relate to and perform in class because of the stated objectives. They learn by how they format their stated objectives and observe that they can witness the change learning creates within their students; that using specific language in the construction of the objectives facilitates learning in their students; that they have created written references that can be used for the creation of examinations and for accountability (i.e., Did I teach what I proposed to teach?). Educators who write behavioral objectives for their courses have noted that the *objective* is as advantageous to the teacher as it is to the student:

- Through your instructional objectives, implant at least one new piece of information, a new technical skill, or a new experience in creative thinking.[7]
- Specify the objectives of each meeting. Have carefully planned them in advance so they are properly related in terms of time and emphasis to the objectives of the entire subject.[8]
- One reason for use of Instructional Objectives is that they are consistent with the concept of accountability.[6]
- College teachers should be accountable . . . they should commit themselves ahead of time to what they are going to accomplish.[5, 6]

A competency	Expressed through ↓	Enforcing ↓	Defines ↓
	Objectives	**Standards**	**Achievement**
A student	Following ↓	Adhering to ↓	Achieves ↓
	Objectives	**Standards**	**Competency**

Figure 3–1 The effectiveness of behavioral objectives.

The purpose is to encourage you to be specific . . . don't get trapped into thinking that the behavior you list is all you should aim for.[5]

The purpose of working out objectives is to facilitate planning, not exhibit it.[5]

The clearer you can become about what you're trying to do, the better.[5]

Our teaching objectives must prepare men and women for a useful life.[9]

With a written objective then, you have a record on which to base later decisions. Are these objectives the best indicators of the intent of the goal? In addition, you may use written objectives for accountability. Here is what we set out to accomplish. Did we do it?[10]

The stated objectives, once written, serve the instructor as a record on which to base later decisions. Further, it will be used for accountability. The student is different after instruction. He/she knows more than he/she knew before . . . understands something he/she did not understand before. He/she has developed a skill he/she did not have before.[11]

See Figure 3.1.

The task then of the instructor is to take a competency and express it as an objective (Table 3–1).

Competency. "Calculates results from test data obtained from laboratory procedures."

Objective. "The student, (doer) having performed a manual red blood cell count,
following the standardized procedure, (conditions)
will calculate the final result (task) within 10% of accuracy, (criteria)
within 5 minutes." (criteria)

Table 3–1

THE ESSENTIAL COMPONENTS OF A BEHAVIORAL OBJECTIVE

Essentials of measurable objectives include the following four major components:

Component	***Example***
1. The *doer*	the *student*
2. The *activity*	*will classify* the red cells
3. The *specified conditions*	*in 10 minutes*
4. The *standard*	*with 100% accuracy.*

1. The *doer:* In stated objectives, if the doer is not specified, the student will assume he/she is the doer.

2. The *activity:* The *activity* must use a verb whose action can be observable: a measurable activity that can be qualified by the instructor. Such words as *know* and *understand* are often used by students: "I really understand this! I know it!"

The instructor's response to this should be, "Show me!" Robert Mager uses the terms *covert* and *overt* in reference to the activity-factor of the objective.

> We say a performance can be covert (mental, internal) as long as there is a direct way of determining whether it specifies the objective. Add, then, to the stated objective, an "indicator" behavior.[12]

The verbs in the box designate an identifiable action be it written, stated aloud, or drawn.

EXAMPLES OF VERBS THAT DESCRIBE OBSERVABLE ACTIVITY		
calculate	identify	report
classify	indicate	restate
compare	illustrate	review
compute	interpret	sketch
diagram	locate	solve
draw	name	translate
dramatize	operate	tabulate
explain	point	trace
estimate	predict	use
extrapolate	repeat	write

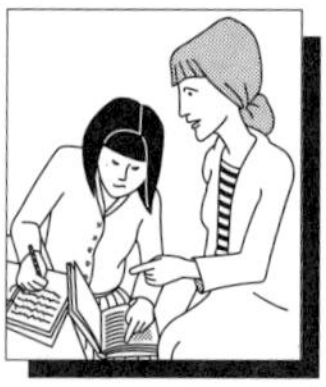

Activity I

Convert the *covert* verb into an action that is observable.

Covert Verbs **Overt Verbs (Observable activity)**

1. consider ________________
2. know ________________
3. understand ________________
4. wonder ________________
5. meditate ________________
6. surmise ________________
7. grieve ________________
8. rejoice ________________

9. decide ______________________

10. deliberate ______________________

11. oppose ______________________

12. delight ______________________

13. happy ______________________

14. hear ______________________

15. imagine ______________________

3. *Conditions:* Factors that define how a procedure is to be performed constitute *conditions* of an objective. Examples of *conditions* include the following:

Time Specifications. Certain procedures designate specific times within the steps that control reactions. Activities such as incubation, mixing, rotating are usually given a specified time frame to bring about an end point or admixing of a specimen and reagent or a bonding culminating in a complex. The *time constraints,* as a condition of a procedure, is one of several essential conditions that contribute to a standardized test. If this condition is not followed, the results of the procedure are not trustworthy.

Examples

- "In performing the glucose determination, incubate the sample for exactly 10 minutes."
- "During this serological slide test, after admixing the serum and the reagent, rotate the slide for exactly 2 minutes."
- "Incubate the sed rate for exactly 1 hour."

Such time constraints as part of a procedure are essential and cannot be changed without affecting the result.

Temperature Specifications. The majority of procedures performed in the laboratory deal with either color development, antibody/antigen reaction, formation of a complex: a variety of activities that are temperature-dependent. Such temperature constraints to a procedure are essential and cannot be changed without affecting the result. In such a situation, a set temperature is used to facilitate a reaction: one that will not take place when subjected to other temperatures.

Examples

- "Perform the crossmatch at room temperature."
- "Incubate the serum at 64 degrees C."
- "Incubate the reagent and serum at 37 degrees C."

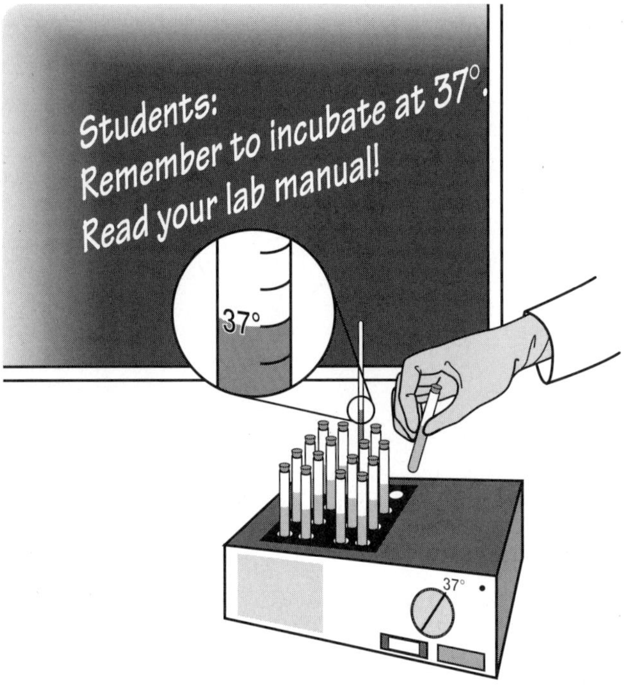
Students:
Remember to incubate at 37°.
Read your lab manual!
37°
37°

Other. Other examples of conditions involved in performing procedures include: the use of controls, standards, calibrated micropipettes, a to-deliver-pipette, equipment, ant the like. Very often, the manufacturer's brochure accompanying a reagent or a kit will specify conditions and standards that are critical to the correct performance of the procedure. Often, it is the order in which reagents are added to a specimen. Those conditions that are necessary for a specific task to be completed should be stated in the objective.

The Standard, Criterion. The *standard* or *criterion* is designated in most laboratory procedures. It may be expressed as 100% accuracy or within a given range of acceptance. If the standard is not stated, the student will assume it to be *100% correct; accurate.* "The result of the red blood cell count will be within the normal range of 4.7 to 6.1 $\times$ 10^{12}/L"; "The glucose result will be within one SD of the normal control."

The expression *providing reasonable care* is emerging in the United States relating to the provisions included within the health care system under consideration for adoption. The implication of the term *reasonable,* when applied to laboratory performance, projects a different *measuring stick* regarding acceptable performance. If and when this is implemented, it will translate to a generated result from a procedure that will not have to be *as accurate* as previously required. Rather, a result can be within a range of certain values that, when used by a physician, would assure "reasonable care." This, then, is the standard of performance that will take precedence in the clinical laboratory. However, in the academic institution, during the training of students, the standard of performance will be *100% accuracy.*

Activity 2

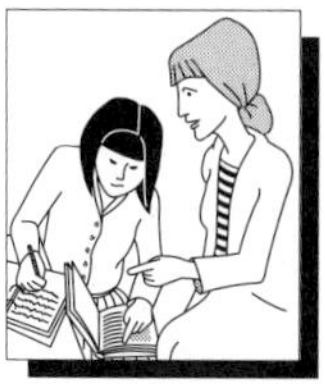

Identify the components of the stated objectives by placing one line under the doer, 2 under the activity, 3 under the conditions, and a circle around the criterion.

1. Given a diagram of a cell membrane, the student will label the outside membrane and the trilipid layer with 100% accuracy.
2. The students, after reviewing the kodachromes on red cell variants, will accurately identify the red cells present on the blood smears.
3. After practicing white blood cell differentials, the junior students will preform a differential in 10 minutes with 95% accuracy.
4. Following exercises drawing a standard curve, the students, using a hemoglobin standard and reagent, will construct a new curve correctly.
5. Referring to the Control and Standard readings, the students will calculate the patients' results within one standard deviation.
6. Using the textbook as a reference, the students will answer the study questions accurately.
7. Given suspended red cells and vials of Anti-A, Anti-B, and Coombs sera, the students will type the unknown blood with 100% accuracy.
8. With supervision, a graduate student will lecture on "The Hookworm" to the class, giving accurate information.
9. Using a flame, a bacterial loop, and sterile blood plates, the student will accurately inoculate a throat specimen onto the blood plate, using correct procedure.
10. Supplied with chemistry data generated from a study performed on newborns, the study group will calculate meaningful statistics accurately and publish their findings in the CLS journal.

Activity 3

Given the following behavioral objectives, identify which component is not present.

1. After incubating the specimen, the students will centrifuge the tubes to determine the presence of or degree of hemolysis.
2. The students are to calculate the amount of gases in the specimen with 100% accuracy.
3. Following the staining of the blood smears, the students will perform differentials.
4. Using the four-headed scope, the students will achieve 100% accuracy.
5. The students will perform the new procedure.

Activity 4

Referring to the course objectives of one of the courses you have taken during the program, paraphrase the objectives of that course.

Activity 5

Referring to the Competencies stated by ASCP regarding "Correlate Laboratory Data," write an objective that states how a student must correlate laboratory and clinical data to assess results.

Summary

The structure of CLS education is based on the competencies mandated by the professional organizations and certifying agency. They represent in totality all the skills that represent *entry-level skills* graduates should demonstrate in order to be recognized as competent laboratorians. Correctly stated objectives are essential in teaching. They provide students with specific directions to acquire knowledge and skills that reflect the competencies for CLS. They offer assurance that the information included in the objective will be consistent with the questions on examinations. They further ensure that cumulative information presented throughout the CLS program expressed in the objectives is indicative of that which will be found on the certifying examination. And upon entering the job market, they will recognize that the objectives prepared them with the necessary knowledge and skills to perform with *entry-level ability.*

There should be no surprises in the system for students who use behavioral objectives properly. The behavioral objectives used in instruction, certifying examinations, and real-world procedures in the hospital and private laboratories should be congruent. The instructor has accountability to himself/herself, the student, the chairperson of the department, the university, the clinical segment of the program, and in fact, "the whole world."

Review Questions

1. True/False: Stated objectives provide the means by which competencies are expressed.
2. It is essential in a stated objective to always include which 3 elements?
3. Read the following objective and determine if it is stated correctly. Comment. If not, rewrite it correctly: Following the lecture on roundworms, the students will understand the manner in which worms enter the body.
4. Using the competencies stated by ASCP, p. 49, write a behavioral objective, expressing this competency.
5. Using the competencies stated by NAACLS confirming abnormal results, write a behavioral objective expressing this competency.

See p. 405 for answers.

References

1. American Society of Clinical Pathologists, Competency Statements Medical Technology. 1994.
2. Mager RF. Preparing Instructional Objectives. 2nd ed. Belmont, Calif, Fearon, 1975, pp 1–4.
3. Faculty Committee of Massachusetts Institute of Technology. American Society for Engineering Educators, 1975, pp 31–37.
4. Beck SJ, LeGrys VA. Clinical Laboratory Education. San Mateo, Calif, Appleton and Lange, 1988, pp 33–53.
5. McKeachie WJ. Countdown for course preparation. *In* Teaching Tips. 7th ed. Lexington, Mass, D.C. Heath and Co, 1978, pp 5–14.
6. Lowman J. Planning course content to maximize interest. Mastering the Techniques of Teaching. Belmont, Calif, Fearon, 1984, pp 146–164.
7. Faculty Committee of Massachusetts Institute of Technology. American Society of Engineering Educators, 1975, pp 13–15.
8. Kebler RJ, Cegala DJ, Watson KW, Miles DT, Barker LL. Objectives for instruction and evaluation. *In* Instructional Objectives and the Instructional Process. Boston, Allyn and Bacon, 1981, pp 1–31.
9. Mager RF. The qualities of useful objectives. *In* Preparing Instructional Objectives. 2nd ed. Belmont, Calif, Fearon, 1975, pp 19–22.
10. Gustafson KL, Tillman MH. Designing the general strategies of instruction. *In* Briggs LJ, Gustafson KL, Tillman MH, eds. Instructional Design Principles and Applications. 2nd ed. Englewood Cliffs, NJ, Educational Technology Publishing Co, 1991, pp 81–117.
11. Green TF. Acquisition of purpose. In Chickering AW et al, eds. The Modern American College. San Francisco, Calif, Jossey-Bass Publishers, 1988, pp 543–555.
12. Mager RF. Preparing Instructional Objectives. 2nd ed. Belmont, Calif, Fearon, 1975, pp 23–48.

Suggested Reading

1. Ballard AL. Getting started writing behavioral objectives. Journal of Nursing Staff Development 1990; 6(1):40–44.
2. Beck SJ, LeGrys VA. Instructional planning. *In* Clinical Laboratory Education. Norwalk, Conn/San Mateo, Calif, Appleton and Lange, 1988, pp 9–28.
3. Davis BG. Tools for Teaching. San Francisco, Calif, Jossey-Bass Publishers, 1993.
4. Green TF. Acquisition of purpose. *In* Chickering AW, et al, eds. The Modern American College. San Francisco, Calif, Jossey-Bass Publishers, 1988, pp 543–555.
5. Hedges WD. Testing and Evaluation for the Sciences in the Secondary School. Belmont, Calif, Wadsworth Publishing, 1956.
6. Hudson MJ, Gordwin BL, Beck CE. Assessment of student affective behaviors in US medical technology programs. Laboratory Medicine 1994, 25(1) 27–31.
7. Mager RF. Preparing Instructional Objectives. 2nd ed. Belmont, Calif, Fearon, 1975.
8. Popham WJ. Instructional objectives. *In* The Teacher-Empiricist. Los Angeles, Tinnon-Brown Inc, 1969, p 3.
9. Yelon SL. Writing and using instructional objectives. *In* Briggs LJ, Gustafson JL, Tillman MH, eds. Instructional Design Principles and Applications. 2nd ed. Englewood, Cliffs, NJ, Educational Technology Publications, 1991, pp 75–121.

APPENDIX 3–A

Competency Statements—Medical Technologist

In regard to laboratory operations and the performance of laboratory tests involving microbiology, hematology, chemistry, body fluids, immunology, and blood bank at career entry, the medical technologist:

APPLIES

- principles of basic laboratory procedures in order to perform tests
- principles of special procedures related to testing
- knowledge to identify sources of error in laboratory testing
- knowledge of fundamental biologic characteristics as they pertain to laboratory testing
- principles of theory and practice related to laboratory operations (management/safety/education/research and development)
- knowledge of standard operating procedures

SELECTS

- procedural course of action appropriate for the type of sample and test requested
- methods/reagents/media/blood products according to established procedures
- instruments to perform test appropriate to test methodology according to established procedures
- appropriate controls for test performed
- routine laboratory procedures to verify test results according to established protocol
- special laboratory procedures to verify test results
- instruments for new laboratory procedures

PREPARES

- reagents/media/blood products according to established procedures
- instruments to perform tests
- controls appropriate for testing procedures

CALCULATES

- results from test data obtained from laboratory procedures

CORRELATES LABORATORY DATA

- and clinical data to assess test results
- and quality control data to assess test results
- with other laboratory data to assess test results
- with physiologic processes to assess/validate test results and procedures

EVALUATES

- laboratory and clinical data to specify additional tests
- laboratory data to recognize common procedural/technical problems
- laboratory data to verify test results
- laboratory data to check for possible source of errors
- laboratory data to determine possible inconsistent results
- laboratory data to recognize health and disease states
- laboratory data to assess validity/accuracy of procedures for a given test
- laboratory data to determine appropriate instrument adjustments
- laboratory data to take corrective action according to predetermined criteria
- laboratory data to recognize and report the need for additional testing
- laboratory data to determine alternate methods for a given test
- various methods to establish new testing procedures
- laboratory and clinical data to ensure safety of personnel
- laboratory operational procedures
- test results obtained by alternate methodologies
- laboratory data to establish reference range criteria for existing or new tests
- laboratory data to make identifications/recommendations

4

Professional Competence: Hierarchical Domains

OBJECTIVES

Upon completion of this chapter, the reader should be able to:

- Recognize the specific hierarchical domains with the accompanying level of performance.
- List the specific hierarchical domains with the accompanying level of performance.
- Combine the correct expression of a behavioral objective with a specific desired level of cognitive/psychomotor/affective domain performance.
- Write behavioral objectives expressing the realms of the domains.

KEY WORDS

cognitive
affective
psychomotor
domain
realm
taxonomy

Introduction

In the previous chapter, the student was introduced to the establishment of goals and the construction of measurable objectives as a means of obtaining the goals. In CLS, the goals are directly related to achieving the competency that characterizes a graduate of an accredited program who has passed the certifying examination given by a CLS agency or association. This chapter introduces the *hierarchical domains* that play an essential role in identifying for the students what level of cognitive/psychomotor/affective performance is expected of them. The verbs used in stating an objective are fine tuned; not only is the activity measurable, as indicated in the previous chapter, but the intellectual level and degree of involvement reflect the level of activity of each domain. The identification and categorical organization (taxonomy) of the three domains were developed by Bloom and associates in 1956. In the educational field, the domains have been used in the development of curriculum as applied to construction of behavioral objectives. Application of the domains extends into teaching, testing, and evaluation. The obvious advantage in expressing behavioral objectives utilizing domains is that the added dimension, *the level*, of performance is clearly indicated and can be measured.

The Cognitive Domain[1]

Perhaps the simplest description of the term *cognitive* is "to come to know." This domain includes the acquisition of knowledge by exercising various levels of capabilities of the intellect. The category identified by Bloom includes the following realms (see Fig. 4–1):

1. *Knowledge* indicates acquiring information by using the lowest, most basic level of mental activity: i.e., through memorization or knowledge acquired through an experience or an association. Ability expressed in this realm is *simple recall.*

2. *Comprehension* encompasses knowledge and expresses ability of understanding acquired information. The student can not only memorize a principle dealing with instrumentation but also is able to explain the process. Ability expressed in this realm is *interpretation*, *explanation.*

3. *Application* is dependent on the two previous realms and drives the process one step further by using the information in a new situation. Ability

	Categorized by CLS
6. **Evaluation** 5. **Synthesis** 4. **Analysis**	III. Problem solving
3. **Application** 2. **Comprehension**	II. Understanding with application to new situations
1. **Knowledge**	I. Recall

Figure 4–1 Cognitive Domains.

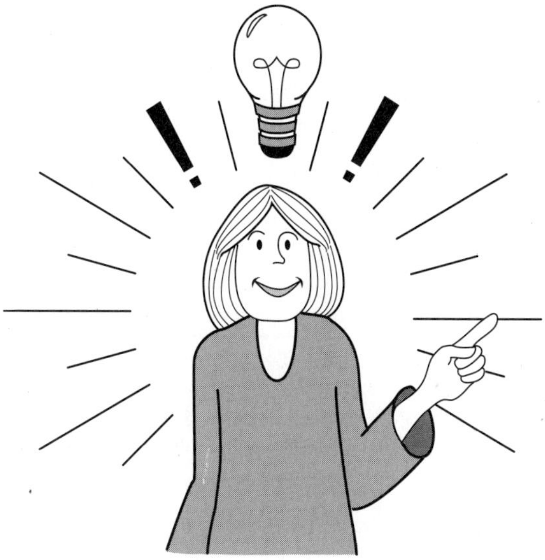

expressed in this realm is *implementation: utilization of* knowledge in various situations.

4. *Analysis* expresses ability to separate components of a statement, a principle, a discussion, with intent of detecting the effect of the relative parts to each other and to the whole. The ability illustrated in this realm is one of *examination, investigation.*

5. *Synthesis* expresses ability of an individual to develop anew, produce a substance, compose, develop a new program, or the like that is original. The key ability expressed is *creation, origination.*

APPLICATION OF DOMAINS TO STATED BEHAVIORAL OBJECTIVES

In the previous chapter, it was stated that objectives provide the mechanism by which competencies are expressed. Reviewing the format of a correctly stated behavioral objective, it was noted that emphasis was placed on the

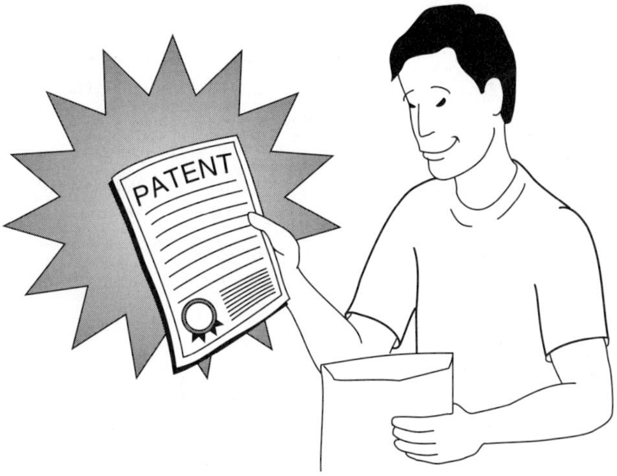

demonstration of the task. The instructor has to *hear* the discussion of information or *see* a list of normal white cells written. In applying realms of domains to a stated objective, a *dimension* of specificity is added, giving the instructor additional information indicating the level of cognitive ability the student exhibits. With regard to the student, identification of a specified task and level of intellectual involvement assists in the achievement of the task. The following examples demonstrate not only the nature of the task, but the cognitive level necessary to achieve it.

EXAMPLE

(Cognitive Domain: Knowledge, expressed as recall)
The student will accurately *list* the five white blood cells found in the peripheral blood on the board.

(Cognitive Domain: Comprehension, expressed as understanding)
The student will *explain* to the class, accurately, the principle of *sample aspiration* used by the various automatic cell counters.

In expressing the activity peculiar to each realm of the Cognitive Domain, a list of verbs that describe specificity is necessary.

VERBS USED IN WRITING OBJECTIVES FOR THE COGNITIVE DOMAIN

1. **KNOWLEDGE** (to recall, to recognize): cite, count, define, draw, duplicate, enumerate, identify, indicate, list, name, point, quote, read, recall, recite, recognize, record, relate, repeat, select, state, tabulate, tell, trace, underline, write
2. **COMPREHENSION** (to translate from one form to another): associate, classify, compare, compute, contrast, describe, differentiate, discuss, distinguish, explain, estimate, express, extrapolate, interpret, interpolate, locate, paraphrase, predict, report, restate, review, translate
3. **APPLICATION** (to use information in a new situation): apply, calculate, complete, demonstrate, dramatize, employ, examine, illustrate, justify, predict, practice, relate, report, solve, use, utilize
4. **ANALYSIS** (to examine and break down into parts): analyze, appraise, categorize, contract, criticize, debate, detect, diagram, distinguish, experiment, infer, inspect, inventory, question, separate, summarize
5. **SYNTHESIS** (to combine, to complex): arrange, assemble, collect, compose, construct, create, design, detect, formulate, generalize, integrate, manage, organize, plan, prepare, prescribe, produce, set-up, specify
6. **EVALUATION** (to make a judgment based on criteria): appraise, assess, choose, critique, determine, estimate, evaluate, grade, judge, measure, rank, rate, recommend, revise, score, select

---

The role of the instructor lies in (1) having students develop an awareness of ascending levels of thinking and (2) providing opportunities for them to use their intellect.

Activity 1: Cognitive Domain

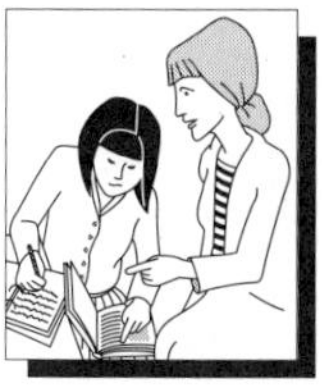

Match the following objectives with the specific realm of the Cognitive Domain.

a. knowledge b. comprehension c. application

d. analysis e. synthesis f. evaluation

_______ 1. Given sufficient control and patient data, the student will be able to evaluate whether or not the calibration of the IL-313 gas analyzer is acceptable or needs to be repeated.

_______ 2. Having studied the various principles of hemoglobin formation, the student will correlate the hemoglobins and their specific pathology.

_______ 3. The student will be able to list all the parameters included in the complete blood count (CBC).

_______ 4. The student will be able to calculate the mean and standard deviation of a given set of values.

_______ 5. Given various pertinent data relating to a hospital lab, its workload and needs, the student will be able to set up a work schedule for the employees of that lab.

_______ 6. Given the results of a patient's glucose tolerance test, the student will interpret the patient's condition.

Affective Domain[2]

Webster defines "affective" as *that which deals with the emotions.* The realms designate the *degree* to which individuals engage themselves in situations involving their morals and values. The domain identifies *attitudes* and *behavior* of the individual.

Realms of the Affective Domain are as follows (see Fig. 4–2):

1. *Receiving* is best described as an individual's *willingness* to listen. It is identified by observing and demonstrating a receptive attitude to a signal. "The student *was open* to the suggestions offered him."

2. *Responding* implies that an individual has taken in a signal and in some observable manner *replies.* "The student, hearing the question, *raised* his hand to answer."

3. *Valuing* encompasses the previous realms of this domain and concludes with the individual identifying with a value, so much so that he/she displays an attitude of acceptance[3]: one of commitment. "Feeling the proposed meeting was important, the student *volunteered* to serve on the committee."

	Categorized by CLS
5. **Characterization**	III. Identifies with the value
4. **Organization** 3. **Valuing** 2. **Responding**	II. Affixes worth to process and internalizes
1. **Receiving**	I. Awareness and reaction of/to stimulus

Figure 4–2 The realms of the Affective Domain.

4. *Organization* further describes an individual who has established his/her own value system and expresses it by internalizing it. "The student, realizing the importance of study, *invests* 4 hours of time every day." The degree of difference between *valuing* and *organization* is one of personal involvement: from one of recognizing value in something outside of himself/herself to embracing that value as his/her own.

5. *Characterization* builds on the previous realms and illustrates a person who has developed a personal value system that now *modifies* that person's behavior. The value system dictates the person's performance; he/she bonds with the system so much that it *characterizes* his/her life. "The student, having performed a procedure in which the standard did not result in the range of acceptance, *typically repeated* the test *knowing* the patient's results could also be incorrect."

In this example, the response of the student to the inaccurate result of the standards *reflects* his/her integrity. The student knows that the procedure must be repeated. He/she knows that the patient values generated from this procedure will be used by the physician in therapy. Much is at risk. It is this type of consistent behavior that contributes to the formation of the *character* of an individual.

APPLICATION OF THE DOMAIN TO THE BEHAVIORAL OBJECTIVES

The desired behavior of students in the CLS profession and that of practicing laboratorians is identified by the various professional and accrediting agencies. In the Code of Ethics written by the American Society of Clinical Laboratory Science, the competencies involving the Affective Domain express the desirable behavior for all associated with the profession.

> Being fully cognizant of my responsibilities in the practice of medical technology, I affirm my willingness to discharge my duties with accuracy, thoughtfulness, and care. Realizing the knowledge obtained concerning patients in the course of my work must be treated as confidential, I hold inviolate the confidence placed in me by patients and physician.
>
> Recognizing that my integrity and that of my profession must be pledged to the absolute reliability of my work, I will conduct myself at all times in a manner appropriate to the dignity of my profession.[4]

And the following stated in the *Essentials of NAACLS:*

> Medical technologists are proficient in demonstrating professional conduct and interpersonal communication skills with patients, laboratory personnel, other health-care professionals and with the public . . . recognizing and acting upon individual needs for continuing education as a function of growth maintenance of professional competency . . . leading supportive personnel and peers in their acquisition of knowledge, skills, and attitudes . . .[5]

Included in the student handbook issued to each individual accepted into the program are competency-based policies. These express explicit desired student behavior. Attributes such as honesty, modest dress, professional attitude, and behavior are listed.

The nature of the Affective Domain makes the task of influencing the adult student in the program difficult. By this time in their lives, students have formed their own set of values, a personal ethical code of behavior influenced by family, friends, religion, and the values of the world. To express "desired behavior" dealing with the Affective Domain relies on the use of specific action verbs that can be used to demonstrate these internal attitudes (covert) and external behavior (overt). These are given in the following box.

VERBS USED IN WRITING OBJECTIVES FOR THE AFFECTIVE DOMAIN

1. **RECEIVING** (accepting): desires, dislikes, enjoys, is willing, is open, likes, loves, shows interest, wants
2. **RESPONDING** (reacts): responds
3. **VALUING** (identifies with): accepts, chooses, commits self, criticizes, declines, participates, praises, prefers, strives, volunteers
4. **ORGANIZATION** (relates to): appreciates, associates with, is dedicated to, invests in, shares values with
5. **CHARACTERIZATION** (identifies with): characterizes, is consistent with, identifies with, typifies

Relevance: The role of the instructor is to provide situations: case studies involving "attitude and value education, moral awareness, and development" as relates to decision-making in the clinical laboratory. Students, through exercises provided in the class, must identify their own value system as applied to laboratory situations in order to understand the value orientations of the profession, the patient, and other persons who are involved or affected.

Activity 2: The Affective Domain

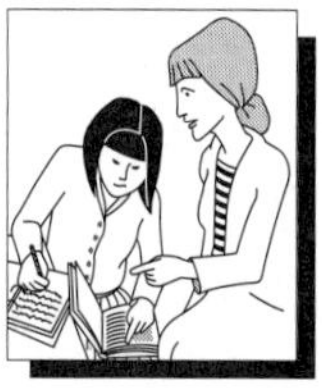

After discussing the following situations, write a short summary reflecting consensus of the group.

1. Within your group, discuss *professionalism*. Include in your discussion the definition, description, and the role professionalism plays in the academic year and in the clinical year.
2. Regarding dress code: How would you deal with a student who attends class dressed inappropriately? Define inappropriate dress. How would you handle this student?

3. Referring to the January 1994 issue of Laboratory Medicine (Vol. 25 No. 1, pp. 27-31), *Assessment of Student "Affective" Behaviors in US Medical Technology Programs* by Hudson et al, read, discuss, and summarize your reactions to the information reported in the article.
4. Every person has been motivated by some force. Discuss motivation within your group, and list the factors by importance of frequency.
5. Research one article on motivation. Write a critique. Upon completion of the group's activities, each member will share his/her findings from the chosen article.

Psychomotor Domain[3]

Realms within this domain describe variability of performance skills dependent on direction or guidance by the mind. An individual exhibiting good psychomotor skills is described as being "coordinated." These individuals know how the limitations of the equipment, instruments, and reagents used can affect the various procedures. The introduction of error to a procedure is constantly being monitored by the mind. It is dictating at every step of performance, cautioning the correct way to pipette . . . the fingers drawing up the fluid to a given level . . . the mind's eye observing and dictating to the hand to wipe the tip and only then to release the aspirated solution into a vial (see Fig. 4–3).

1. *Perception* refers to the person who *observes* the steps of a procedure demonstrated by the instructor and makes *mental notes* on what is to be done, how it is to be performed, what reagents and equipment are to be used, and why.

2. *Set* refers to a response by the learners resulting in their being ready to perform the procedure just observed. The person organizes the necessary reagents, checks out the equipment, reviews the procedure, and is *prepared* to start. He/she is *ready.*

3. *Guided response* describes the student repeating the demonstration, imitating the instructor's technique. The student imitates.

	CLS Categorizing
7. **Origination** 6. **Adaptation**	III. Modify, invent
5. **Complex overt response** 4. **Mechanism** 3. **Guided response**	II. Proficient through practice
2. **Set** 1. **Perception**	I. Aware and ready to respond

Figure 4–3 Realms included in the Psychomotor Domain.

4. *Mechanism* expresses the ability to repeat a procedure with ease and *proficiency* and without error in the required time. This level of performance reflects time spent on extended practice.

5. *Complex overt response* refers to ability to perform *many highly coordinated* motor activities accurately.

6. *Adaptation* describes extremely well developed motor skills and the ability to *modify* and use them in new situations.

7. *Origination* encompasses all six realms and culminates in the development of new movement pattern skills that enhance an existing procedure or are employed in a newly designed test.

Psychomotor skills are the basis of most work that laboratorians will use in the clinical laboratory. This domain is at the heart and soul of program training: to instruct and train students to perform tasks accurately while understanding the importance of each step. It is not uncommon to have students who excel in the cognitive portion of the program and fail in the psychomotor area. They understand the theoretical aspects but lack coordination.

A stated competency statement selected from the Task Document of ASCP reads as follows: "The Medical Technologist will prepare instruments to perform tests." A stated objective expressing this competency reflects Realm 2: *Set* and read as follows: "The student, having learned how to prime the Coulter STX, will, following the manufacturer's instructions, *prepare* the instrument for the morning runs."

To perform this will involve running standards and adjusting the necessary controls to generate accurate readings. It is assumed that the student has had demonstrations and practice time to master the skill with and without supervision. Specific verbs, then, must be used in expressing objectives dealing with the performance tasks. See the following box.

VERBS USED IN WRITING OBJECTIVES FOR THE PSYCHOMOTOR DOMAIN

1. **PERCEPTION:** hear, see, smell, taste, touch
2. **SET:** adjust, approach, locate, place, position, prepare
3. **GUIDED RESPONSE:** copy, determine, discover, duplicate, imitate, inject, repeat
4. **MECHANISM:** adjust, build, illustrate, indicate, manipulate, mix, set up
5. **COMPLEX OVERT RESPONSE:** calibrate, coordinate, demonstrate, maintain, operate
6. **ADAPTATION:** adjust, conform, change
7. **ORIGINATION:** build, construct, create, design, fabricate, invent, produce

RELEVANCE

The role of the instructor involves providing opportunities through laboratory exercises for the students to master the skills currently used in the clinical laboratory. Practical examinations following supervision should be part of the course.

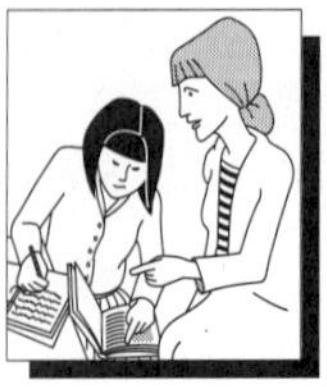

Activity 3: Psychomotor Domain

1. Within your group, discuss the type of *skills* necessary to function in the field of CLS. List by importance.
2. Write objectives for the following realms: A, Guided response; B, Adaptation.

Activity 4: Summary

After reviewing the levels of achievement in each domain of the following students, identify the one student whose levels of accomplishments are not in synchronization. Discuss this student's achievement levels, as well as those of the others.

Student No.	Cognitive	Affective	Psychomotor	
1.	Knowledge	Receiving	Perception	______
2.	Analysis	Valuing	Adaptation	______
3.	Evaluation	Organization	Origination	______

Summary

The Behavioral Objectives, using the domains, establish the *matrix* of the professional program upon which all instruction is based. The instructors design lecture and laboratory exercises in such a way that provide for development and mastery of these realms.

Several considerations regarding the domains must be made: (1) The relationship of domains indicates a pattern of ascending complexity and personal involvement. (2) There is a transcending relationship of the domains from one to another illustrating a synchronous development. This is highly desirable but not always realistic (see Fig. 4–4). One domain can influence the expression of another for good or for bad. Attitudes (affective domains) such as a closed mind, rejection, charged emotions, and dislike, can end an academic experience in a very short time. *Motivation* and a positive attitude are crucial when engaged in such a demanding program as CLS. (4) The advantages of using objectives indicate specific requirements for the student regarding knowledge and skill that must be mastered to succeed. For the instructor, objectives constitute a *reference* that dictates construction of lectures, emphasis given to specific subjects, and construction of laboratory exercises, quizzes, and exams. For certifying agencies, they constitute a guideline to the taxonomy of questions that make up the certifying exams.

Review Questions

Identify the domain and realm of each of the following stated objectives:

1. After studying a stained blood smear, the clinical laboratory scientist accurately identified the child's type of leukemia.

2. Having run the laboratory for 10 years, the CLS manager evaluated and revised all lab procedures in order to meet the standards of NAACLS.

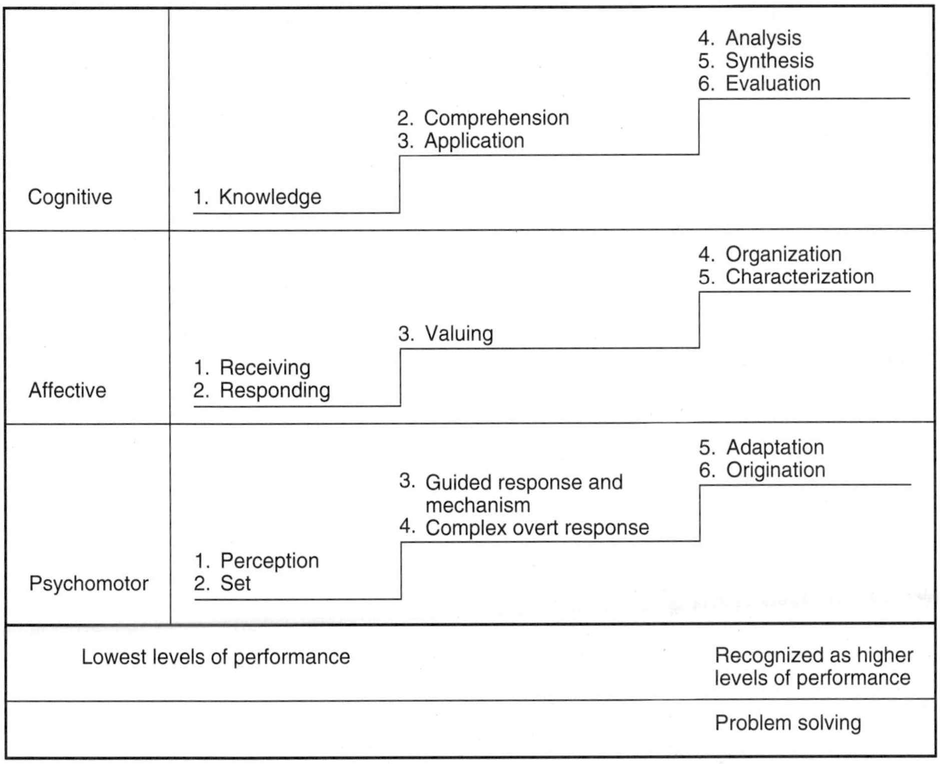

Figure 4–4 Relationship of the Cognitive, Affective, and Psychomotor Domains.

3. The chemist, after repairing the multichannel instrument, reviewed and analyzed 100 samples according to the manufacturer's standards.

4. The students, having viewed a video on immunology, accurately explained the content to the audience.

5. Identify the domain involved in the following situation and comment on how you would handle the situation if you were teaching the class. *The student sat down in the back of the class, in the very back row. She was so small, she could barely be seen from the front. When you began the lecture, she took out a novel and began to read, looking up occasionally at you. You knew she was taking this class for credit and was enrolled in the professional program. This class was to be followed by a lab in which information given in the lecture explained the laboratory exercise.*

See p. 405 for answers.

References

1. Bloom BS. Taxonomy of Educational Objectives: The Classification of Educational Goals. New York, David McKay, 1956, p 18.
2. Krathwohl DR. Taxonomy of Educational Objectives: The Classification of Educational Goals. New York, David McKay, 1964, p 35.
3. Harrow AJ. The classification of the educational objectives in the psychomotor domain. *In* Kibler RJ, Cegala DJ, Watson KW, et al, eds. Objectives for Instruction and Evaluation. 2d ed. Boston, Allyn and Bacon, 1974, p 104.
4. American Society of Clinical Laboratory Science. Code of Ethics. Unpublished Data. 1988.
5. National Accreditation Agency for Clinical Laboratory Science. Guide to Accreditation. Chicago, NAACLS, 1992.

Suggested Reading

1. Bloom BS. Taxonomy of educational objectives. *In* The Classification of Educational Goals: I. The Cognitive Domain. New York, David McKay, 1974.
2. Blocher DH, Rapoza RS. Professional and vocational preparation. *In* Chickering AW, et al, eds. The Modern American College. San Francisco, Jossey-Bass Publishers, 1988, pp 212–231.
3. Developing Better Test Questions with the Blooms: Taxonomy. The Teaching Professor. Madison, Wisc, Magna Publications, 1993.
4. Eble KE. The Craft of Teaching. 2nd ed. San Francisco, Calif, Jossey-Bass Publishers, 1988.
5. Gottsching C. Limits of preventive health care and health education. Offentliche Gesundheitsweses 1990;52(8-9):361–367.
6. Hedges WD. Testing and Evaluation for the Sciences in the Secondary Schools. Belmont, Calif, Wadsworth, 1966.
7. Kibler RJ, Cegala DJ, Watson KW, Barker LL, Miles DT. Objectives for Instruction and Evaluation. 2nd ed. Boston, Allyn and Bacon, 1981.
8. Knapp D. Career preferences of clinical laboratory science graduates: influence of personality type and other factors. Clinical Laboratory Science 1992;5(2):117–121.
9. Krathwohl DR, Bloom BS, Masia BB. Taxonomy of Educational Objectives. Handbook II: Affective Domain. New York, David McKay, 1973.
10. LeGrys VA, Beck SJ. Clinical Laboratory Education. San Mateo, Calif, Appleton and Lange, 1988, ch 3.
11. Lowman J. Mastering the Technique of Teaching. San Francisco, Jossey-Bass Publishers, 1984, pp 119–145.
12. McKenna A, Ledfetter M, Ramalkeo L. Integrating values education into an allied health curriculum: Part I. Journal of Radiologic Technology 1989;60(6):499–502.
13. McKenna A, Ledbetter M, Ramalkeo L. Integrating values education into an allied health curriculum. Part II. Journal of Radiologic Technology 1989;61(1):41–46.
14. Perry WG. Cognitive and ethical growth: the making of meaning. *In* Chickering AW, et al, eds. The Modern American College. San Francisco, Jossey-Bass Publishers, 1988, pp 76–116.
15. Posner GJ, Rudnitsky AN. Course Design. A Guide to Curriculum Development for Teachers. New York, Longman, 1986: ch 7.
16. Yelon SL. Writing and using instructional objectives. *In* Briggs LJ, Gustafson KL, Tillman MH, eds. Instructional Design: Principles and Applications. Educational Technology Publications, 1991, pp 75–121.

5

Teaching Methodologies: Matching Style to Need

OBJECTIVES

Upon completion of this chapter, the reader should be able to:

- Identify Gagne's "Preparatory Steps to Teaching" and discuss their value in using any type of teaching method.
- Discuss the types and description of teaching methodologies available for instruction.
- Demonstrate the use of specific instructional methodologies with a designated competency to be acquired.
- List the advantages and limitations of each methodology.
- Develop a short teaching unit demonstrating utilizing stated objectives and an instructional methodology in fulfilling a competency.
- List the advantages and disadvantages of each method.

KEY WORDS

lesson plan
educational methodologies
discussions
questioning

Introduction

You have just about thought of everything that has to be in place before you actually start teaching. How many hours have you put into preparation? And you haven't even taught 1 hour. This chapter deals with the variability of educational methodologies for you to consider in preparing your *lesson plan.* It is essential to use a methodology that will best assist the students in acquiring the knowledge and skills stated in the competencies. In fact, the factors determining the teaching methodology used by instructors in CLS education should reflect (1) changes in the workplace that relate to advanced technology and skills of personnel, (2) the changing role of the laboratorian, (3) the curriculum identifying *new* technology and skills, (4) the variability of student learning abilities (You haven't met your class yet to find this out!), and (5) the knowledge of the learning process by the instructor and his/her ability to use the instructional method for optimal learning.

The Lesson Plan

Earlier, you were prompted to look at the specific discipline you were asked to teach and to organize your topic into presentations covering a semester (usually 14 weeks of instruction). The Course Syllabus establishes the course content that instructors project will be covered in that designated time together with a calendar designating the dates specific topics will be presented. The *Lesson Plan* deals with the instructor's organization of the individual presentation and includes the following considerations for organizing the lesson plan:

- Make a careful written record of what you expect to accomplish.
- Check the objectives of the subject.
- Be sure of the order of the presentation.

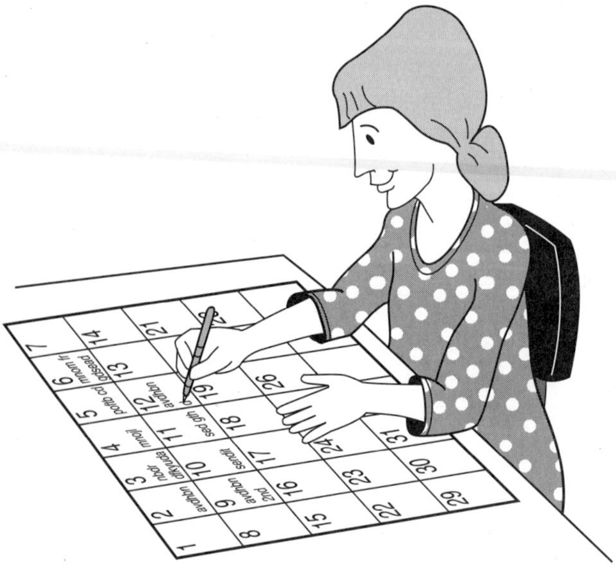

- Prepare adequate notes and master them, so that an occasional glance at the notes is all you need.
- Rehearse.
- Never read.
- Collect and organize all teaching aids.
- If you have taught the subject before, look for different approaches to the subject.
- Make a considered selection of material; no lecture can possibly cover everything pertinent.
- Prepare provocative questions illustrating problems and situations to stimulate the interest of the students.
- Stimulate the students with unsolved problems of the present day.[1]

The lesson plan comprises your *immediate preparation* or your *planning of the lesson.* Take nothing for granted; be overprepared.

Strategy in Preparation

Once the instruction begins, no matter the choice of method, there is an established sequence of "Instructional Events" that the teacher should initiate.[2]

- Gaining attention (engaging the interest of the student)
- Presenting the objective (identifying the knowledge/skill the student will gain)
- Stimulating recall of prerequisite learning (reminding the student what was previously learned)
- Presenting the stimulus material (providing the stimulus to the student, whether it be verbal or demonstration)
- Providing learning guidance (facilitate learning by using checklists and outlines for display of sequential steps)
- Elicit the performance (causing the student to perform a task)
- Providing feedback about accuracy of performance (informing the student of improvements to be made)
- Assessing the performance (determining if the student achieved the objective)
- Enhancing retention and transfer (assisting the student to apply knowledge from one situation to another).[2]

For new graduates who will be instructing the senior students in the clinical laboratory, the planning process is no different. A syllabus of the material should be obtained from the department chair. This will give you the overview of material and skills to be covered. The calendar the department chair gives to you designates the exact dates students will be with you to learn designated subject content and skills. This enables you to format your *lesson plan,* which follows the scheme just outlined. Your availability for the students will be determined by the patient load of the day. Always have "activities," study cards, and so forth for your students to use in situations that take you out of the instruction mode and place you back into the working mode. This has the advantage of contributing to the independent learning of the students.

The Various Educational Methodologies

THE LECTURE

The lecture, by definition, involves the dissemination of information by an "authority" on a subject with the sole objective of having students listen and understand the material in order to use and apply it in new situations. The lecture is best suited for large groups and covers subjects that do not involve learning massive amounts of new information. Developments regarding an already established topic, research findings related to a known disease state, explanations, and discussions of difficult concepts relating to previous knowledge are examples of correct use of the lecture. Weimer lists the many advantages of getting students more actively involved in the lecture by using discussions.

> Discussion (1) cultivates the kind of involvement that leads to learning functions as a feedback, identifying what the students do and don't understand; (2) brings members of a class into a closer working relationship with each other and with an instructor; (3) teaches students to listen and respect the opinions of their peers; (4) and can be used to further understanding, both in the students and in the instructor.[3]

The lecture has survived and remains the primary teaching method in educational institutions. Overheads, Kodachromes, and even case studies (when applicable) have contributed to the interest and variability of presentation. However, educators should remember their response to and behavior after the various lectures they attended. We have all slept during a lecture, been bored, felt trapped, had negative reactions, and felt uninvolved in a presentation. Sometimes it provided us a chance to escape into our own world. That always seems such a better place to be. How do we present a more successful lecture than those we have experienced? Why are we expecting and demanding a better response from our students? Udolf reminds us of the following:

> Preparing a lecture is the work part of the job; delivering it is the fun part. If you've done a good job of preparation, you can have confidence that the lecture will go well. If you haven't, you will discover that the best teacher in the world is no better than his material.[4]
>
> The most important thing to remember in delivering a lecture is that you must interact with your audience, not just talk at them. This is why it is so ineffective to read lecture notes. Interacting with a class means not only answering questions when they arise but observing your students and getting feedback as to how they are following the lecture. Without having to be told by student questions, a good lecturer knows if a class is following him intently or is bored and confused. He not only notices this but responds to it by slowing down, backtracking, or elaborating when necessary. He keeps his class actively involved in the lecture by rhetorical or actual questions and by his response to student

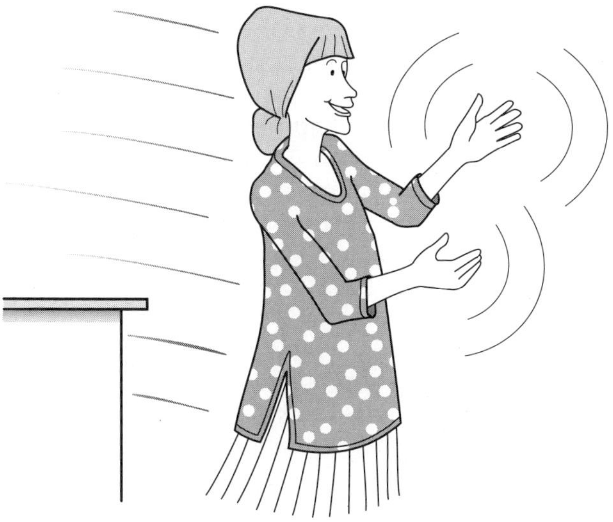

> reactions. He makes even a lecture an active participatory experience for all members of the class.[4]
>
> Interacting with a class in its fullest means considering the needs of *every member of the class.* This can tax the skill of the best of lecturers.[4]

And perhaps now you can realize the importance of what was stated in Chapters 1 and 2: that you know your material so well that you can spend classroom time watching responses and nonresponses of the students. Udolf continues:

> Thus, a good lecture must be a compromise between the requirement of the best student, who may be bored with too rudimentary an explanation or too slow a pace, and the poorest, who may be overwhelmed by anything more. The instructor must give something to each and at the same time consider the requirements of the other. This is why teaching never gets boring; it presents a challenge to attain a standard that the best of us can only hope to approximate in practice.[4]

Clarke[5] in "Building a Lecture that Really Works," states the following:

> Successful lecturers often succeed because they leave room for students to react, encourage reaction, and scan the audience for clues about the health of the interaction. Develop a question that serves as a guide. Pose your questions at the start of your lecture, then answer it at the end.

Johnson[6] states the following:

> Know your subject. You must reflect a knowledge of your discipline. Remain current; throw out the old, add the new. Speak slowly, loudly, and clearly, aiming your words at all areas of the room. Vary the pitch of your voice. Look at the students. You pick up cues from expressions on their faces. Be prepared, but be alive and spontaneous. There is something positive about spontaneity in the classroom that keeps students attentive. . . . Move your body as well as your mouth; don't take a fixed posture at the podium.

The case studies provide a vehicle by which the lecturer either presents or summarizes a focus of the lecture. There are many advantages of case studies. They can be used skillfully by the lecturer and students can become involved in all parts of the study. Case studies involve the students in the higher cognitive activities including analyzing, synthesizing, and judging. The teacher supplies the students with ample background and data, attaches the problem, and applies basic concepts and information.[7]

The lecture is facing tremendous ongoing criticism as a very ineffective teaching method. It is not the lecture that is at fault but rather the *lecturer* who has abused this form of instruction by reading from a prepared script, a book, or notes and has not included the students in the presentation.

The lecture as a method of instruction has many advantages, but its disadvantages, or rather limitations, warrant an alternate method that designates an active role by the learner (Table 5–1). When the objective specifies the exercise of decision making, problem solving, and the development of interpersonal communication skills to be achieved, the teaching method must provide the means of accomplishing the objective. Hansen suggests that the emphasis should be placed on encouraging *learning,* instead of stressing the *teaching* aspect of the activity.[8]

You're beginning to get the picture. It is a given that you know the material; that is important. What the students learn through their own mental activity, by themselves or within a group, is what is really important (Fig. 5–1).

Summary

The success of the lecture as a teaching/learning instrument is based on how it is utilized by the instructor. It has the potential for involving the students

Table 5–1
REVIEWING THE LECTURE

Advantages	Disadvantages
Gives all students the same information	Constitutes a passive group of students
Covers much information in a short time	Creates the illusion that presence is indicative of listening and learning
Includes material that can stimulate discussion	Loses the individual student in the mass
Provides the opportunity for the instructor to view students for indication of grasp of the material	Neglects to engage the higher thought processes of the students (most of the time)
Enables the instructor to emphasize what is essential regarding the lecture subject	Establishes the instructor as the object and subject of all attention
Constitutes relatively easy preparation and delivery of material	Limits the learning of gifted students
Provides a "springboard" for further learning processes	Limits the learning process of students with different learning patterns
Provides the instructor with **ultimate control** over all processes and activities	Intimidates students as members of a large group to ask or answer questions or to make contributions to the class
	Assumes all students have the same base knowledge before lecture
	Provides noninvolved students the vehicle to escape into their own world
	Gives the working student extra time to rest when the lights are dimmed for showing of Kodachromes
	Limits interrelationships involving self-expression, sharing of ideas, explanations by the students
	Impedes students from discovering knowledge for themselves

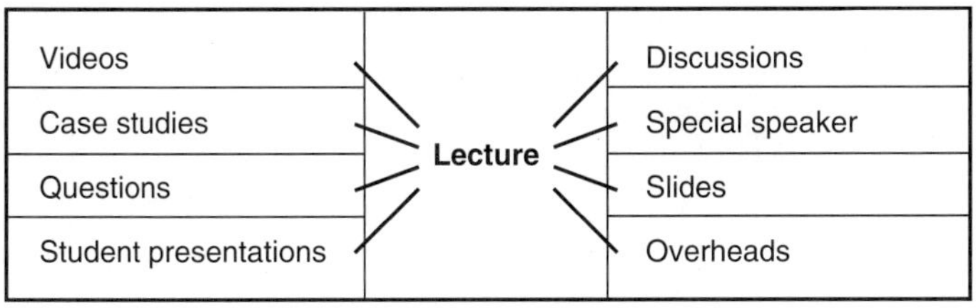

Figure 5–1 Enhancing the lecture.

in high-level critical thinking. When necessary, its function will be dispersion of knowledge that should include involvement with the learners. Review of the objectives, the nature of what is to be taught, and design of the learning tool to facilitate and optimize the specific learning process are essential.

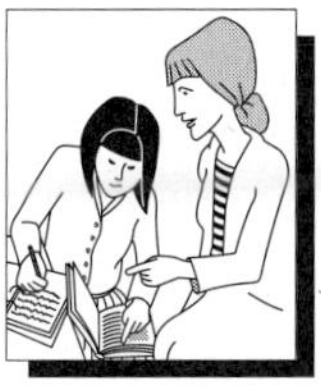

Activity 1

Within your group, discuss lecturers that you have been exposed to in your various classes; include the approach, the format of the lecturer, the qualities you best remember (both good and bad), and your response during those lectures. Provide suggestions on how the instructor could have improved the lecture.

Activity 2

Within your group, choose a lecture topic that can be easily divided into natural components (example: *The Weather*). One person can introduce the topic and define *weather.* Certain types of weather can be presented by each member. The sixth member of the group can summarize the presentation. Present the topic to the entire class. Remember to engage members of the audience during the presentation. Record your organization of the topic outline and the information to be covered by the group members. Do not forget to present your objectives at the start of the "team-taught" lecture. The instructor can videotape your performance, which can later be studied by the group to gain insight and positive feedback on the presentation. Summarize your experience.

SMALL GROUP FORMATION

In presenting small group formation involving either *problem-based solving (PBS)* or *cooperative learning (CL),* experience has established factors that are identified with both modes of instruction.

1. The role of the instructor becomes one of moderator, facilitator, organizer of the learning module, and reference person.
2. The students become the focal point of the learning activity.
3. Groups are composed of no more than six individuals. The instructor organizes the composition of each group in order to ensure a diversity of students, preventing the possible formation of a "social group."
4. The students assume a role within the group. The facilitator encourages involvement by all members; keeps the discussion ongoing and the recorder

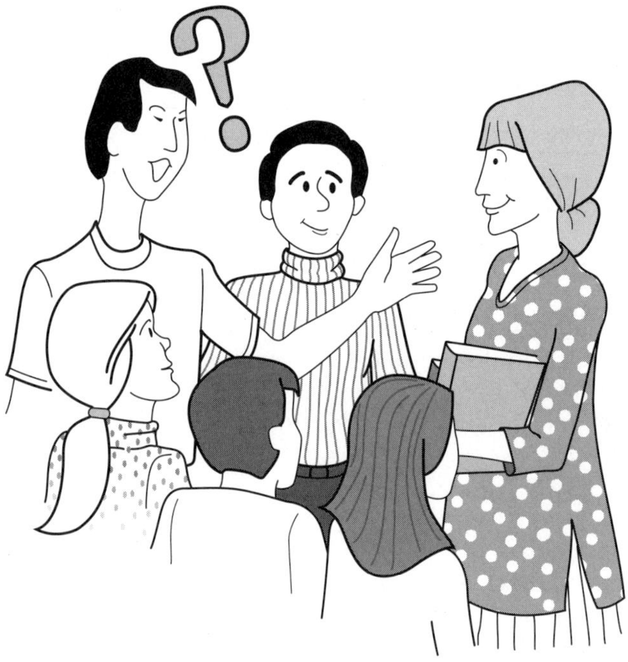

keeps a log of the learning activity within the group. All students are potential resource persons.

5. Students engage with each other in presenting ideas, listening to those of others, compromising, and resolving differences in order to agree on a solution or establish a mode of action. These *negotiator skills* best describe those used when one is involved in discussion in the laboratory or while attending meetings in the professional world.

6. Students are provided with an arena that gives the opportunity to practice expressing and explaining thoughts and points of view. These *technical communication skills* focus on developing *expression, verbalization* of concepts and ideas. Precision (vocabulary) and clarity (thought process) are skills needed to be developed and fine tuned.

7. The small group lessens anxiety by creating a friendly learning environment.

8. Students learn to use each other as resources, to take responsibility for their own learning, and to build support systems.

9. Collaborative learning can be extended and used in all areas of instruction. The advantages of versatility of implementation have been borne out by the literature. Statistics support using the *small group* to improve composition, computer-designed programs, science, and mathematics, and so forth.

Problem-based solving is concerned with group involvement working through difficult or complex situations and arriving at a solution. The popular vehicle used in CLS for problem-based solving is the *case study*. This type of learning emphasizes the input from all members of the group (employing higher cognitive levels) with the objective of resolving the problem.

> PBL provides a means for developing the skills needed by today's professionals as independent learners, problem solvers, team players, and group participants. The facts of science will change, but the need for self-reliance in learning and the need to be a group contributor will not.[9]

Cooperative learning does not involve the members of the group in "solving problems." Its objective is to encourage the exchange of ideas and, when needed, provide explanation within a group in order to assist one another in learning. It uses students with varying backgrounds and abilities to explain concepts and translate difficult information for those who express different learning patterns. A positive interdependence is established among the members of the group, and each student assumes accountability for learning; this is essential.

Summary

The advantages of learning through the small group have been recognized and are being used in educational programs for allied health professions, nursing, and medicine. Statistics indicate that students who use this method retain more information, developing better reasoning, critical thinking, and communication skills, than those who use other modes of learning.

A good combination of methodologies, if time allows, would be to combine lecture and small group learning, which at the end of the group activity, involves individuals sharing their results with the entire class.

Activity 3

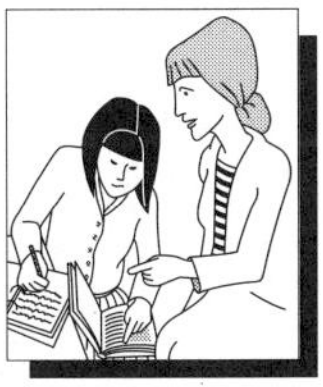

Within your group, discuss how you would change the oil in your car. Keep notes of how many students contribute to the correct sequence of procedure. (No, you may not say that you would take it to a gas station!) Do not forget to state what you would do with the used oil. Ask within the group if there is anyone who could do it on his/her own. This type activity demonstrates cooperative learning, a sharing of information, so that all members of the group learn and contribute to the learning.

TEACHING VIA ELECTRONIC MEDIA

Computer-Assisted Instruction (CAI) or Computer Tutorials

The versatility of programs available through computer software companies reflects advancement in the presentation of technical knowledge, program design, and the engagement of a higher cognitive level by the students. CAI accomplishes the following goals:

1. Provides reinforcement and application of lecture information
2. Engages students with the application of higher cognitive skills when dealing with a presentation such as a "Case Study" approach
3. Enables students to learn independently and at a rate that reflects their needs
4. Decentralizes the instruction, freeing the instructor and fostering independent learning.[9]

The use of software by a small group provides numerous advantages in that each person contributes reinforcement and support by sharing different background information, understanding of the subject, computer skills, and language and again exercising and developing communication skills. Gagne's approach to the use of CAI identifies and categorizes the type of "learning outcome" by examining the objective of the lesson. The categories identified by Gagne[10] are as follows:

1. Verbal information: Recall
2. Intellectual skills
   A. Discrimination
   B. Concrete concept* Identity properties of an object previously unencountered
   C. Defined concept* Learn and define a concept and apply the definition to one or more other learning instances
   D. Rule* Demonstrate the application of the rule
   E. Problem solving* Confront a situation problem by analysis of given information; apply rules, deduce the solution.
3. Cognitive Strategies
4. Motor skills
5. Attitudes

Careful selection of computer programs by the instructor is crucial so that the specific information is technically correct and updated. Several companies have their programs tested and evaluated by students before dissemination. Despite the time factor involved in producing home CAIs, those instructors involved in their production note that the end product—reflecting control of design, selective subject matter, activities, and their "persona"—has resulted in desirable and effective software. Because the field of CLS represents a small market of potential buyers only a limited number of software companies are involved in producing programs for this discipline. However, one company has developed seven programs for CLS with plans for further production.

Summary

The value of CAI or computer tutorials, establishes an additional medium for learning. It provides an opportunity for students to learn material related to the objectives stated by the instructor at their convenience. CAI challenges faculty to discover *how* and *what* is involved in creating CAI programs.

TEACHING USING THE INTERNET

Before utilizing the Internet as another mode of teaching/learning, the instructor should realize that the degree of computer skills varies among students. When making an assignment using the Internet, place the students in small groups, making sure that there is one with a high degree of computer literacy in each group.

Regardless of the make of computer system universities have adopted, all are equipped with access to the Internet. The Internet has quickly developed from an information highway to one of worldwide communication.

*More commonly applied to CAI.[13]

When students are given web-based assignments, an easy and efficient way to locate information on the web is to use one of the many servers (free search services) available. Once the user is onto the program, the item WWW (World Wide Web services) appears, which lists a summary of WWW servers alphabetically by continent, country, and state. Within the United States, the various servers differ only in the direction and extent of information they offer. Alta Vista, Excite, Infoseek, Lycos, Webcrawler, and Yahoo are among the better servers. Yahoo offers many unique features, making it popular among students.

To enter Internet, Netscape, one of the engines for gaining entrance, is clicked. As the user scrolls down using the mouse, the directory "Other World Wide Sites" appears. Signaling this prompt reveals a list of many directories. One directory includes the topic "Learning Tools." Through this program, instructors can communicate with their students, giving assignments, reading lists, and the like. Students likewise can communicate with their instructors via E-mail.

Clicking Yahoo and scrolling down also introduces many directories. Under Education is found the lists of universities and colleges; upon clicking, the program presents them alphabetically. Each specific university admits the user to specific information regarding the college. When entering the various departments, specifically CLS, one can find, for example, a blood cell atlas in color within the University of Washington; California at Irvine presents various case studies to discuss and solve.

Examples of programs that have been described as available on the Internet, including direct communication (No. 3 below), are:

1. CLS education: Enter universities and departments and view programs.
2. Hemophiliacs: Various coagulation abnormalities are presented.
3. Johns Hopkins: Communication with patients with specific disease states is possible. This communication is monitored by an attending physician.
4. Pharmacy: Drug searches including drug interactions.
5. Disease states: Found through topic or author if known (Telmet, Trumpet). Abstracts are viewed on the monitor and can be printed by the user.

At conventions, many speakers advertise their E-mail address on their handouts for those who seek further information regarding the topic presented. The advantages of using the computer in CLS education are many. Assignments dependent on computer/Internet assist those students who will enter professions and businesses that require computer literacy.

ROLE PLAY

Role play provides an effective medium to generate a provocative and unrehearsed expression of learning, usually related to the *affective domain.* The instructor, whether using a situation in an educational or managerial setting, involves at least five to six students in a given situation. Each student is provided a sheet of paper with sufficient data to indicate the role the student is to assume. The role each student plays (what has happened to him/her or what he/she has done and to whom) establishes the situation and the problem. Each student reacts to the situation as if he/she were the person involved. When students take role playing seriously and enter into the roles as described, those involved in the given situation begin to understand each other's viewpoint and circumstances a little more clearly. It contributes to an appreciation for what others experience throughout life. Also, students learn something about themselves—their viewpoints of problems and how they themselves would react as opposed to the reaction of the character they played.

Summary

The purpose of role play as a learning experience is to provide students the opportunity of (1) understanding the feelings and emotions of others expressed in highly stressed or tense situations; (2) realizing the importance of understanding the facts that contribute to such situations; and (3) realizing the necessity of modifying one's behavior accordingly.

Role play videos referred to as Trigger Tapes are of great assistance in dealing with the affective domain. The University of Kentucky has professionally produced a series of videotapes, one in particular dealing with ethics/moral topics. Each tape contains many professionally acted-out scenes. An accompanying set of questions that should trigger discussion is included. These tapes make the discussion of sensitive topics much easier.

DEMONSTRATIONS

When the instructor is dealing with complex instruments, detailed procedures, and procedures requiring manual dexterity, demonstration based on sequential steps is essential. Guidelines include (1) limit the number of students to a number that allows clear visibility for all; (2) have a step-by-step narrative prepared for logical and sequential presentation; (3) stimulate discussion when identifying parts of an instrument or movement associated with a manual procedure; (4) provide diagrams for easy reference and study related to the subject presented; and (5) assign a written summary or a paraphrase defining function, principle, and the reagents utilized by the instrument. Follow up.

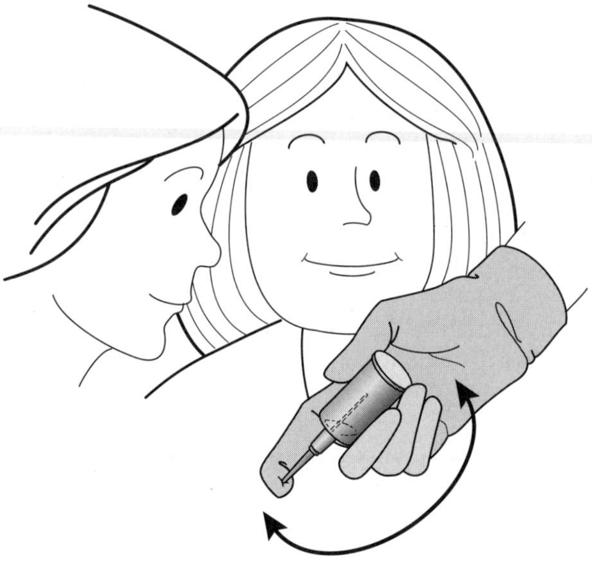

Summary

A well-prepared demonstration is worth a million words.

USE OF VIDEOS

Several years ago, a major hematology company sent a representative to our department and demonstrated their new cell counter to a large group of students and laboratorians. Following the demonstration and question/answer period, the technical representative played a video that summarized the function, procedure, and principle of the counter and the instrument's capability. The colors, graphics, flow cytometer, generated parameters, and histograms were vividly depicted. The running time of 12 minutes was packed with well-paced information. Best of all, the video was left with our department as a gift.

Companies involved in designing various pieces of instrumentation for the clinical laboratory produce videos that are available and suitable for educational as well as promotional purposes. The number of publishers who supply videos with the purchase of a textbook is on the increase. Their advantages are similar to those of CAI.

1. Objective: Describes the function of the instrument with accompanying explanation of methodology
2. The viewers: Designed for individual or small group
3. Construction: Produced professionally
4. Message: Delivers a vivid, moving, exciting, colorful, clear message and presents specific and limited information in a stimulating form
5. Usage: Used by need (review, replay, difficult sections), accompany group discussion and clarification, with student input
6. Cost: Negotiable, rental, free?

The professional organization ASCP recently advertised a video on "Blood Collection: The Pediatric Patient," which presents a complete agenda of subject matter. Depending on the *objectives* of the lesson in regard to the use of this video, it appears that instructors present their objectives to the students, show the video, and have prepared discussion questions pertaining to the set objectives and other pertinent subject matter covered. Response to the questions would allow additional time and opportunity to those who need to view the video again.

Summary

Use of the video as a primary or supplementary learning tool offers advantages similar to those of CAI. These include usability by an individual or small group at a comfortably paced rate and the opportunity for interactive learning and immediate feedback. When applicable, videos can engage the student at a higher cognitive level.

TAPES

It has been the practice of the professional organizations to offer taped copies of presentations given at annual conventions. Topics range from the politics of health care reform (involving the laboratory), specific technical areas, laboratory administration, and education. The advantage of these tapes is that they provide *recent* information regarding the topic. The cost is minimal.

DISTANCE LEARNING

The use of advanced communication technology through which an educational activity at one geographic site is transmitted to another best describes *distance learning.* Advanced electronic technology has culminated in the provision of innovative communication through the *electronic blackboard.* "Chalk talk" is converted to signals, transmitted, and visualized on an *interactive television monitor* providing immediate audio and video feedback over small or large geographic distances. Microwave and cable delivery modes are the most frequently used methods.

Summary

Educators in CLS now have the opportunity to use and develop multiple educational media owing to an explosion in the development of technology as applied to education and communication. The statement once made by a teacher, "You can't beat the blackboard," is being challenged. A philosophy of caution must be exercised in the use of methodologies that are becoming available to every educational institution. The use of media for optimal learning must be the reason why it is used. It must be better than, or at least equal to, whatever methodologies are being used. The objectives and the need must dictate its use, and educators must roll up their sleeves and learn the process well before it is used.

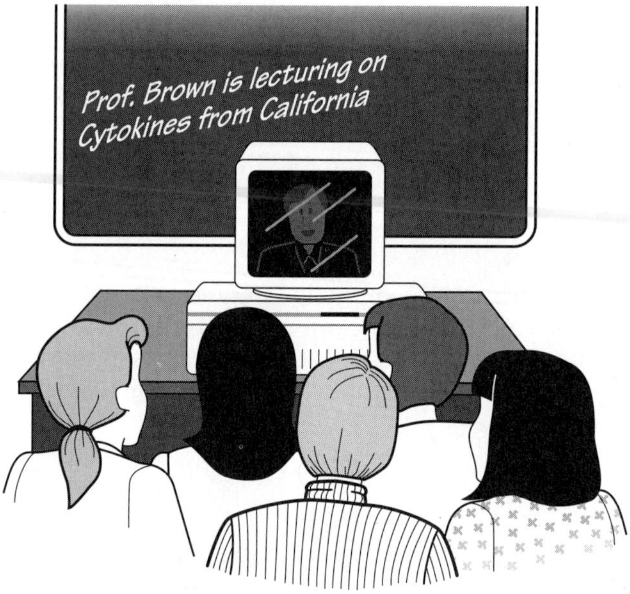

Review Questions

Directions: Fill in the blank with your choice of teaching methodology that best fits the skill to be taught/learned.

1. ______________ Performing a manual procedure.
2. ______________ Developing interpersonal skills.
3. ______________ Learning new information regarding a disease state.
4. ______________ Exercising critical thinking.
5. ______________ Helping/receiving assistance in understanding concepts.
6. ______________ Discussing and working out solutions.
7. ______________ Interpreting, discussing test results with a doctor.
8. ______________ Receiving instruction from a nearby university.

See p. 406 for answers.

References

1. Faculty Committee of Massachusetts Institute of Technology. Technique of teaching. *In* You and Your Students. Washington DC, The American Society for Engineering Education, 1975, 16–30.
2. Aronson DT, Briggs LJ. Models of Instruction in Instructional-Design Theories and Models: An Overview of Their Current Status. Reigeluth H, Charles M, eds. Hillsdale, NJ, Lawrence Erlbaum Publishers, (Abstr): July 1993.
3. Weimer ME, Neff RA. What Can Discussion Accomplish in Teaching College? Madison, Wisc, Magna Publications, 1990, p 97.
4. Udolf R. *In* Preparing and delivering good lectures. The College Instructor's Guide to Teaching and Academia. Chicago, Nelson-Hall, 1976:45–57.
5. Clarke J. Building of a lecture that really works. Education Digest Oct 1987; pp 52–57.
6. Johnson GR. Enhancing the Lecture in First Steps to Excellence in College Teaching. 2nd ed. Madison, Wisc, Magna Publications, 1990, pp 19–23.
7. McLeish J. The Lecture Method in the Psychology of Methods, 75 Yearbook of the National Society for the Study of Education. Part I. Chicago, University of Chicago Press, 1976, pp 43–47.
8. Hansen AJ. Suggestions for seminar participants. *In* Christensen CR, ed. Teaching and the Case Method. Boston, Harvard Business School, 1987, pp 54–59.
9. Doig K. Problem-based learning: developing practitioners for today and tomorrow. Clinical Laboratory Science 1994; 7(3) 172–177.
10. Gagne RM, Wager W. Computer-assisted instruction lessons. *In* Briggs LJ, Gustafson KL, Tillman MH, eds. Instructional Design Principles and Applications. 2nd ed. Englewood, NJ, Educational Technology Publications, 1991, pp 221–226.

Suggested Reading

1. Albanese MA, Mitchell S. Problem-based learning: a review of literature on its outcomes and implementation issues. (Abstr) Academic Medicine 1993; 68 (7): 545.
2. Blake WE. Four points of a good speech: from the students' perspective. *In* The Teaching Professor. Madison, Wisc, Magna Publications, 1994, pp 1–2.
3. Bruce JM, Bruce AW. Distance learning: a learner-centered paradigm. Clinical Laboratory Science 1994; 7(3):178–182.
4. Bruhn JG. Problem-based learning: an approach toward reforming allied health education. Journal of Allied Health 1992; Summer: 161–173.
5. Dastur F. Meditations on teaching. The Teaching Professor. Madison, Wisc, Magna Publications, 1994, p 1.
6. Davis BG. Tools for Teaching. San Francisco, Jossey-Bass Publishers, 1993.
7. Doig K. Problem-based learning: adopting and adapting it for clinical laboratory science. Laboratory Medicine 1993; 24(7): 411–416.
8. Doig K. Risk-taking: deciding what not to teach. Clinical Laboratory Science 1992; 5(2):79.
9. Doyle K. Introducing clinical laboratory science students to computer technology. Clinical Laboratory Educators' Convention, Rhode Island, 1994.
10. Freeman V. Multi-Media and Computer Fo-

rum. Clinical Laboratory Educators' Convention, Rhode Island, 1994.
11. Hargrave CA. Developing a more effective training program. Medical Laboratory Observer 1993; 25(9):50–56.
12. Held MS, Snyder JP, Castleberry B, Mauck K. Evolution or revolution: MT curriculum review. Laboratory Medicine 1993; 34(24): 396–398.
13. Kantrowitz B. The Group Classroom. Newsweek May 10, 1993, p 73.
14. Kiob DA. Learning styles and disciplinary differences. *In* Chickering AW, et al, eds. The Modern American College. San Francisco, Jossey-Bass Publishers, 1988, pp 232–255.
15. McEnerney K. Quality-teams: the foundation of quality improvement. Clinical Laboratory Science 1994; 7(2):103–107.
16. McEnerney K. Cooperative learning in clinical laboratory science education. Clinical Laboratory Science 1994; 7(3):166–171.
17. Menges RJ. Instructional methods. *In* Chickering AW, et al, eds. The Modern American College. San Francisco, Jossey-Bass Publishers, 1988, pp 556–581.
18. Michels E. Enhancing the scholarly base: the role of faculty in enhancing scholarship. Journal of Allied Health 1989; 129–142.
19. Prawat RS. The value of ideas: problems versus possibilities in learning. Educational Researcher Association 1993; 22(6): 5–16.
20. Richards J. Computer tutorials getting high marks. Augmenting MT Classroom Lectures. Advance 1994; 6(27):8–15.
21. Stasz C. Lecturing is not dead: a nature hike through effective teaching. *In* Weimer M, Neff RA, eds. Teaching College. Madison, Wisc, Magna Publications, 1990, 69.
22. Symposium: Consensus on strategies to teach professional skills. Laboratory Medicine 1993; 24(7):434–437.
23. Symposium: Opportunities to apply problem-based learning. Laboratory Medicine 1993; 24:417–419.
24. Teshima DY, Morton K, Taylor P. Problem-based learning in clerkship training at the University of Hawaii. Clinical Laboratory Science 1994; 7(4):209–211.
25. Theriot BL. Energizing Allied Health Educators Through Creative Teaching Strategies. Rhode Island, Clinical Laboratory Science Educators' Meeting, 1994.
26. Weimer M. What can discussion accomplish? *In* Weimer M, Neff RA, eds. Teaching College. Madison, Wisc, Magna Publications, 1990; pp 95, 96.

Videos

University of Kentucky. Role Play: Ethics and Morals.

6

Testing: How Well Did They Do? How Well Did *You* Do?

OBJECTIVES

Upon completion of this chapter, the reader should be able to:

- Discuss the necessity of "testing" in various aspects of society.
- Identify the responsibility that accompanies "passing an exam" in an allied health profession such as CLS.
- Compare the responsibility of a student passing an exam in biology with that of one passing an exam in an applied science such as hematology, immunohematology, and immunology.
- Differentiate *norm-referenced* from *criterion-referenced* tests.
- Identify and discuss the various types of objective tests; include their advantages and disadvantages in testing the realms of the cognitive domain.
- Recognize the *attributes* of test questions and their application in test construction.
- Recognize the aspects of a well-stated test question.
- Analyze and recognize a correctly constructed and an incorrectly stated test question (true/false, multiple choice, matching, short answer).

KEY WORDS

competencies
objectives
quiz
exam
responsibility

Introduction

Several months ago, a pharmacist was discussing with a peer group the performance of his students in a class dealing with pharmaceutics (drugs). The class had just taken a mid-term exam, and the instructor mentioned that the class average was 76%. His face showed concern. A professor within the peer group smiled, commenting, "That's not a bad average for a cumulative exam, Henry. You should be pleased with that result—you teach a difficult course." Henry responded, "It's not the 76% that worries me. It's the 24% that represents lack of knowledge about administration of drugs that troubles me."

CLS instructors—academic and clinical—experience the same concern regarding students who "just get by." It's not the 70% required information they know; it is the 30% of knowledge and performance of skills *not demonstrated* that worry us all. Testing is a fact of life. No matter which career individuals enter, demonstration of proficiency by testing will take place at the end of the training period. However, educators must ensure that the testing instruments used have the qualities that designate the test as reliable and valid.

This story is important, especially as you have finished selecting an instructional methodology, presented the material to the students, and now are ready to evaluate how much and how well the students learned the material/skills. This chapter presents practical issues regarding test construction and administration by instructors and test-taking by students. It is essential that "homemade" tests measure as accurately as possible that which they attempt to measure. Remember the story.

Testing

Testing in the academic segment of a CLS program is crucial in that it measures whether or not students have achieved the *stated objectives* and to what degree. This involves knowledge and skills that instructors know are utilized in the clinical laboratory. *They* know what students have to know first-hand. They meet regularly with the educators at their clinical sites to become aware of advanced technology, instrumentation (procedures and principles), and further information that is being introduced in their area of expertise. Instructors are attuned to the professional organizations regarding what constitutes entry-level knowledge and skill with accompanying cognitive taxonomy level of performance. The instructor uses the body of knowledge and standards of performance set forth by these organizations and translates them into *stated objectives*. All testing, no matter the type, is *objective-based*.

The importance of testing is essential in that CLS programs prepare *students capable of understanding as they perform accurately* for the clinical

Table 6–1
RELATE STATED OBJECTIVES/COMPETENCIES TO TESTING[1]

Stated Objective		Competency	
recall	separate	to know	to analyze
explain	combine	to comprehend	to synthesize
transfer	judge	to apply	to evaluate

sites. This contributes and strengthens the clinical laboratory's link in the health care system (see Table 6–1).

Activity 1

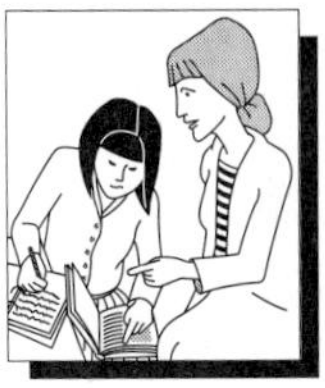

Discuss within your group the attitude of students regarding the reaction following a test. Do the majority of students attempt to learn the questions they were not able to answer, or is it just enough to pass and continue to the next section?

CONSIDERATIONS REGARDING STUDENTS IN TEST-TAKING

Many students state that they do not test well. Whatever the cause, this statement has been accepted by educators as reality; therefore, a university, through its student center, managed by the Academic Development Unit of University Counseling Services, offers assistance in "Test-Taking" and "Test Anxiety." This service is brought to the students' attention through a required competency course during the first 2 years of undergraduate studies.

Activity 2

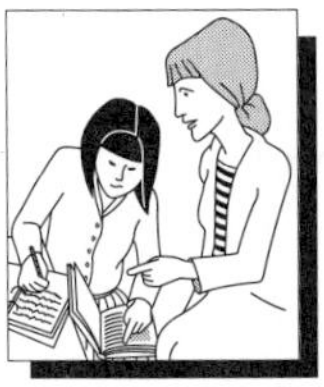

Can anyone in the group identify with the above problem? What, specifically, have you experienced that has interfered with your ability to take a test? How have the students handled the situation?

There is an attitude in test-taking during the undergraduate years that once courses are finished and tests taken, the mental "tapes" can be removed, the material forgotten, and new "tapes" put in. The reality of being held responsible for remembering, retaining, explaining, interpreting, and relating the information to other classes being taken simultaneously during the professional academic year comes as *a shock*! Furthermore, after a "cumulative exam" (so marked on the schedule of exams) was given, the remark made by many students was, "The exam was unfair." This is the era that has often been labeled The Era of Irresponsibility; this attitude carries over into education.

Activity 3

Can you identify with the above practice? Discuss learning/testing during the first 2 years of college and contrast with that carried on in the professional program.

The words multicultural, multiethnic, and multiethical (different value systems) describe the diversified population of the United States and of students entering our programs. There is no easy way to prepare for this diversification. The impact of this phenomenon affects the way we teach, the terminology we use, the way we communicate (most carefully), *the way we test, and the way they test.* Do their test results display how well they understand the information covered or how limited their understanding is of our language and of how to express themselves? As an example, one student would take home notes taken in English, translate them to her native language, learn the material, and rewrite the information in English.

Activity 4

Discuss a "multicultural" student body. Discuss both sides: that is, students born, raised, and educated in the United States and students born in a foreign country and continuing to be educated in this country, specifically, in a CLS program. Include "being tested" in your discussion. List at least four concerns generated from your discussion.

Preparing for the Test: The Review Session

The review session fulfills a necessary function for both instructor and student: that is, it focuses on essential information contained within an extensive presentation of factual material. Review of the objectives associated with the unit should start the process. All essential information relates to these statements. If time warrants, the instructor should prepare a review paper outlining topics of importance. Students feel secure with a confirmed list giving specifics from which to study. They use it as a check-off list. This also serves those students who say, "I studied so hard, but it was the wrong material."

THE TEST GRID: THE INSTRUCTOR

The review exercise also provides the instructor with an opportunity to construct a test grid on which test items are plotted along the *x axis*, with consideration given to the material, the time used in teaching, and the percentage of total content covered in the unit, against the *y axis* representing the

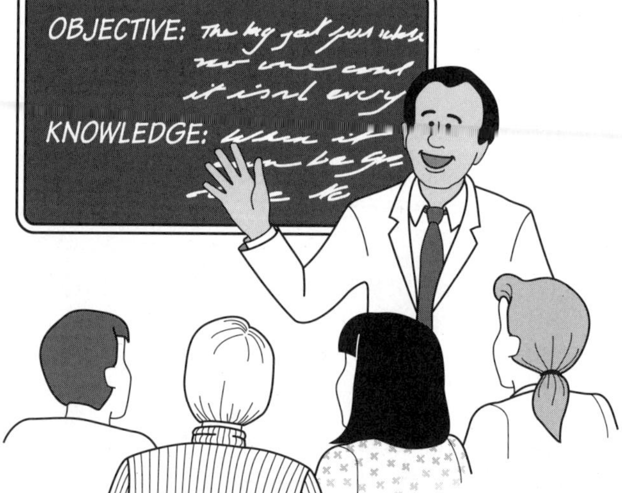

cognitive level, type of question, and number of questions dedicated to the item. The difficulty of content covered within a unit and the type of exam given determines the nature and number of questions asked.

It would be an interesting project for student groups to prepare a test grid in preparation for a scheduled exam from their point of view. How would the composition of their test grid compare with that of the instructor? Figure 6–1 presents input into the test grid; Figure 6–2 shows an example of a test grid.

If time permits, students needing individual assistance should be encouraged to meet with the instructor. Students often bring concerns they do not feel free to discuss with anyone except the instructor. Instructors should try to reserve a few *open hours* for such students before an exam.

Composing/Constructing the Test

TYPES OF TESTS

Depending on the purpose for testing students, various types of tests can be used.

Pre-test. Before beginning a unit, an instructor might choose to assess the knowledge or skills a student has in a particular subject before it is taught. Often, before teaching the venipuncture procedure, the instructor administers a pre-test involving the procedural steps, the vacationer system, and the actual drawing of blood. The results identify MLT students and those who have been taught the procedure in private laboratories. Once checked, they will not need the same supervision the other students do every time blood is drawn. They often volunteer to assist the instructors in supervising those learning the procedure, and in the process, themselves develop teaching and interpersonal skills.

Norm-Referenced Test. A norm-referenced grade compares the individual

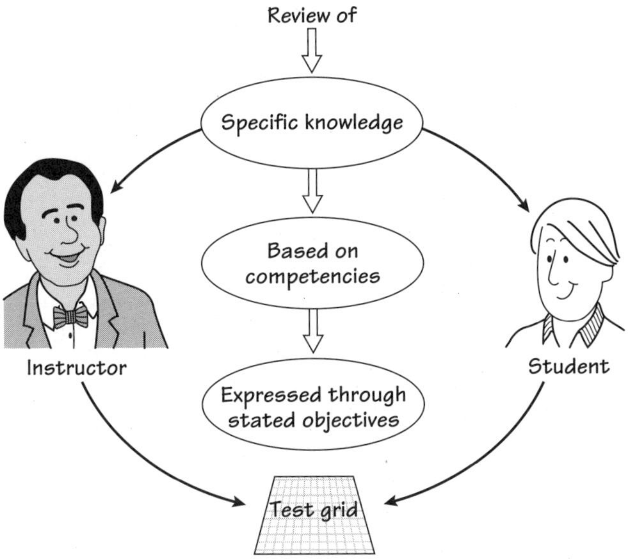

Figure 6–1 Input into the test grid.

Topic: Hemoglobin

Cognitive Level
(Problem solving)

Content: Hemoglobin (Hgb) Structure/function	Knowledge	Comprehension	Application	Analysis	TOTAL QUESTIONS
1. Primary Hgb ID Hgb by chains %:	12 8M 3TF 1MC	6 4MC 2SA	2 1MC 1SA		
2. Primary Hgb Normal Hgb %:	6 6MATCH	6 4MC 2SA	1 1MC	2 2MC	
3. Secondary Hgb Helices/function %:		1 1SA			
4. Tertiary Helices/function %:	2 2TF	5 5MC			
5. Quaternary Hgb Chain relation %:	1 1MC		2 2MC	3 3MC	
6. Oxygen dissoc. Curve %:	6MC 6		3 2MC 1SA	3 3MC	
TOTAL	27	18	8	8	61

Figure 6–2 Example of a test grid.

student's achievement to that achieved by the members in his or her class rather than judging against a rigid set of external standards.[2] The *norm* involves the total number of students having taken a test and the ranking of their grades from highest to lowest results. This type of exam can involve *curving*. Given that the highest result is 85%, the instructor uses this as the norm, which translates to an "A." Consideration has to be given to the competencies measured in regard to their standard of performance.

Criterion-Referenced Test. The competency stated as an objective becomes the *criterion* to which all students' scores are compared. If the highest result is 85%, it remains a "B" grade, if the departmental numerical scale so designates. The criterion or criteria of success are carefully spelled out in terms of minimum levels of acceptable competence: levels that can be demonstrated in specific behavior or performance.[3] Criterion-referenced tests communicate *mastery*.

Quizzes, either norm- or criterion-referenced, test for limited information. The value of quizzes when regularly administered is that they highlight important concepts and facts from several lectures. The aspect of the amount of information they are responsible for encourages the students to study consistently, thus indirectly fostering good study habits. It also establishes a base of information that can be referred to for exams. Both instructor and students like quizzes because they keep them on track. Furthermore, it gives the students immediate feedback on performance.

Exams deal with testing a larger information bank that bridges from simple knowledge (memorization of reagents, principles, symbols) to the analysis of a case study involving information and problem-solving. They can be cumulative: testing information from several units and applying information from one unit to another for purposes of analysis.

Activity 5

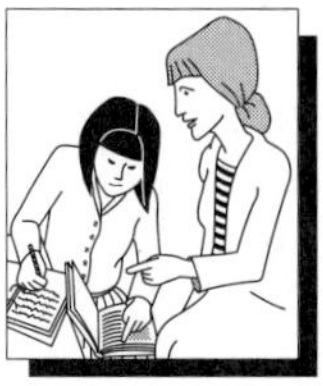

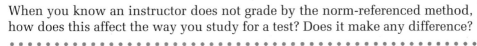

What is the reaction of students when an instructor is known to grade by the norm-referenced method?

When you know an instructor does not grade by the norm-referenced method, how does this affect the way you study for a test? Does it make any difference?

TEST ATTRIBUTES

Attributes are defined as inherent characteristics that connote quality to a person or thing. The attributes associated with tests are reliability, validity, objectivity, fairness, and practicality. A test, based on the stated objectives and possessing the five attributes, measures (as accurately as any finite instrument can) the knowledge and skills acquired and demonstrated by the learner.

Reliability. Reliable tests are based on their consistency and stability. *Consistency* is generated from the administration of the test with the results near to constant, year after year. Instructor-made tests are said to have reliability of about 0.60, whereas examinations composed by writers of standardized tests achieve a reliability as high as 0.90. Instructors evaluate their exams after each administration, conduct an item analysis, and reword or eliminate and substitute for the "bad questions." The greater the consistency, the higher the reliability. Consistency of scores generates a *stable* testing instrument. Reliability studies are performed on all manufactured, standardized tests.[3] CLS programs constructing exams for the purpose of evaluating students both at the end of the junior (academic year) and at the end of the clinical year before graduation are submitting these exams for statistical analysis—specifically, reliability.

Instructors usually do not deal with analysis of their exams; rather, they try to improve them through item analysis and increasing the objectivity of

ATTRIBUTES OF A TEST
RELIABILITY
Consistency
Stability
VALIDITY
OBJECTIVITY
FAIRNESS
PRACTICALITY

the question. Factors that instructors control that contribute to the consistency of a test are as follows:

1. *Quality:* Well-composed, carefully written, clearly expressed with correct usage and spelling, objective in nature; using higher cognitive levels.

2. *Adequate number of test items:* A general rule regarding statistics is, the greater the number, the more reliable the generated result. The greater the number of questions, the more likely a student will achieve a higher score (assuming he/she has studied).

3. *Objectivity of test composition:* Instructors should make sure all questions deal with fact. No room should be left for expression of feeling or attitude. Incidences involving conflicting information sometimes appear at testing time. It is imperative that the instructor has detected statements that conflict with information contained in the lecture notes. Differences *MUST* be brought to the attention of the students during lecture when dealing with that specific topic. Prevention of this type of situation is imperative. Many times, it is not a discrepancy but is information that was available at the time in contrast to more recent knowledge generated by advanced technology.

Instructors should realize that *stressed physical and emotional state of students during test-taking* could generate an unrealistic score that would affect the students' overall average and, in turn, the reliability of the test. Instructors have no control over students who choose to be tested while experiencing stressed physical or emotional states. There will always be instances related to health or situations out of control in students' lives that make it impossible for them to be tested at the same time with the class. It is advisable that instructors have several forms of exams that test for the same material but use a different set of questions.

Validity. Validity indicates that the test gives a true measure of what it was

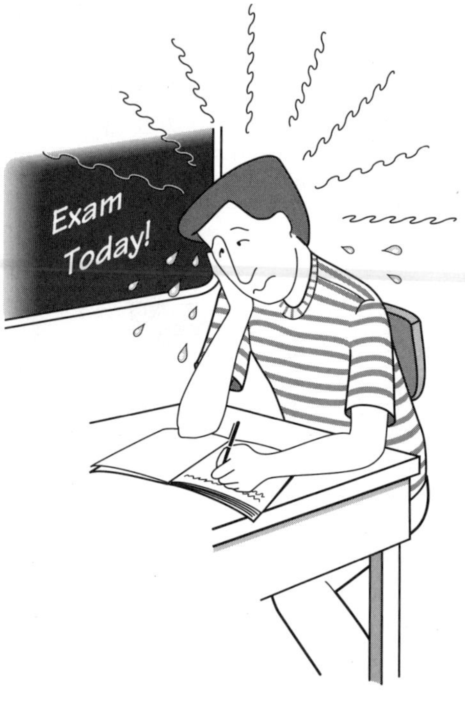

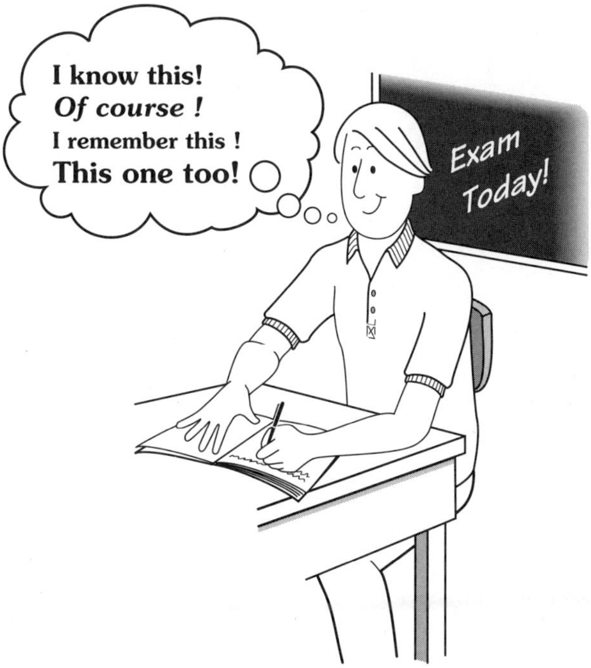
I know this!
Of course !
I remember this !
This one too!
Exam Today!

intended to measure. It focuses on the intended objective.[4] A *valid* test is such when it tests *specific* information or procedure the instructor has designated to be mastered. An example is a practical exam performing a reticulocyte count that reflects a stated objective included in the students' laboratory exercises.

Objectivity. Test scores should be as free as possible of variations due to factors other than the exact behavior being measured.[5] Examples of factors that deter objectivity include clerical errors, ambiguity in either the test questions or answers, a preconceived idea of a student's performance, a student's writing and composition skills, the instructor's mood, and possible scoring errors.

Fairness. The quality of a test that by far is reacted to more often when not applied is fairness. What are the factors that contribute to a "fair" test? There are many. A fair test reflects the following:

- Questions that use stated objectives, from both cognitive and psychomotor domains.
- Material emphasized during lecture and laboratory; that which is essential to understanding concepts or principles of procedure.
- Number and types of questions appropriate to essential versus nonessential, ambiguous material (refer to test grid); They do not test ambiguous, irrelevant material.
- Clear and concise directions.
- Legibility, clarity of printing, adequate space for short and long answers.
- Adequate time given to complete the exam.

- Impartiality shown to all students by not giving preferential treatment when answering questions before or during the administration of the test.

Probably the two greatest sources that have labeled test items unfair are "trick items" and "teachers' biases."[5]

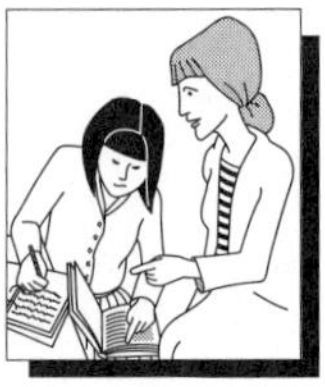

Activity 6

Can you remember situations before, during, or after an exam that you thought were unfair?

Practicality. This attribute involves factors related to both the instructor and the student. Five practical considerations that contribute to this quality of a test are ease of administration, ease of scoring, ease of interpretation and application, low cost, and proper mechanical make-up. In short, any test you make must be a compromise between the high quality expected of commercial instruments and the time and effort you can realistically expend toward test development.[5] Marshall-Hales expressed this quality as "The test questions reflect the economical use of both the instructors' and students' time in test construction, administration, and scoring."[6]

STRUCTURE OF TEST QUESTIONS

The subject matter determines the type and format of the stated question. After reviewing objectives, the material is organized from the easy to the difficult. For subject matter that can be covered by asking the questions who, what, where, when, and which, the popular objective forms of questions can be used. Some instructors choose to group their material in sections: that is, first section pertaining to red blood cells, second to platelets, and last, the white blood cells. This helps students to think along a certain line.

The objective types of questions utilized in exams include true/false, multiple choice, matching, short answer, and essay. Each has the capability to test both simple and complex, difficult material. This includes all directives within the stated objectives that deal with the following:

- *Recognition* of terminology, definitions, principles, functions, components, formulas, normal values, and the like
- *Differentiation* of cells, enzymes, reagents, stains, conditions, disease states, and so forth
- *Organization*: listing by sequence chemical activities, maturation of cells, functions within a cell, and so forth
- *Classification* by various attributes
- *Application* of knowledge
- *Explanation* of cause and effect
- *Evaluation* of normal/abnormal processes
- *Interpretation* of information, test results, values

- *Deduction* of information from given facts
- *Development* of new concepts and theories

FORMAT OF TYPES OF TEST QUESTIONS

True/False

Instructors should consider the limitation of this item format and select from among instructional objectives those that are amenable to measurement with items of this type.[6] Recommendations that assist in constructing reliable true/false items include the following:

- Expressing statements as *totally* true or false
- Expressing the question in a positive manner
- Including necessary information to present facts as they are
- Avoiding the use of "determiners" (always, never, sometimes, often)
- Using quantitative versus qualitative descriptors (numbers versus the words, many, few, large, small)
- Eliminating the use of nonessential information
- Planning a balanced number of true/false items on the test
- Decreasing the 50% guess-factor by giving total credit to only those students who correct the *false* statements with an accompanying explanation; provide a lined page at the back of the test booklet for this purpose
- Including sufficient questions to sample the material

True/false items have those *advantages*: (1) they are easily constructed, objective by nature, and quickly scored; (2) are geared to using less time for completion; and (3) are efficient in testing low cognitive domains.

Examples: True/False

1. Hemoglobin contains four atoms of iron.
2. Hemosiderin is visualized when stained with Prussian blue.
3. Drabkin's reagent converts sulfhemoglobin to cyanmethemoglobin.
4. Monocytic leukemia expresses itself clinically both as an acute and chronic malignancy.
5. ADP, released by the platelet, causes further aggregation of platelets.

Activity 7

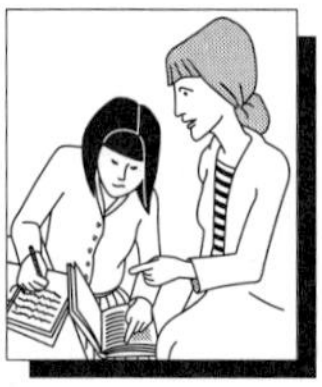

Discuss the following true/false items. Identify the *abuse* to the recommendations given for their proper construction. Rewrite those test items stated incorrectly.

1. Carboxyhemoglobin can never be measured by the cyanmethemoglobin procedure.
2. Often, the hematocrit will be off by 3%.

3. The glycoproteins responsible for aggregation in the platelet are Glycoproteins IIa and IIIb. Sometimes glycoprotein Ia assumes the function.
4. All the leukemias clinically exhibit an acute and chronic phase.
5. Hodgkin's and non-Hodgkin's lymphoma clinically share a similar prognosis: one of short duration.

Multiple-Choice Items

Multiple-choice testing has great versatility in its adaptability for use in essentially all subject matter areas. When constructing this type of test, review the purpose of the test and the items specific for testing the stated objectives.[7] This type of question is difficult to construct. Thorough knowledge of the subject is essential when constructing the "stem" and "distractors" that relate closely to the material and the right answer. Many published test booklets written by MTs/CLSs consisting of standardized questions are available and are of great assistance. Many textbooks include multiple-choice questions at the end of each chapter as a review for the students. The exams administered by ASCP and NCA essentially conform to this format. Recommendations that assist in constructing reliable multiple-choice items include the following:

- Establishing the "question" in the stem (The stem is the statement; the *distractors* are the variable answers provided from which to choose the correct statement.)
- Providing logical distractors along with the correct answer
- Constructing the distractor statements at about the same length as that of the correct answer
- Varying the placement of the correct answer throughout the test
- Limiting the use of the distractors "all the above" and "none of the above"
- Stating the question in a positive format
- Clarifying the directions: "Choose the best answer"
- Providing distractors dealing with numerical values, ranges, that do not overlap

The *advantages* of using multiple-choice items are their versatility in measuring all levels of the cognitive and affective domain and the ease of scoring the items, which provides immediate feedback to the student, enabling evaluation of student performance by the instructor.

Examples of Multiple-Choice Questions

1. Which of the following white blood cells produce immunoglobulins?
   a. Neutrophils
   b. Monocytes
   c. T lymphocytes
   d. Eosinophils
   e. B lymphocytes

2. The chemical pathway within the mature red blood cell responsible for regulatory distribution of oxygen to tissues is the
   a. Embden-Meyerhof pathway.
   b. hexose monophosphate shunt.
   c. methemoglobin reductase.
   d. Luebering-Rapaport pathway.

3. The biochemical stain used to identify a myelomonocytic leukemia is
   a. Sudan black.
   b. peroxidase.
   c. alkaline peroxidase.
   d. muramidase (lysozyme).
   e. acid phosphatase.

4. The following red blood cell parameters—Hgb 6 gm/dL, 18% Hct, RBC 2.5 $\times$ 10^{12}/L, with an MCV of 70 fl—are most consistent with which type of anemia?
   a. N/N
   b. Hypo/micro
   c. N/hypo
   d. Hypo/macro
   e. N/hypo

5. An older man presented with a clinical history of increasing fatigue and irregular breathing. The ordered lab work revealed RBC 1.5 $\times$ 10^{12}/L, Hct 15%, Hgb 5 gr/dL. The peripheral blood smear revealed "bizarre" red blood cell precursors and scanty numbers of all white blood cells. The result of the special stain, PAS, was positive. These findings best describe
   a. Blackfan-Diamond anemia.
   b. Iron deficiency anemia.
   c. Polycythemia vera, third phase.
   d. Fanconi's syndrome.
   e. DiGuglielmo's syndrome.

Activity 8

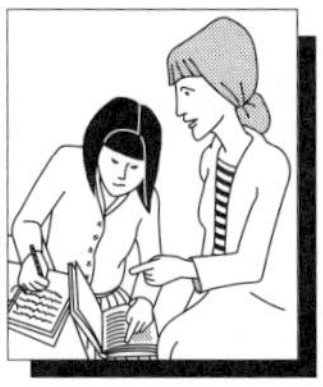

Evaluate the following multiple-choice questions.

Identify the *abuse* covered in the Recommendations given for their proper construction.

1. Calculate a red blood cell count using standard factors and having counted a total of 587 red blood cells. Match the correct answer given to that which you have calculated.
   a. 3.87 $\times$ 10^{12}/L
   b. 4.87 $\times$ 10^{12}/L
   c. 5.87 $\times$ 10^{12}/L
   d. 6.87 $\times$ 10^{12}/L
   e. 3.87 $\times$ 10^{12}/L

2. Which of the following are Romanowsky stains?
   a. Wright's
   b. Giemsa
   c. Jenner
   d. Leishman
   e. May-Grunwald
   ab. None of the above
   ac. All the above

3. Which of the following biochemical processes do not occur in the mature red blood cell?
   a. DNA synthesis
   b. RNA synthesis
   c. Protein synthesis
   d. All the above
   e. None of the above

4. Sickling of red blood cells in Hgb SS is
   a. Related to the age of the red blood cell.
   b. Related to the amount of oxygen bound by the red blood cell.
   c. Controlled by the Golgi apparatus.
   d. Caused by the substitution of lysine for glutamic acid on the sixth site of the beta chain.

5. Which of the following functions is *not* attributed to the platelet?
   a. Adhesion
   b. Aggregation
   c. Secretion
   d. Support
   e. Fibrinolysis

Matching Format

The matching test, by design, uses one list of terms or short phrases that are related to other terms or short phrases of another list. On the previously established relationship or associations, a matching set of questions can be composed. The mental process utilized in taking matching tests is one of recognition; that is, recall. It is a very convenient way to test for cell/function; stain/purpose; component of cell/function; terms/definition; units/symbol; enzyme/substrate; and the like. Again, its limitation of focus is not a disadvantage because every applied science taught includes immeasurable material that has to be stored in memory. An obvious advantage is that of simple construction regarding time and space on the exam proper.

Recommendations that assist in writing matching questions are as follows:

- Use at least six, but seldom more than 12, responses in each exercise.
- In your directions, define the basis for matching.
- Include at least three or four extra choices as distractors.
- Use related items in the matching exercise.

- Place the list containing the longer statement on the left hand side of the page.
- Use capital letters to identify the options.
- Confine the exercise to one page.

Examples of Matching Items

Directions: Match the hemoglobins listed below with their Greek letters. Place the letter of the option on the appropriate line provided before the hemoglobin.

______ 11. Gowers I	a. alpha 2, epsilon 2
______ 12. Portland	b. zeta 2, epsilon 2
______ 13. Hgb F	c. zeta 2, gamma 2
______ 14. Hgb A2	d. alpha 2, beta 2
______ 15. Gowers II	e. alpha 2, gamma 2
______ 16. Hgb A	f. gamma 4
______ 17. Hgb Barts	g. beta 4
	h. alpha 2, beta 2 ly6
	i. alpha 2, beta 2 val6

Activity 9

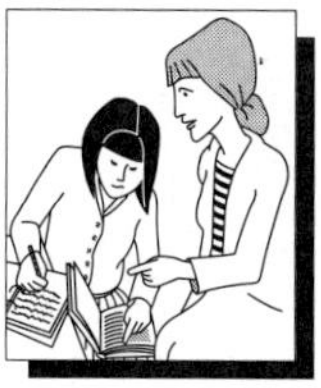

Evaluate the following matching test. Identify those features that abuse the recommendations given.

Matching Test:

______ 1. Prussian blue	a. Iron
______ 2. New methylene blue	b. Screening stain
______ 3. Eosin	c. Component of Romanowsky
______ 4. Crystal violet	d. DNA
______ 5. Methylene blue	e. RNA

Short Answer/Completion Items

In contrast to true/false and multiple-choice items, students are completely dependent on their memory to generate the short answer. There is no guess factor involved, no answers from which to choose. This type of item is best used in testing for multifactual aspects of CLS information: reagents and their functions, normals of all parameters, component of cells, and the like. There is no limit to the minutia of information students are responsible for in both all lectures and the laboratories. Completion test items can also be used to test a higher cognitive ability (example: test calculations. Given several red blood cell parameters, calculate the MCV).

Thus, even though they measure low cognitive abilities, short answer/completion items are valid. The material has to be mastered along with the more challenging subject content. *Recommendations that assist in* constructing reliable short answer/completion questions follow:

- Exact wording of the statement given should not be copied verbatim from the text.
- Compose the statement in such a manner that the specific answer sought is the only possible answer. However, if the student answers a question in a way not foreseen by the instructor, credit should be given the student for the answer.
- Avoid "giveaways" such as the articles "*a*, *an*" or *the*; and singular/plural forms and tense of verbs—these are clues to the answer.
- If a multiple answer question is constructed, all the blanks supplied should be numbered, designating the number of multiple answers.
- The length of the blank should be adequate for the word sought. All blanks should be of equal length.
- Sufficient space should be given if the answer is a phrase.
  When constructing the test format, leave a blank by the number preceding the statement to be completed. This would align the answers for convenient correction.

Examples of Completion/Short Answer Test Items

Directions: Place the answer to the question on the line before the question.

1. ______________ The Greek notation for Hemoglobin F is

2. ______________ Given a hematocrit of 40% and a hemoglobin of 15 gm/dL, calculate for MCHC.

3. ______________ Lack of synthesis of these globin chains in the first trimester of pregnancy causes stillbirth.

4. ______________ The substance within immature granulocytes that reacts with Sudan black to produce a brown-black color is

5. ______________ The glycoprotein on the platelet's membrane that is responsible for the function of *adhesion* is

The Essay Question/Exam

When considering testing for application, analysis, synthesis, and evaluation, the essay question/exam is appropriate. Engaging the abilities of students to express themselves and organize material—with correct usage and grammar—following directions, the essay question indicates to the instructor where students stand. Writing an essay is like building a house. There must be an obvious plan or theme that flows: the integral parts that give it substance.

Recommendations for Constructing Essay Questions

Perhaps the most important aspect in administering an essay question is the *wording of the directions*. The task must be presented so *exactly* that there is a control on what can be expressed. Through the directions, instructors should limit the area of a topic they wish the students to develop.

Determine the scoring on the essay before it is administered: material, facts presented, comparisons made, and the weighing of these elements. Communicate the scoring procedure to students taking the test. Correct the essay question of each exam before going on to the next question. Try to ignore the student's name as the essay is read and corrected.

Examples of Essay Questions

- Compare the cause of and effectiveness of oxygen exchange in red blood cells containing normal but decreased hemoglobin to those red cells containing hemoglobins such as Hgb SS, Hgb CC. Include the construction of an oxygen-dissociation curve to illustrate the mechanism of delivery of O_2.
- Compare the structure of the red blood cell membrane to that of a platelet. Include the three layers of each, their component parts, and their functions.
- Analyze characteristic karyotypes associated with Blackfan-Diamond anemia and Fanconi's syndrome. Explain the effects the karyotype has on the morphology and function of the red blood cells in these conditions.
- Interpret the clinical and laboratory parameters in the following case study. Analyze the accompanying Kodachromes, noting the normal/abnormal features of the cells. Give the specific disease state(s) that are associated with these findings.
- Indicate the characteristics of *stages* in chronic granulocytic leukemia (CGL) and polycythemia vera. Give possible explanations as to the similarities. Include all cell lines in the discussion.

The Oral Examination

This type of examination is best used to assess the depth and extent of a student's knowledge of and understanding regarding a specific topic. The questions used by the instructor must be prepared in advance in order to test a higher cognitive level of understanding. The advantage of individual testing is that it affords the instructor the luxury of establishing a comfortable nonthreatening atmosphere in which the student can be extensively tested.

The obvious disadvantage is the amount of time involved in such a testing methodology. We have used the oral examination format in cases of student absenteeism on the day of a scheduled exam, if the student has presented an acceptable excuse. Much of the same material given on the exam can be covered in the oral exam. The distinct advantage is better testing of the

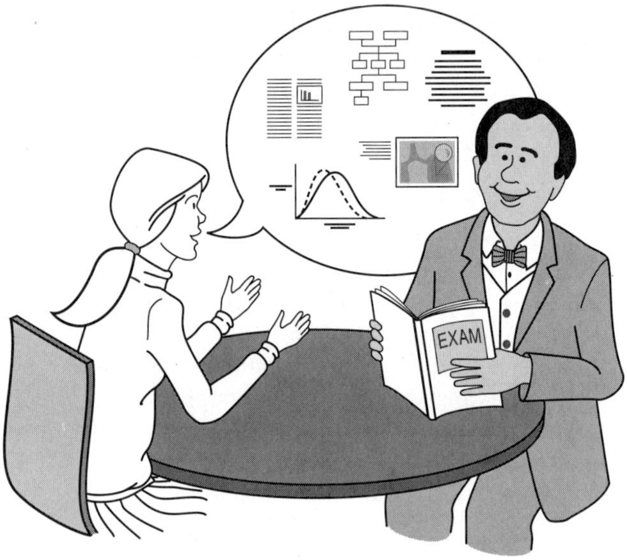

student's understanding and application of knowledge. When students tell instructors that they will be absent, the instructors can then inform the students of the substitute method of testing.

Designated Weight of Test Items

The material covered in the applied science courses varies according to the index of difficulty. Every course contains difficult information. It cannot be memorized; it has to be read, reread, and discussed in order to be learned. Some information is complex; various formulas and calculations become involved. Such material should be weighted differently than tests of lower cognitive levels. Students should be alerted to the weighting system before the examination.

IMMEDIATE PHYSICAL PREPARATION BEFORE THE TEST

- Choose a room large enough that the students are separated (at least two yards apart). (This program uses the laboratory to test students for exams.)
- Provide adequate number of proctors per student.
- Control the light and temperature so that the students are comfortable.
- Supply a pencil sharpener close to the testing room.
- Check for adequate numbers of test booklets and answer keys. Place one test booklet at each station where you plan for students to sit.
- Have students check the number of pages in the booklet.
- Announce the time given to take the test. Write it on the board.
- Give the students a 10-minute warning before the end of the test.
- At the given time, collect all test booklets.
- Check to see that students' names are on the booklets.

A FUNCTION OF THE CLASS REPRESENTATIVE: CHECK-PLUS

For about the last 5 years, the author has used the class representative as a "quality control" over the exam. Once all students have finished the exam and all papers have been collected, the students are encouraged to meet with the representative and list any questions they thought were not fair or were ambiguous or not covered adequately. They are also asked to state the reason why.

They are then given the exam key that contains the answers and the instructor's explanations to the answers. Following thorough review of the exam, they meet with the instructor, who listens, reviews the questions from their point of view, and takes action. This has proven to be most effective in that (1) the students realize a function of their class representative is to represent their viewpoint to the instructor; (2) it obliges class representatives to listen openly to their peers' concerns and represent them in a nonaggressive manner to the instructor; (3) it provides opportunities for the class representative to practice and develop "listening skills and negotiating skills"; and (4) it provides a peaceful mechanism through which the instructor deals with the entire class through their representative. It works, and it works well. This activity obviously is related to testing and the formulation of questions, just to get back on track.

CORRECTION OF TEST ITEMS

Have you ever watched students go to their mailboxes in the department to retrieve corrected test papers? They look for their grade, and then they begin to search each page to see where there is writing! If they don't find it on the first page, they go to the second, then the third, and on to the last to see if there are any remarks about the work they did or comments regarding expression on the test. Finding none, they glance back at the items missed and then put the test paper away. Correcting papers is an art. It can be a chore, but there are ways to cut down the negative aspect by the construction of the test, providing a format conducive for correction, and by balancing the type of test items used. Whatever the construction of tests, students deserve some type of critical evaluation, including, when appropriate, some comment regarding their writing, grammar, and correct usage. Words of praise go a long way; the word "good," written alongside a difficult, complex question correctly answered boosts the ego. Students need constructive and honest feedback. Rather than using a negative approach, "Don't use, don't say . . . ," encourage them to "try using this term to better express the condition you are studying." Such remarks will improve subsequent scientific expression in writing and oral presentations.

Retesting (Retention)

Is there a reason why, when an exam is given early in the semester, that the information included must to be learned by a certain date and the grade carved in stone? In some cases, yes; there is prerequisite information for what follows. But students who are slow learners, foreign-born, culturally disadvantaged, or handicapped should be allowed to demonstrate that they can indeed learn the material at their own rate. Reviewing the material with these students, discovering the reason why they did not achieve, and making it possible for them to do so provides us with an opportunity to help them succeed. Establish the grading system of retesting so that it reflects their true knowledge. Retest and regrade, but open it up to the entire class. All students must be treated the same and given equal opportunities to improve. This relates to retention of students. Consideration has to be extended to those who performed well on the first administered test.

Summary

The exercise of witnessing the achievement of competencies both through written and practical tests is essential to guarantee the graduation of "competent clinical laboratory scientists" through an accredited program to the health care team. Instructors should work at constructing exams, following the protocol necessary, to produce a precision-measuring instrument based on the stated objectives. It is essential that the achieved grades reflect and demonstrate the knowledge and ability of the students. Consideration must be given to those students who evidence different rates of learning. Additional support given these students will often reflect their true learning capabilities.

Review Questions

Place your answer to the question on the blank provided.

1. ________________ is that quality of a test which results in close scores year after year.

2. Place the word True/False on the line provided. If False is marked, make the necessary correction.

   ______ Criterion tests do not utilize curving of the results.

3. Match the following Test Attributes with their description. Place the letter of the description on the line provided before the number.

   ______ 1. Reliability

   ______ 2. Validity

   ______ 3. Objectivity

   ______ 4. Fairness

   ______ 5. Practicality

   a. measures specifically what it was meant to test

   b. economic in preparation, administration, and correction

   c. reflects clearly material emphasized during lecture

   d. characterizes standardized tests

   e. is short and concise in what it tests

   f. based on clear and concise presentation; not biased by instructor

   g. consists of a variety of types of questions

4. Encircle the letter which precedes the correct answer to the following question.

   1. A test question which asks students to explain, in detail, the 02 Dissociation Curve, is an example of which stated objective (competency) given below?

      a. knowledge
      b. comprehension
      c. interpretation
      d. analysis
      e. synthesis
      f. evaluation

5. Discuss the planning of a review session. Include in your discussion, review of the material in the unit to be tested, the stated objectives, and the test grid.

See p. 406 for answers.

References

1. Jacob LC, Chase I. Developing and Using Tests Effectively: A Guide for Faculty. San Francisco, Jossey-Bass Publishers, 1992.
2. Marshall JC, Hales LW. Planning Achievement Tests in Essentials of Testing. Menlo Park, Calif, Addison-Wesley, 1972, pp 7–22.
3. Green JA. 9. Assigning Grades and Course Marks in Teacher-Made Tests. New York, Harper and Row, 1975, pp 157–178.
4. Hedges WD. How to make a good science test. *In* Testing and Evaluation for the Sciences. Belmont, Calif, Wadsworth Publishing, 1966, pp 3–24.
5. Green AJ. Planning measurement instruments. *In* Teacher-Made Tests. New York, Harper and Row, 1975, pp 19–41.
6. Marshall J, Hales L. Principles of Educational Measurement. *In* Essentials of Testing. Menlo Park, Calif, Addison-Wesley, 1971, pp 1–6.
7. Marshall J, Hales L. Construction and use of true-false tests. *In* Essentials of Testing. Menlo Park, Calif, Addison-Wesley, 1971, pp 68–75.
8. Marshal J, Hales L. Construction and use of multiple choice tests. *In* Essentials of Testing. Menlo Park, Calif, Addison-Wesley, 1971, pp 45–67.

Suggested Reading

1. ASCP Medical Technology Examination Content Outline. Chicago, American Society of Clinical Pathologists, 1992, pp 1–6.
2. Briggs LJ, Gustafson KL, Tillman MH. Instructional Design Principles and Application. Englewood, NJ, Educational Technology Publications, 1992.
3. Davis BG. Tools for Teaching. San Francisco, Jossey-Bass Publishers, 1993.
4. Eble KE. The Craft of Teaching. 2nd ed. San Francisco, Jossey-Bass Publishers, 1990.
5. Green JA. Teacher Made Tests. 2nd ed. New York, Harper and Row, 1975.
6. Hedges WD. Testing and Evaluation for the Sciences. Belmont, Calif, Wadsworth Publishing, 1966.
7. Jenkyns T. Tactics for tests. The Teaching Professor (Vol. 9, No. 1). Madison, Wisc, Magna Publications, 1995.
8. LeGrys VA, Beck SJ. Clinical Laboratory Education. San Mateo, Calif, Appleton and Lange, 1988.
9. McKeachie WJ. Teaching Tips: A Guidebook for the Beginning College Teacher. 7th ed. Lexington, Mass, D.C. Heath, 1978.
10. Popham WJ. The Teacher Empiricist. Los Angeles, Tinnon-Brown Inc. Book Publishers, 1970.
11. Reigeluth CM. Instructional Design and Models: An Overview of Their Current Status. Hillsdale, NJ, Lawrence Erlbaum, 1983.
12. Schneider H. Effective Test Construction in the Health Professions. Jackson, Miss, H & B Hess Co, 1984.
13. Udolf R. The College Instructor's Guide to Teaching and Academia. Chicago, Nelson-Hall, 1976.

7

Grades, Evaluations: Necessary Feedback

OBJECTIVES

Upon completion of the chapter, the reader should be able to:

- Relate specific performance to a fixed grade.
- Discuss the *need* for a grading system.
- List the advantages and disadvantages of grades.
- Research and report on what factors contribute to an objective grade.
- Differentiate between grading and evaluating a student.
- Discuss the use of "Instructor Evaluation Questionnaires."
- List and discuss the advantages and misuse of instructor evaluation forms.

KEY WORDS

grade
objective
subjective
evaluation

Introduction

The tests have been administered, collected, and now need to be graded. Your department in the university might have an electronic instrument that corrects the answer sheets as they are fed through their instrument, performs an item analysis (marks how many times a question is missed), and generates the average grade. If not, both in the university and in the clinical site, the exams will be hand corrected, and a grade affixed to the paper.

This chapter deals with the primary function of grades and the message they communicate to the instructor and the student (and to those who are in a position to view them). Additional benefits are experienced by using grades for constructive learning.

You, as the instructor, are then evaluated. How well did you do your job? *Grades* did not always exist in the educational arena. When fewer students were on campuses, the instructors grew to know each student in a more "complete" way. The student's capabilities, efforts, struggles, and achievements were intimately known by the instructor. In those days, deportment and decorum were as formative as academic attainment in **sharing** the grade. It was not until the late 1880s that the grading system utilizing A through F with pluses and minuses was devised.[1]

In a competency-based educational program, grades are essential. Whether in the hospital clinical laboratory or the university academic segment of the educational program, the grades earned by students must reflect their competency regarding entry-level knowledge and skills. The goals of Chapter 6, which dealt with reliability and accuracy in constructing exams and quizzes, are now brought into sharper focus. The grades students achieve through test-taking must measure and reflect, as accurately as possible, the abilities and achievements of that student. The test itself cannot take away from the true measurement of the student performance.

Grades

Grades, by definition, are letters or numbers to which a value has been affixed; grades represent the quality of achievement, of performance. Grades, therefore, indirectly reflect the ability of an individual to achieve. When an educator studies a student's transcript, giving attention to the grades affixed to the various classes listed, the grades immediately translate and reflect the capabilities, the abilities, achievement, and the discipline of an individual student. Information, then, is gleaned from a transcript that enables an educator to admit or not admit a student into a program based on academic evidence.

THE NECESSITY OF GRADES

Grades tell us much more than *how well* students have achieved in their classes. Eble comments:

> Both students and teachers should share the recognition that grades play a part in the students' learning and, (grades aside), that knowing how one is doing is a necessary part of learning. Although I have stressed the vexations of grading, I think that students place reasonable demands on teachers; that is, they want to know what the teacher's expectations are, they want to feel that they are being

evaluated fairly with respect to those expectations, and they want a final grade to give an accurate and unbiased reflection of how well they have met the expectations.[2]

For students, grades:

1. Identify what they have mastered
2. Provide recognition for a job well done
3. Provide records of their performance
4. Encourage a better performance
5. Pinpoint specifically what is known/not known
6. Serve as a motivational force to achieve more
7. Help students assess themselves
8. Indicate the consistency of students' performance
9. Identify a trend in performance
10. Identify valuable learning patterns

For instructors, grades:

1. Provide evidence of student performance
2. Indicate what should be reviewed/re-taught
3. Identify students who perform well/not so well
4. Review the objectives in the course outline
5. Provide praise and recognition to those who deserve it
6. Encourage those who need to be encouraged
7. Help construct an honor roll for the dean's list
8. Promote desirable learner growth and behavioral changes in learners
9. Indicate good and poor learning patterns
10. Serve as statistics for future studies
11. Assist faculty in making program admission decisions

In higher academic institutions, and for prospective employers, grades on a transcript demonstrate the caliber of graduates and their academic history throughout their university years. On the transcript is found the translation of the letter system, and the number values included in the letter-grade groups.

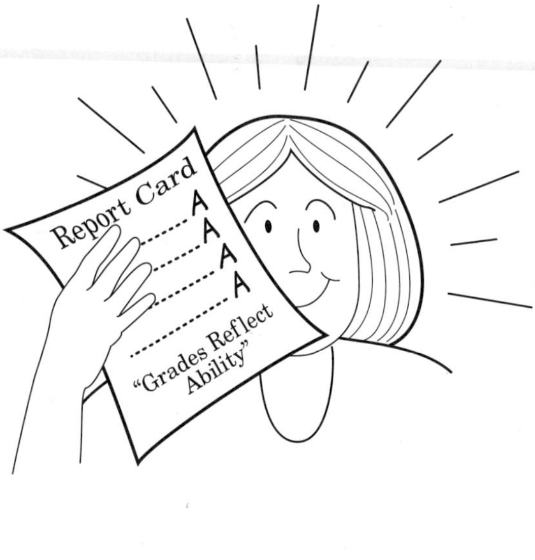

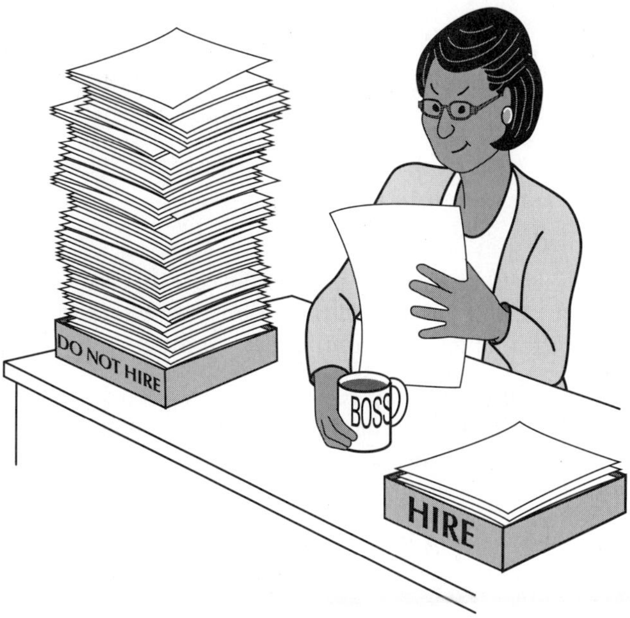

Activity 1

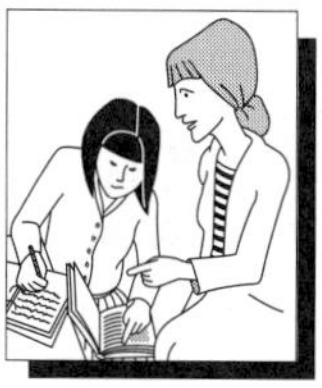

Within your group, discuss the above lists and comment on the items with which you can identify. Have you experienced other feedback from grades you yourself have received? How have you *used grades* in your learning situation?

GRADES: THEIR INTERPRETATION

Whether you teach in a clinical laboratory program or in an academic setting, it is essential for the students that you include, in the course syllabus, the grading system that you use in your course, together with the interpretation of each letter grade. If the educational program is competency-based, the criteria for grades are simplified. That is, all grades are dependent on the achievement of the objectives. Instructors must identify the major and minor objectives and then devise a grading system that can identify whether a student has or has not achieved them. In 1950, Travers proposed one set of absolute standards[3]:

- A: All major and minor objectives achieved
- B: All major objectives achieved; some minor ones not
- C: All major objectives achieved; many minor ones not
- D: A few major objectives achieved, but student is not prepared for advanced work
- E: None of the major objectives achieved[3]

To this, Williams, in *The Teaching Professor*, adds the following[4]:

The "A" Student: An Outstanding Student

- *Attendance*: "A" students have virtually perfect attendance. Their commitment to the class resembles that of the teacher.
- *Preparation*: "A" students are prepared for class. They always read the assignment. Their attention to detail is such that they occasionally catch the teacher in a mistake.
- *Curiosity*: "A" students show interest in the class and in the subject. They look up or dig out what they don't understand. They often ask interesting questions or make thoughtful comments.
- *Retention*: "A" students have retentive minds. They are able to connect past learning with the present. They bring a background with them to class.
- *Attitude*: "A" students have a winning attitude. They have both the determination and the self-discipline necessary for success. They show initiative. They do things they have not been told to do.
- *Talent*: "A" students have something special. It may be exceptional intelligence and insight. It may be unusual creativity, organizational skills, commitment—or a combination thereof. These gifts are evident to the teacher and usually to the other students as well.
- *Results*: "A" students make high grades on tests—usually the highest in the class. Their work is a pleasure to grade.

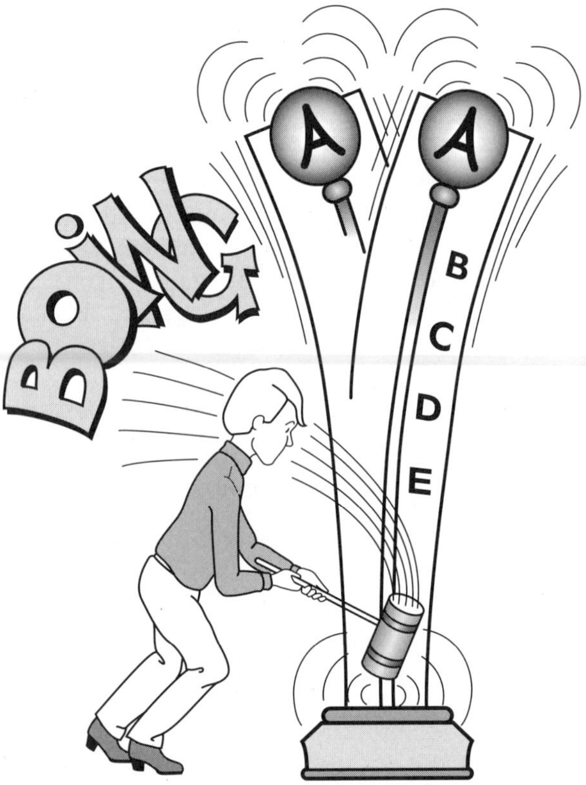

The "C" Student: An Average or Typical Student

- *Attendance*: "C" students miss class frequently. They put other priorities ahead of academic work. In some cases, their health or constant fatigue renders them physically unable to keep up with the demands of high-level performance.
- *Preparation*: "C" students prepare their assignments consistently but in a perfunctory manner. Their work may be sloppy or careless. At times, it is incomplete or late.
- *Attitude*: "C" students are not visibly committed to the class. They participate without enthusiasm. Their body language often expresses boredom.
- *Talent*: "C" students vary enormously in talent. Some have exceptional ability but show undeniable signs of poor self-management or bad attitude. Others are diligent but merely average in academic ability.
- *Results*: "C" students obtain mediocre or inconsistent results on tests. They have some concept of what is going on but clearly have not mastered the material.

The author adds that "these profiles help communicate his values to the students." He adds, "While they are not the profiles any and every professor might write, *they do serve to acquaint students* with my expectations and to prepare a successful semester in my class."[4]

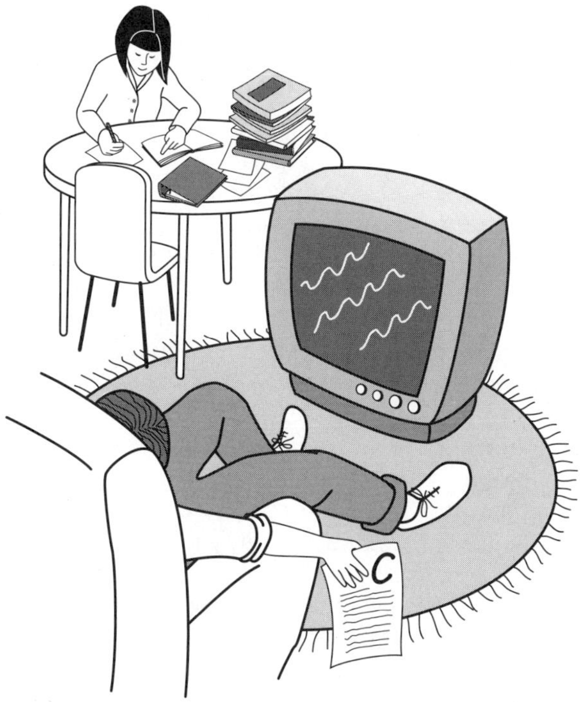

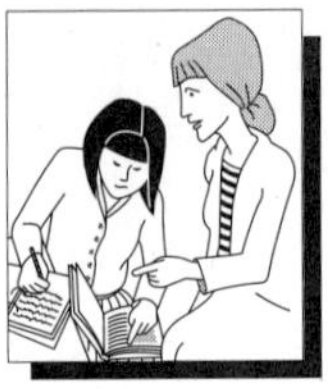

Activity 2

Using the above characteristics regarding the outstanding and average student, can you identify students in past classes that exhibit the above qualities of each category?

One other consideration deals with the variability of the inclusion of number grades within the A group (Table 7–1).

Not all institutions follow the scheme in the table. In the academic portion of our program, we do use this value system; however, in our clinical setting, the letter grades represent a different numerical grade: A (100–93), B (92–85), C (84–75), D (74–70), E (below 70).

Table 7–1
CONVENTIONAL INCLUSIONS IN THE A GROUP

A	represents the number grades	100–90 inclusive
B		89–80
C		79–70
D		69–60
E or F		below 60

Evaluating the Student versus Grading the Student

By now you have received the message that grades are meant to reflect the academic achievement of students. In many programs, points are taken off the final grade for absenteeism, continual tardiness, and lack of effort displayed. Le Grys and Beck make a strong point in differentiating between grading and evaluating the student. They note that evaluation is a judgment of the student's attempts to meet the acceptable level of performance and it involves observing the student, collecting data and giving feedback to the student. Evaluation is used to help students improve their performance.[5]

Many educators advise keeping logs on students for this purpose: to establish a record of dedication to improve by increasing study time and practice needed to develop required skills. A high grade does not communicate how it was achieved, either by a very intelligent student who exerts little effort or by one who struggles and learns the hard way. Remember, the primary function of grades is to translate the degree of academic mastery.

The inclusion of negative behavioral patterns affecting the final grade masks the interpretation of the true meaning of a grade. There are no easy solutions. It is usual for all clinical and academic programs to have set policies regarding the subject. It is wise to discuss any questions that might arise with your director/chair.

Students should realize that when they seek a letter of recommendation from one of the instructors from a specific university, the forms used have a section that deals with nonacademic factors; this is a personal evaluation that prospective employees are very eager to see. The responding instructor is directed to mark one of the columns on the form: below average, average, above average, good, outstanding, or unable to comment. Examples of traits included in the form are (1) self-reliance and independence in scientific work, (2) motivation toward a scientific career, (3) emotional stability and maturity, (4) responsibility, (5) ability to communicate via speech and writing, and (6) compatibility with fellow students and staff. There is always a space provided for comments.

YOUR GRADING SYSTEM

The grading system you have adopted, contained within your Course Syllabus, should be given to and discussed with the students the first day of class. This system provides the *exact* mechanism by which they are graded. If you use "weighing" in the calculation of students' grades, an explanation should accompany your handout. Students should know how their final grade is determined. Overheads, demonstrating the grading system with written-in grades, work very well. Along with the class schedule, the author includes an exact copy of a student's grade sheet and advises students to keep their copy current, placing their grades on the appropriate lines, so they can keep current with their overall grades, progress, and achievement.

The Grading System

In the following form (Fig. 7–1), the weighting system attributes 30% to quizzes. If you are asked why the weight is so high, have an answer ready.

Student's name: ____________________ Year ______ Semester ______

1. Quizzes **(30%)**

Student's points   Possible points   Total

Quiz 1. ____________________

Quiz 2. ____________________

Quiz 3. ____________________

Quiz 4. ____________________

Quiz 5. ____________________

Quiz 6. ____________________

Quiz 7. ____________________

Quiz 8. ____________________

Quiz 9. ____________________

Quiz 10. ____________________

____

2. Exam I **(20%)** ____________________

3. Exam II **(20%)** ____________________

4. Final exam **(30%)** ____________________

Final grade: __________

Figure 7–1 Hematology grade sheet CLS 305.

One good reason is that the weekly quiz grade reflects the continual effort students exert to achieve a good grade. It represents consistency that students attain throughout the course. To determine the final weight that *Quizzes* contribute to the final grade: (1) total the possible points affixed to a quiz; (2) total the points achieved by the student; (3) divide the student's number by the possible points, which will generate a percentage grade; and (4) multiply the percentage grade by the weight put on the quizzes. This final number represents the total points the student achieved out of 30.

In the example above, total points possible were 97; the student achieved 83. Using the simple formula, the calculations given above demonstrate the points generated by each weighted factor (quizzes, exam I, and so on) and how they contribute to the (total) final grade of the student. This type of grading system is straightforward, communicating to students exactly how their grades are calculated. It is wise to affix each student's grades to a separate sheet. The reason for this is that when students ask to check their grades with the instructor, the grade book can be opened to their page; all that is seen are the grades achieved by that particular student. It affords students the privacy they should have. The format also affords the instructor ample room to record the grade and to include the calculation for each separate and final grade, which the students can see and calculate for themselves. It is the author's policy to have students calculate their grades prior to the administration of the final exam *together with the instructor.* This helps students realize where they stand in terms of achieving a specific grade and how well they have to perform in order to do so.

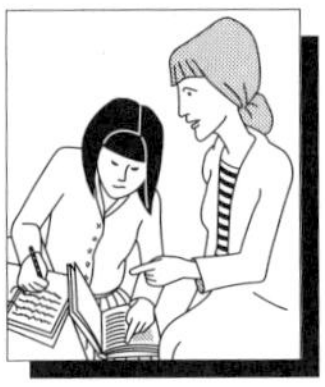

Activity 3

Discuss and summarize other examples of a grading system that you have experienced throughout your courses. Has the final grade represented your academic achievement? If they were *objective* in format, list the factors that contributed to that system. If not, list the activities that contributed to your final grade.

With this in place, let us discuss some grade strategies. Davis, in her chapter on Grades, states the following:

> Grade on the basis of students' mastery of knowledge and skills; restrict your evaluation to academic performance. Eliminate other considerations, such as classroom behavior, effort, classroom participation, attendance, punctuality, attitude, personality traits, or student interest in the course materials, as the basis of course grades. If you count these nonacademic factors, you obscure the primary meaning of the grade, as an indicator of what students have learned. Avoid grading systems that put students in competition with their classmates and limit the number of high grades. Try not to overemphasize grades. Keep students informed of their progress throughout the term.[6]

This practice contributes to the *reliability of the grade.* It ensures that the grade (1) is based on the achievement of the student on designated tests that are included in the course syllabus schedule; (2) is based on academic achievement of the student; and (3) is listed in the instructor's grade book, has been recalculated together with the instructor, is identical to the student's own copy; and (4) reflects the competency of the student in regard to the achievement of the stated objectives.

When you stop to think about it, instructors are merely recorders! They correct exam papers and calculate and record grades onto the students' pages in their grade books to later calculate the final grade. Every number that is recorded is student-generated.

This type of objective grading eliminates *teacher's bias*, which considers previous knowledge of a student—a good student or a not-so-good student entering a new class, a fast learner or a slow learner. The teacher is *very aware of the previous achievement of the student and can become biased because of that knowledge*. It would be difficult for an instructor with a bias toward a student to alter an objective-type grading system, such as the example given above.

Activity 4

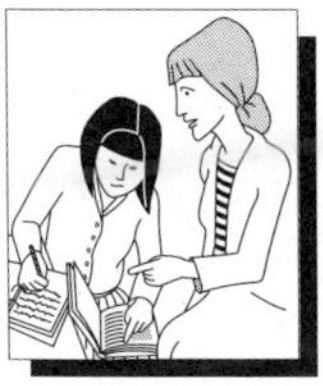

Calculate a student's final grade given the category and its weight, and the student's grades:

	Student's Points	**Possible Points**	
Quizzes (25%)			
Quiz 1 =	12	16	
Quiz 2 =	10	16	
Quiz 3 =	6	10	
Quiz 4 =	9	12	
Quiz 5 =	11	15	
Quiz 6 =	14	16	
Quiz 7 =	12	18	
Quiz 8 =	5	5	
Quiz 9 =	18	20	
Quiz 10 =	7	10	
	______	______	
Exam I (20%)	35	40	______
Exam II (20%)	15	35	______
Final Exam (35%)	85	100	______

Final Grade ____________ %________

In conclusion, be able to account for every grade that is recorded in your grade book: to the student, to the chairperson, and to the students' parents. Have the calculations that were used to determine the grade available for all parties to view. It is good practice to have every *D* and *E* checked and recalculated by another faculty member—"safe-check."

MISCELLANEOUS CONSIDERATIONS REGARDING GRADES

Meaning of Grades

What an instructor communicates by a grade depends on the meaning of the grade to the student receiving it and the effect that it has on that person.

An instructor cannot change the meaning of grades unilaterally. While the grade may have a new meaning for the instructor, those reading the grade will interpret it in terms of the meanings they have traditionally assigned to grades, unless the instructor explains his/her views, specifically interpreting for them the meaning.[7]

Posting of Grades

It is a good idea to post grades without names, and not in alphabetical order. Post grades from the highest mark to the lowest. Indicate the average calculated from the grades. In some classes, students are assigned a number that is then posted with the grade.

When to Grade Exam Papers

Some of the most effective learning by the student takes place after the test. *Grade the test as soon as possible* and discuss the results with students during the first class meeting afterward. Keep individual test results confidential; you do not want to embarrass students who did poorly on the test, or, at the opposite extreme, students who did well by pointing them out in class.[8]

Various Methods of Grading

Davis discusses the various mechanisms for generating grades: Criterion-refer-

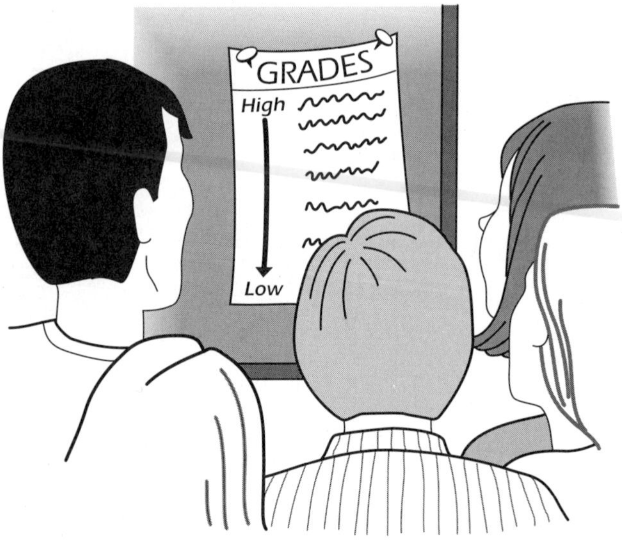

enced grading versus norm-referenced grading based on improvement; some faculty allow students to grade themselves and give reasons to justify the grade, grading according to the mastery of the objectives.[6] Programs that are competency-based are just that! The stated objectives must be achieved.

Abuse of Grades

More up-to-date studies are needed on *grading reliability.* It is fairly safe to assume that numerous errors still creep in. Tests are not precise measurement instruments such as yardsticks, scales, or thermometers (although even these instruments can be in error). *Just because you translate the results into numbers does not mean that the precision has been increased.* Use your grades; do not allow grades to use you.[9] A practice of "inflating grades" is common in some educational institutions; that is, a lower-than-standard work is given a grade that does not represent the low caliber of the work. For example, a project that is of "C" caliber is graded "B" by the instructor. This discrepancy is often discovered when students transfer to another university where grades earned there realistically reflect the capabilities of the student.

Characteristics of a Good Grading Scheme

A good one should have the following characteristics:

- It should be based on adequate sampling.
- It should be equitable and fairly applied.
- It should be consistent but not so inflexible that special circumstances can't be handled.
- The students should be informed of it at the beginning of the term.[10]

Practical Statistics

Several statistical tools for analyzing both *tests* and *test results* use the measures of central tendencies, mean, median, and mode. These statistics measure the *group*, not the *individuals* comprising the group.[11]

The *mean* is calculated by dividing the sum of all the individual grades and dividing them by the number of students who took the test. The *median* is determined by listing the grades in order from high to low (or low to high) and identifying the central value. The *mode* identifies the grade most often achieved by the students. Example: Individual grades of 15 students on an exam were as follows:

100	100	100
100	100	100
99	99	99
98	98	98
98	98	98
92	92	92
90	90	90

89	89*	89
85*	85	85
85	85	85*
85	85	85
82	82	82
75	75	75
72	72	72
60	60	60
*Mean: sum = 1310/15 = 87.3	*Median: 89	*Mode: 85

The mean is a useful measurement if the group results follow a bell curve. The median is a better measurement if the grades are skewed; that is, if there are too few high or low scores. The mode is useful in identifying the most frequent response in an objective test.[12] However, the mean is sensitive to extremes, whereas the median is not. The median can characterize the group adequately; however, the median tends to ignore useful information. This value concentrates on the central value only. The mode has one possible advantage to the mean and median in that it describes several individual results; it fails in that it provides little information regarding the group.[11]

These central tendencies are so easily determined that all three values can be generated within seconds. Reap the benefits from them all. It is essential, in using these statistics, to identify and assist students who fall short of the mean, median, and mode and to further challenge those who exceed them.

Faculty Evaluations

Faculty evaluations are as important to instructors as grades are to students. The feedback that instructors are eager to receive from students is the answer to these questions: "Am I helping you to learn and how well? How can I assist you to achieve?"

Faculty evaluations did not always exist in academic and clinical settings. According to Eble, since the 1960s, student evaluation has become a formalized part of the reward system in a majority of collegiate institutions.[13] In most higher-education settings, the agreement between the university and the union resulted in their mandatory use for a number of years. Faculty look upon these evaluations as necessary feedback and welcome them. The university uses them as part of a reward system for good teaching.

As evaluations are used today, students, after finishing a clinical rotation or a class in the university, are asked to complete the questionnaire. Protocol requires the procedure to be carried out in the absence of the instructor and the process to be entirely conducted by the class representative, with total anonymity ensured. In time, the instructor receives the evaluation forms to read and study. It is the practice at this university that all evaluations are printed into a book (per semester, by course number and instructor) and are available to *anyone* to review. This book includes the questions asked and the *mean* of the responses.

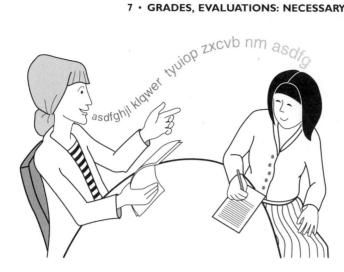

In Chapter 2, the three aspects that were exhibited by the teacher that contribute to the quality of instruction were technical knowledge, teaching skills, and personal qualities. Faculty evaluation forms cover these three areas. The following represents frequently used statements used to rate faculty. The rating scheme used progresses from 7 to 1, 7 being excellent, 1 representing poor.

1. Rate the course content.
2. How would you rate this course?
3. How would you rate the instructor's teaching in this course?
4. All things considered, would you recommend this course?
5. Appropriate attention was given to course organization.
6. At the beginning of the course, the overall class plan was clearly presented.
7. At the beginning of the course, my responsibilities as a student were made clear.
8. All things considered, the instructor was available to students.
9. This instructor respected me as a person.
10. The instructor provided prompt feedback on my performance on assigned activities.
11. The grading procedures were clearly explained at the start of the course.
12. The material presented in class and in the assignments was fairly represented in examinations.

Evaluation regarding laboratory instruction:

13. Was the instructor prepared for lab? (*yes* or *no*)
14. How good was the instructor's knowledge of the laboratory instruments, test methods, and procedures?
15. How was the lab instructor's attitude toward questions and/or requests for help?
16. How clear were the instructor's answers to questions?
17. How accessible was the laboratory instructor for answering questions?
18. Was the instructor helpful to you in learning the appropriate instruments, test methods, or procedures in laboratory experiments?

19. What did you like most about this instructor? (Write in)
20. What suggestions would you offer this instructor to make him/her a more effective teacher? Be specific.

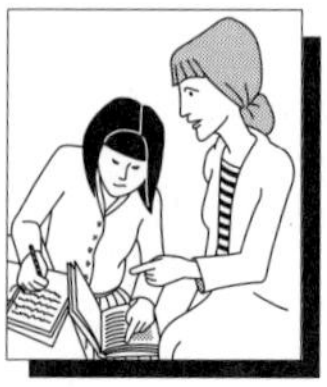

Activity 5

Beginning with number 3 of the evaluation form, categorize the area of the question asked in the appropriate line given below:

Questions	Knowledge and Skills	Teaching Skills	Personal Qualities
3.			
4.			
5.			
6.			
7.			
8.			
9.			
10.			
11.			
12.			
13.			
14.			
15.			
16.			
17.			
18.			
19.			
20.			
Totals:			

Discuss and comment on your findings. Do the questions represent a balance of an instructor's attributes? What suggestions would you make?

In his Appendix B, McKeachie includes the evaluation form used by the University of Michigan. An obvious advantage is that the questions are categorized for students. The heading on the evaluation form reads: "Student Perceptions of Learning and Teaching."

Impact on students:

1. My intellectual curiosity has been stimulated by this course.
2. I am learning how to think more clearly about the area of this course.
3. I am learning how to read material in this area more effectively.
4. I am acquiring knowledge about the subject.
5. The course is contributing to my self-understanding.
6. The course is increasing my interest in learning more about this area.

Instructor effectiveness:

1. The instructor is enthusiastic.
2. The instructor gives good examples of the concepts.
3. The instructor goes into too much detail.
4. The instructor is helpful when students are confused.
5. The instructor seems knowledgeable in many areas.

Rapport:

1. The instructor knows students' names.
2. Students discuss each other's ideas.
3. Students feel free to disagree with the instructor.

Difficulty:

1. The instructor makes difficult assignments.
2. The instructor asks for a great deal of work.

Structure:

1. The instructor plans class activities in detail.
2. The instructor follows an outline closely.
3. The instructor keeps students informed of their progress.
4. The instructor tells students when they have done a good job.
5. Tests and papers are graded and returned promptly.

STUDENT SELF-EVALUATION

- I had a strong desire to take this course.
- I actively participate in class discussions.
- I try to tie-in what I am learning with my own experience.
- I attend class regularly.
- I use all the learning opportunities provided in the course.
- I have created my own learning experiences in connection with the course.
- I have helped classmates learn.
- Overall evaluation:

1. Rate the instructor's general teaching effectiveness for you.
2. Rate the value of the course as a whole to you.[14]

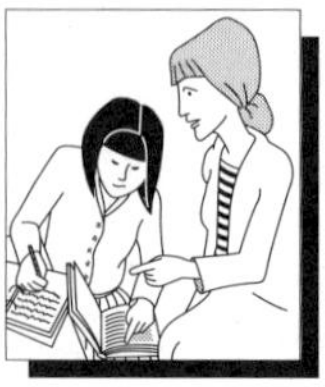

Activity 6

Discuss, evaluate, and comment upon the content and format of this evaluation form.

Clinical Instruction Evaluation

As students enter the clinical segment of the CLS program, they take with them theoretical and laboratory skills that need to be tested, refined, and perfected. Their knowledge should be tested with a greater degree of application exercises. They enter with a good knowledge and skill base. The obligations of the clinical instructors are similar to that of the university faculty. Clinical sites provide lecture series, teleconferences, guest speakers, and slide/tape presentations to reinforce the theoretical knowledge base established by the university. The clinical instructors also introduce new instrumentation and procedures to the senior students. Together with the university faculty, they are responsible for strengthening the Cognitive, Affective, and Psychomotor Domains and bring the students to achieve and perfect the entry-level knowledge and skill base. They, together with the university faculty, are evaluated by the students as they finish rotating through their departments. In reviewing the factors for review given below, keep in mind the three categories that reflect the instructors' abilities and attributes. The following are excerpts taken from a Clinical Instructor Evaluation form. (The following represents *only* those items that reflected the obligations and responsibilities of the clinical instructor.)

The classroom

- Atmosphere is relaxed and conducive to learning
- Students receive help from personnel other than instructor
- Space is provided for student to work
- Supplies and equipment are provided

Rotation coordinator

- Has interest in students
- Is patient with students
- Has time available for students when needed
- Has ability to impart knowledge of material
- Gives periodic, constructive appraisal of student progress
- Keeps students informed of teaching schedule
- Informs students of any schedule change

During rotation, the student

- Performs technical procedures with direct or indirect supervision
- Performs technical procedures without supervision
- Studies during *assigned* study periods with no specific activity assigned

Types of instruction provided

- Demonstrations
- Lectures and/or discussions
- Reading manuals
- AV guides
- Study questions
- Case-study discussions

Provision of reference material

- Insufficient
- Sufficient
- Organized

Correlations of exams and objectives

- Yes/No/sometimes

Were you informed of your progress after completing each task?

- Always
- Usually
- Sometimes
- Rarely[15]

Activity 7

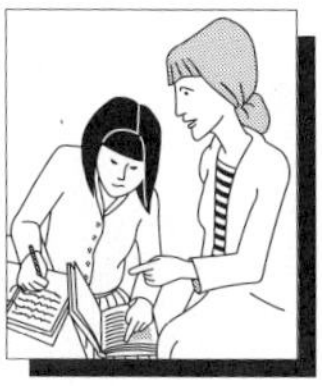

On the balance of the items in the evaluation form, comment on the performance of the clinical instructor. What similarity do you observe regarding clinical/academic evaluation?

Summary

Grades are indispensable for any profession preparing students to enter the health care system. It is the responsibility of the academic and clinical site to use the grading system to eliminate those who do not meet the standards set by the profession identified as "entry-level skills."

Therefore, the grades have to identify, as accurately as possible, the true abilities of graduates. Equally important, the evaluation of faculty engaged in CLS instruction has as its focus constructive criticism. Faculty need feedback on improving the various facets of instruction. Teachers are not born, they are made, and students play a vital role in this "making" of a teacher.

Review Questions

1. Factors contributing to the grade of a student in a CLS program should be
   a. academic achievement, behavioral patterns.
   b. the number of times absent and tardy.
   c. a combination of a and b.
   d. academic achievement alone.
2. Differentiate between grading and evaluating.
3. Summarize what can happen when a student with inflated grades is accepted into a CLS academic program.
4. Which of the three central tendencies provides the most practical information that can be used by both instructor and students?
5. You have all taken laboratory courses during the academic portion of the program. Design a grading system using a weighing system.

See p. 407 for answers.

References

1. Pollio HR, Humphreys WL. Section 4: Grading students in teaching college. *In* Collected Readings for the New Instructor. Madison, Wisc, Magna Publications, 1990, pp 109–116.
2. Eble KE. Grades. *In* The Craft of Teaching. 2nd ed. San Francisco, Jossey-Bass Publishers, 1990, pp 153–163.
3. Travers RMW. Appraisal of the teaching of the college faculty. Journal of Higher Education 1950; 21:41–42.
4. Williams JH. Clarifying grade expectations. The Teaching Professor 1993; 7(7): 1.
5. LeGrys VA, Beck SJ. Clinical teaching. *In* Clinical Laboratory Education. San Mateo, Calif, Appleton and Lange, 1988, pp 115–139.
6. Davis BG. Grading policies. *In* Tools for Teaching. San Francisco, Jossey-Bass Publishers, 1993, pp 282–287.
7. McKeachie WJ. Grades. *In* Teaching Tips. 7th ed. Lexington, Mass, D.C. Heath, 1978, pp 174–186.
8. Johnson GR. Testing and evaluating students. *In* First Steps to Excellence in College Teaching. 2nd ed. Madison, Wisc, Magna Publications, 1990, pp 61–63.
9. Hedges WD. Assigning grades. *In* Testing and Evaluation in the Sciences. Belmont, Calif, Wadsworth Co Inc, 1966, pp 203–215.
10. Udolf R. Testing and grading. *In* The College Instructor's Guide to Teaching and Academia. Chicago, Nelson-Hall, 1976, pp 81–95.
11. Remington RD, Schork MA. Descriptive Statistics. *In* Statistics and Applications in the Biological and Health Sciences. Englewood Cliffs, NJ, Prentice-Hall, Inc, 1970, pp 18–58.
12. LeGrys VA, Beck SJ. Test Development and Analysis in Clinical Education. San Mateo, Calif, Appleton and Lange, 1988, pp 89–114.
13. Eble KE. Being a teacher. *In* The Craft of Teaching. 2nd ed. San Francisco, Jossey-Bass Publishers, 1990, pp 214–226.
14. McKeachie WJ. Appendix B. *In* Teaching Tips. 7th ed. Lexington, Mass, D.C. Heath, 1978, pp 391–295.
15. Faculty Evaluation Forms, CLS Program, Detroit Receiving Hospital, Detroit, Michigan.

Suggested Reading

1. Davis BG. Tools for Teaching. San Francisco, Jossey-Bass Publishers, 1993.
2. Eble KE. The Craft of Teaching. 2nd ed. San Francisco, Jossey-Bass Publishers, 1990.
3. Green JA. Teacher-Made Tests. 2nd ed. San Francisco, Harper and Row, 1963.
4. Hedges WD. Testing and Evaluation for the Sciences. Belmont, Calif, Wadsworth, 1966.
5. Kebler RJ, Cegalo DJ, Watson KW, Barker LL, Miles DT. Objectives for Instruction and Evaluation. Boston, Allyn and Bacon, 1981.
6. LeGrys VA, Beck SJ. Clinical Laboratory Education. San Francisco, Appleton and Lange, 1988.
7. Lowman J. Mastering the Techniques of Teaching. San Francisco, Jossey-Bass Publishers, 1984.
8. Magnan B. 147 Practical Tips for Teaching

Professors. Madison, Wisc, Magna Publications, 1990.
9. Marshall JC, Hales LW. Essentials of Teaching. Menlo Park, Calif, Addison-Wesley, 1972.
10. McKeachie WJ. Teaching Tips. 7th ed. Lexington, Mass, D.C. Heath, 1978.
11. Neff RA, Weimer M. Classroom Communication. Madison, Wisc, Magna Publications, 1989: ch 5.
12. Weimer M, Neff RA. Teaching College. Madison, Wisc, Magna Publications, 1990.
13. Udolf R. The College Instructor's Guide to Teaching and Academia. Chicago, Nelson-Hall, 1976.

8

The Adult Learner: Factors Affecting Achievement

OBJECTIVES

Upon completion of this chapter, the reader should be able to

- List and discuss the *responsibilities* of students enrolled in a professional program of the academic year.
- List and discuss the rights of students enrolled in a professional program of the academic year.
- Define multiculturalism and discuss its impact on education.
- Research and submit one paper on factors affecting "adult learning."
- Identify and discuss among your group what has motivated and continues to motivate your learning.
- Discuss within your group "how you learn."

KEY WORDS

adult learner

learning

motivation

diversity

multiculturalism

Introduction

The *educational process* has presented you with step-by-step directions in preparing to teach. The process consists of sequential steps leading the student to the acquisition of knowledge and skills, demonstrated through examinations and demonstrations.

Students are *contracted customers* who exist outside the educational process and as graduates are the *product* of that process. At the onset of a course, a few students demonstrate their commitment to serious learning. This population of students has developed the discipline necessary to achieve competence, and competence is essential to the possession of purpose, because competence defines the individual's potential and because it is experienced by that individual as self-worth—an important characteristic of all people who are purposeful. Discipline and practice are essential because competence is always expressed through some practice, *to which discipline gives order or structure.*[1] These students will be characterized as competent despite unforeseen demands placed on their already full calendar of commitments and obligations.

This category of student usually includes a few of every class; the remainder, for one reason or another, do not achieve at their level of potential. Why not? The factors that affect the performance of students are many and need to be reviewed.

Instructors need to (1) Understand the "person" of the student, how he/she is coping with the peculiar demands that are part of his/her life. These demands reach into the energy, time, finances, and behavior of the student with a resultant performance that usually does not reflect the potential of that student. (2) Identify those students with less ability and give them individual help, and develop study guides to assist these students. It is essential to identify, as early as possible, those students who need assistance.

Student Responsibilities

As mentioned in an earlier chapter, the instructor should be aware of students' responsibilities and rights. Some of these are printed in the university catalog, a publication that very few students ever see. It is advisable to copy these statements and include them in the student handbook. When students are admitted into the university and then into a professional program, they are given materials that contain and spell out for them their responsibilities, first as a student admitted into a university student body, and then as a member of a professional program. Located in the front section of every undergraduate university catalog is printed a list that enumerates the responsibilities of students:

1. To inform themselves of and to fulfill all requirements of the university and those of the college and department from which they expect to receive their degree
2. To fulfill conscientiously all assignments and requirements of their courses
3. To attend classes regularly and punctually
4. To maintain a scholarly, courteous demeanor in class
5. To uphold academic honesty in all activities

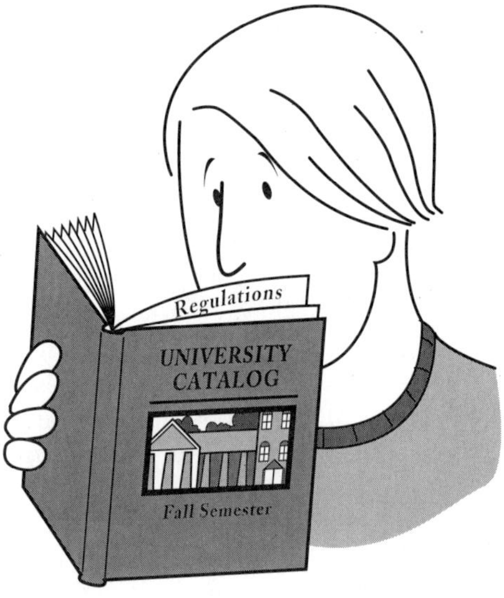

6. To notify the instructor as early as possible if prevented from keeping an appointment or carrying out an assignment

7. To discuss with the instructor any class-related problem and follow established procedures in the resolution of these problems

8. To adhere to the instructor's and general university policies on attendance, withdrawal, or other special procedures[2]

Analyzing these responsibilities, it is noted that they all pertain to the *Affective Domain*: Did you read those over carefully? Read them over again and again. It pertains to the students you are going to teach. This is important. This is going to cost *them*. There's a message here, telling the prospective student: "Look hard at what responsibilities you are going to assume together with those that already exist in your life. Can you internalize these attitudes and modify your behavior to conscientiously fulfill these superimposed obligations? Can you internalize and identify with those aspects that are specific to the code of ethics that pertain to Clinical Laboratory Science? Can you discipline yourself to carry this off? This is quite a commitment!"

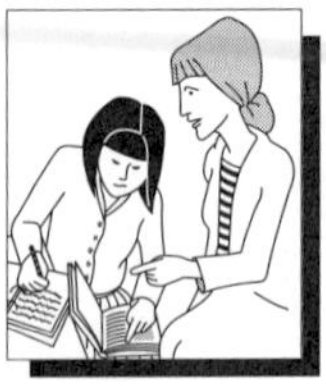

Activity 1

Within your group, discuss what type of exercise you would develop for your students to make them aware of their responsibilities.

The Rights of Students

When the rights of individuals are considered, the points of reference in acknowledging these rights include (1) their persona, their being; (2) their national citizenship; and (3) their role in society, whether they are in the academic arena, are preparing to enter the workforce, or are already a part of

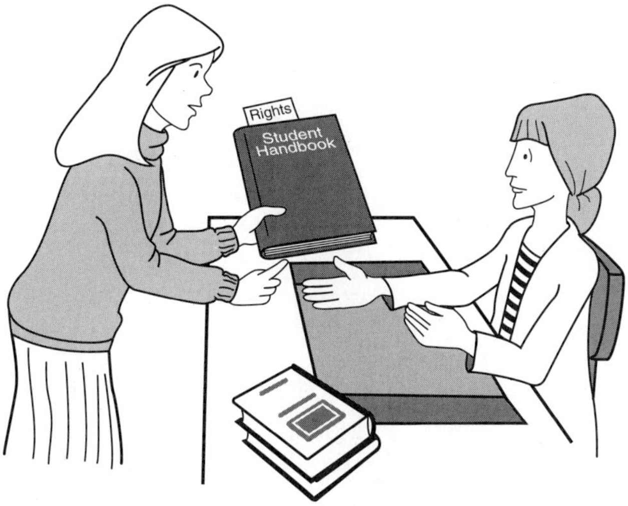

it. As persons, we and students share the right to be respected. To respect deals with having and showing a high regard for each other—to esteem, to consider worthy of high regard. Basically, it involves recognizing people for who they are and for their individuality, and acknowledging it by how one communicates and behaves with them.

The first consideration is listed as one of the items in the faculty evaluation forms. "Did the instructor show you respect"? What can a faculty member do or fail to do to receive a negative response from a student? When you examine all the possible explanations in the dictionary for the word "respect," they deal with building up, giving to, bestowing upon. When a faculty member does not show respect to a student, he/she treats that student as a nonperson, and takes away from the person by either belittling (to cause a person to feel less), or embarrassing (to cause to experience a state of self-conscious, distress), or intimidating (to take away self-confidence). Instructors do these things, whether they realize it or not. If they continue to receive negative responses on their evaluation forms regarding this item, they should begin to ask themselves, "What am I doing to generate this type of evaluation? Am I aware of my actions?" Some questions they could entertain are as follows:

- Do I correct a student in front of other students?
- Do I respond to students' questions as less than *good* questions?
- Do I ever use the word "stupid" when responding to a student's remark?
- Do I ignore students when they are motioning for assistance?
- Do I put a student "on the spot" with a difficult question in front of the other students?
- Do I use negative body language when dealing with a student?
- Do I ever indicate that an answer to a question was not a good answer?
- Do I treat all students equally?
- Do I learn the names of students in my class?
- Do I give equal time to students who need help?

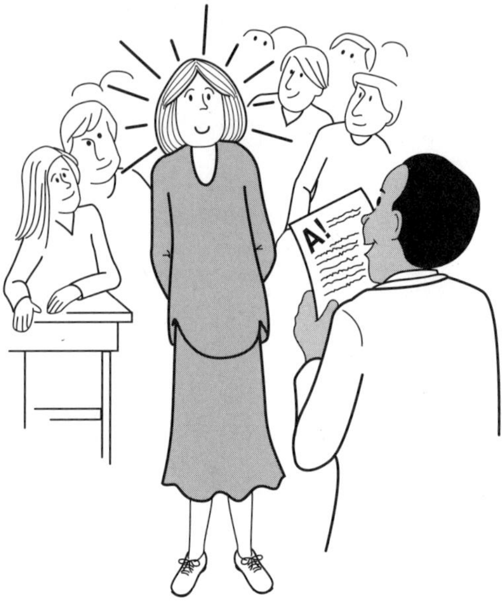

- Do I acknowledge students' differences and show appreciation for them?
- Do I make an effort to become acquainted with students as individuals?
- Do I treat the students as responsible adults?
- Do I give equal recognition for work well done?
- Do I provide all students with equal feedback on their exams?
- Do I give recognition to students as I pass them in the hallway?
- Do I publicly acknowledge students' ideas as good ones or deny building up their self-esteem? Do I claim their ideas as mine?

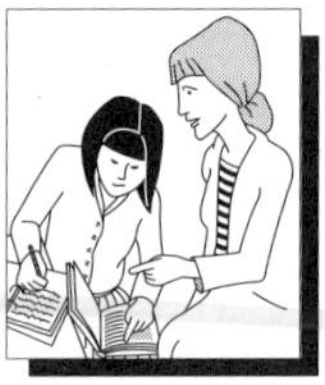

Activity 2

Within your group, discuss the items above and possibly other ways that instructors inadvertently or advertently deny students the respect they are due. What could be some reasons why instructors behave this way?

Instructors, intent on improving their relationships with students, can use this list to perhaps spur their recollection of how they have treated students in the past to earn a negative evaluation at the end of their courses.

As citizens of the United States, our basic rights to life, liberty, and the pursuit of happiness are guaranteed us in the Constitution. As a member of the university student body, the student assumes basic rights as established by the Board of Governors of the University:

> The association of a student with a university brings with it certain rights and privileges and likewise imposes obligations and responsibilities. For instance, a student has the right to competent instruction, good counseling, and adequate facilities, and in all areas he has the right to expect the highest degree of

excellence possible within the resources of the University. A student also has the right to protection from unreasonable and capricious actions by faculty, administration, and student organizations. He has the responsibility to devote himself to the serious pursuit of learning and to respect the rights and opinions of others, including faculty, the administration, and his fellow students. In addition to such general rights and responsibilities, the following specific student rights and responsibilities are held to be indispensable to the full achievement of the objectives of a university in a free society.

1. Each student has the right to be considered for admission, advancement, honors, and all academic and co-curricular activities and benefits without regard to ancestry or religious, political, or country origin.
2. Each student has the right to know the rules by which he (or she) is governed . . . insofar as a written set of specific rules is possible . . . through the medium of a clear and precise written exposition of the rules, given proper publicity. Each student has the right to advocate changes in any rule by which he (or she) is governed.
3. Each student has the right to be advised in writing of charges that might lead to disciplinary action in nonacademic matters. Each student has the right to a fair hearing before final disciplinary action is taken.
4. Each student has the right to free inquiry and scholarly investigation and the right to discuss, exchange, and publish any findings or recommendations, either individually or in association with others, provided he makes no claim to represent the university without due authorization.
5. Each student has the right to organize, join, and participate in recognized campus organizations, subject to the university rules governing such organizations.[3]

The Class: Diversification

The author remembers teaching a class in 1955 composed of all white students, typically Americanized, giving only subtle clues to original ancestry. In November, a young Polish student was admitted to the class, immediately becoming the center of attention. He spoke differently, he even appeared "different," and he looked at us in such a way that *he* literally made *us* feel different. Before the admission of that student to the class, diversity among the students did not exist. Today as then, factors (*variables*) that contributed to this diversification are buried deeply within the personality of each student; these variables affect the *process* of learning for each individual. Student behavior indicates the existence and influence of these variables and to what degree they affect the learning process.

THE ADULT LEARNERS

The concept of the adult learner, at first appearance, seems so simple—as if *age* were the only identifying characteristic factor. Every text on education attempts to explain the various factors that expand this group into a complex patchwork quilt, with each student contributing complexity to an already diverse group.

1. The typical American adult learner, historically, has been described as single and white, attending a prestigious university (with a football team), boarding at the university, and having the cost absorbed by parents.
2. The urban universities identify typical American adult learners as working part time or even full time, attending classes during the day, night, and weekends—whenever they can fit them into their schedule. Their families

are unable to contribute toward their education; these students absorb the total cost.

3. Add to this group the responsibilities of a marriage and children.

4. Reentry students, adults over the age of 25 who have been away from formal education for at least 2 years, make up an increasingly large proportion of the student body. These students represent a wide range of ages, attitudes, and interests and no longer conform—if they ever did—to the stereotype. In general, they tend to be less involved in the social and extracurricular life on campus and are more likely to treat their professors as peers, are intrinsically more motivated to learn, have a more practical problem-solving orientation to learning, and are clearer about their educational goals. These students are motivated, interested, and excited about learning.[4]

5. Include in the group the handicapped student—those in wheelchairs, with crutches—who are disabled in body but perhaps intellectually equal to or above the average student.

Multiculturalism

There are further complexities to the class composition, with religious and cultural differences contributed by an overwhelming number of culturally and ethnically diverse students now attending our universities, bringing with them a value system often unlike the "traditional American way." The result is diversity upon diversity upon diversity. Depending on the specific area of the country in which you teach, the nationality and the culture of the students vary. Bernstein, in his book, *Dictatorship of Virtue*, contends that all these groups should not lose their identity as they become one with the nation. Members of each group must contribute their uniqueness to the fabric of the patchwork quilt, that it is visible, *equal* to all the other patches but not the same, yet all integral and essential.

The CLS instructor should be grateful that class size makes it possible to work with, enjoy, and learn from those with diverse backgrounds. The statement made in Chapter 1, "Know your material so well that you can concen-

FACTORS THAT DIVERSIFY

Age	Father	Minority
Aloofness	Friendly	Motivation (non)
City (home)	Full-time student	Mother
Economic background	Gender	Religion
Economic status	Handicapped	Sheltered
Educational ability	Learner, quick	Suburb (home)
Educational background	Learner, slow	Work (full time)
Ethnicity	Marital status	Work (part time)
Experience	Maturity	

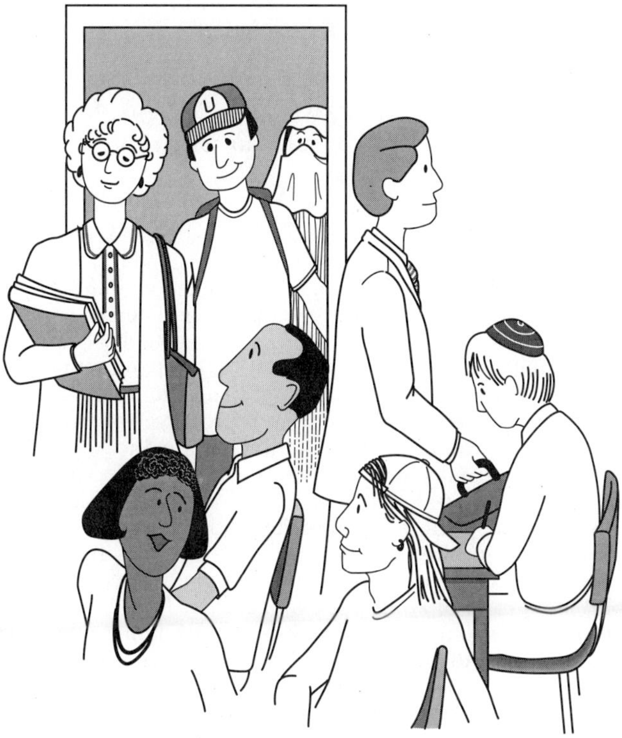

trate on the needs of your students as you teach," should make more sense to you now.

INSTRUCTOR RESPONSE TO STUDENT ATTRIBUTES/BEHAVIOR

Intelligence

McKeachie stresses that most faculty members have to work with large groups in which personalization of education depends on sensitivity to individual differences among students. Knowing student differences in intelligence is not important in itself, but recognizing that highly intelligent students need to be taught in some way different from students of less intelligence is. Of concern here are interactions: that is, *characteristics differentiating students for whom different kinds of teacher behavior are differentially effective.*[5]

For these students, journals and various texts of the subjects that they are involved in during their training should be available to further their depth of knowledge. Critiques of the various articles could be assigned with the objective that these students sharpen their writing, analytical, and evaluation skills.

Students who have different learning rates must be identified for the same reason. The instructor should pursue that type of teaching/learning methodology that would enhance acquisition of knowledge/skills. The first group will learn in spite of you; the second group will learn because of you. Your function here is one of facilitator.

Ethnic, Gender, and Cultural Diversity

Davis states "that there are no universal solutions or specific rules for responding to these diversities in the classroom. Perhaps the overriding principle is to be thoughtful and sensitive and do what you think is best."[6] She offers the following general strategies:

> Recognize any biases or stereotypes you may have absorbed. Do you assume that most African American, Chicano/Latino, or Native American students are enrolled under special admissions programs? Treat each student as an individual, and respect each student for who he/she is. Rectify any language patterns or case examples that exclude or demean any groups. Do your best to be sensitive to terminology. Terminology changes over time, as ethnic and cultural groups continue to define their identify, their history, and their relationship to the dominant culture. In the 1960s, for example, the term *Negro* gave way to *black* and *Afro-American.* In the 1990s, the term *African American* gained general acceptance. Most Americans of Mexican ancestry prefer *Chicano* or *Latino* or *Mexican American* to *Hispanic.* Most Asian Americans are offended by the term *Oriental* and prefer Japanese American, Chinese American, and so forth. In California, *Pacific Islander* and *South Asian* are accepted by students from those regions. Get a sense of how students feel about the cultural climate in your classroom. Don't try to "protect" any group of students. Don't refrain from criticizing the performance of individual students in your class on account of their ethnicity or gender. This, on the part of the student, is seen as patronizing, and the rest of the class will resent the preferential treatment. Be evenhanded in how you acknowledge a student's good work. It is good practice, once all papers are corrected, to compare your responses to specific questions to ensure that your responses are equal in praise to all students. Convey the same level of respect and confidence in the abilities of all your students.[6]

Every September, soon after classes start, the author holds a "Diversity Lunch" for which every student prepares a *dish* of their country. During the lunch, students talk about their background, their beliefs, and so on. Experience has shown that the members of the class are pleased with this manner of introduction and recognition of the diversity of the class. Attending the same basic CLS program, experiencing the same frustrations and demands from various classes, and experiencing the establishment of "small learning groups" provides a comfortable turf on which to work together. The university setting is a microcosm reflecting the diversity graduates will experience in the workplace.

The Emotional Student

McKeachie in his chapter "Problem Situations and Problem Students (There's Almost Always at Least One)" describes the following:

- *The angry, aggressive student* who seems to have a chip on his/her shoulder . . . who conveys both verbally and nonverbally hostility toward you and the whole enterprise: The author suggests trying to better understand the student through his/her writings, inviting that student to come to the office and discuss how he/she feels about the course. If the anger is evidenced in class, he suggests, "Ignore him/her."
- For the *attention seeker,* who dominates discussions, the author suggests the following strategies when students dominate the class through asking questions or prolonging a response:

    1. Suggest that you want everyone's ideas . . . that each student has

a unique perspective . . . that it is important that we bring as many perspectives and ideas as possible to bear on the subject under discussion.

2. If the problem persists, ask to see the student outside the class and mention that you are concerned about class discussions—that it would be helpful for him/her to hold back some comments until everyone else has been heard.

3. The *silent student*: Outside of small groups and pairings, these students remain silent in class discussions. Assigning brief reference papers dealing with the subject at hand may "break the ice" for them. Have questions ready to ask the student; encourage the class members to direct their questions to those students. Then, give praise in moderate terms.

4. The *inattentive student:* This usually involves two or three students in the back of the room carrying on their own conversation during lecture. This is annoying to the lecturer and to the students sitting near them. To remedy this, break the class into small groups with an assigned question to solve or answer. This usually works, at least for one class. If the situation persists, give an assignment to write a "minute paper" on a subject related to what is being taught and call on those students who persist in talking.

5. The *chronically unprepared student*: Review your syllabus to see if it is specific in its assignments: i.e., specific page numbers for the readings.[6] If this is not the cause, meet with the student and discuss the problem to uncover the possible reason.

The various examples of student *behavior* listed here, together with others not covered, are indications of *attitudes* that reside within students. If these behavior patterns begin to characterize a student, the problem is deeply rooted, and that individual may need counseling. It is advisable to try to uncover the reason for the behavior early in the semester so that the student can modify it and prevent it from emerging in the workplace.

Motivation

The fact that students were accepted into the program indicates a high degree of motivation on their part. Once classes begin, student achievement indirectly communicates to the instructor not only something about the level of their basic intelligence but also about the *force* of their motivation. The definition of the word *motive* is "something (a need or desire) that causes a person to act." Instructors will observe the students' results, which can be used as indicators of the degree of their motivation but which generate no information regarding the *reason* behind the motive.

It is essential that you recognize the various levels of motivation of your students. Your motive as their instructor is to stimulate students to become *self-motivated.* Davis states: "Whatever level of motivation your students bring to the classroom will be transformed, for better or worse, by what happens in that classroom." She notes that there is no single magical formula for motivating students.[7] She offers many suggestions as to how instructors can encourage students to become self-motivated and independent learners:

- Give frequent, early, positive feedback that supports students' belief that they can do well.

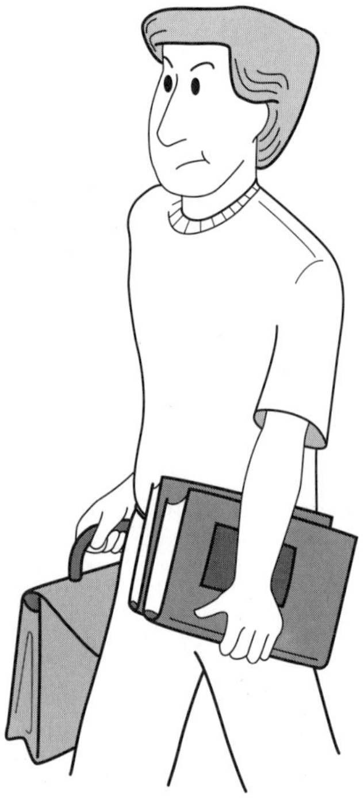

- Ensure opportunities for students' success by assigning tasks that are neither too easy nor too difficult.
- Help students find personal meaning and value in the material.
- Create an atmosphere that is open and positive.
- Help students feel that they are valued members of a learning community.[7]

As you start to teach, read to find out what others have learned through their teaching experiences regarding motivating factors that affect student performance, although your *rough days* and *hard knocks* will be among your best teachers. Years of teaching have borne out (for the author and confirmed by other educators) that most students react positively to and are further motivated by the following:

- An enthusiastic instructor that presents a syllabus with the specific information for which they will be responsible, and a calendar of events: material to be covered, reading assignments, exam schedule. If for any reason a scheduled exam has to be changed, allow the students to vote on the new date for the exam.
- The relevance of a course made clear during instruction. ("You will see these disease states in this city! Recognize their characteristics while doing your microscopic studies.")
- An active class with involvement by the students in a learning situation (use the small group approach when possible).
- The use of variable teaching methods that enhance the understanding of a difficult concept.
- An instructor who avoids intimidating students by how he/she presents or displays his/her knowledge of a subject (this can be overwhelming to the student).

An instructor who treats students as you would have liked to have been treated; and praise, praise, praise sincerely when warranted.

During laboratory exercises, the author will sometimes announce: "The first student to find a Cabot ring will be given a prize." It is clear in this situation that the prize equals the *motivation* to search for and identify an unusual structure associated with a specific disease. Mager, using delightful humor in the introduction to his chapter on "Sources of Influence," gives a short discourse between two children to prove a point about motivation. The main players consist of two small boys: one empty-handed and one holding and licking a huge lollipop. The empty-handed boy speaks first:

"Hi. Where'd you get the sucker?"

"My mommy gave it to me as a reward for crying."

"You mean your mommy wants you to cry?"

"I guess so. Whenever I cry, she gives me a lollipop."

"Gee, I'd cry a lot more often if I always got a sucker."

"Of course. It's elementary psychology."[8]

Activity 3

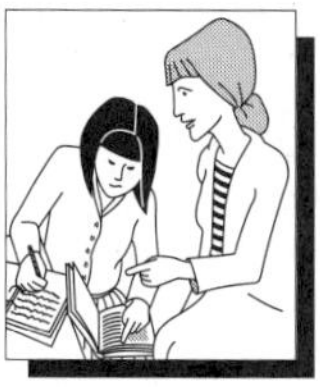

Discuss among your group the above story as related to "external motivation." What lesson can be learned here?

Activity 4

Discuss among your group the factors that have contributed to the development of your self-motivation and those factors that are identified as external motivators. Include the experiences you have had that have affected your motivation as a student.

About Learning

Instructors must realize that their role in the learning process of students is limited to (1) guidance (identifying the subject matter/skills, the competencies students must master; (2) encouragement; (3) developing various assignments and laboratory exercises in both the theoretical (lecture) and practical (laboratory areas) through which knowledge/skill is acquired; and (4) providing students with feedback in identifying what they know well and, specifically, what they do not know well. Also, if they recognize that certain students do not possess good study learning skills, assistance can be given. *Learning* was defined earlier as *to come to know, to realize.* The current view of learning is that memory refers to some properties of an information processing system. This system involves nerve cells in activities having to do with learning and retrieving meaningful relationships. Learning and remembering are active processes. Because understanding and learning involve adding previously learned relationships of meanings, students differ in what and how they learn in a particular lecture or assignment."[9]

In applying this theory, students in the CLS Program take basic anatomy and physiology in one of the first 2 years of the undergraduate studies. When students are admitted to the professional program, specialty courses, such as urinalysis, chemistry, and hematology, make up the curriculum of the junior year.

Applying the theory of learning, students should see the relationship of the specifics of one specialty science—urinalysis—and relate it to the kidney, which was a subject presented in physiology. The theory should work. If a student can link that which is being taught to something that he/she already knows, it is more likely that it will be understood and remembered.

McKeachie makes two general statements that help us to analyze the process of learning. First, he notes that human beings are learning organisms . . . seeking, organizing, coding, storing, and retrieving information all their lives: building on cognitive structures to continue learning throughout life, seeking meaning. Secondly, human beings can remember images; they can remember transcriptions of the exact words that were used in a lecture or textbook and they can remember meanings, depending on the demands of the situation. Meanings tend to be recalled more easily than exact words. The meanings a student gets depends not only on the student's past experiences but also on the student's learning strategies.[9] McKeachie is saying that no one can accomplish learning for the student, and the student best learns by understanding the meaning of what he/she is studying. The small group learning approach assists students in achieving understanding by the contribution the other students make regarding experiences they have had that the others have not.

When discussing *learning strategies* with students, many of the students stated that their learning methodology varied with the subject being studied. For subjects such as microbiology and parasitology, the small index card format was used. Some students would tape large computer sheets together in order to see the entire scope of what they had to learn. Others said they would pace up and down a walkway repeating words that meant nothing to them until at last the meaning would come through. One student would use different colored pens in designating the variability and sameness of the meaning of various categories.

An external evaluator of our program once told us that she had been a salesperson before her present job. She recalled that as part of her training, she was told the number 7 was important. Statistics had borne out that if a customer heard about or saw consumer goods seven times, he/she probably would make the purchase.

She told us this should apply to education. That students hear or write a fact seven times, they will probably learn it. But remember, it has to have meaning for them.

Summary

Students are the most important persons in the lecture room or the laboratory to receive consideration. They are there to acquire the knowledge and skills necessary to be hired into the clinical laboratory and thus enter the health care field. Instructors can facilitate this learning process by better understanding adult learners with whatever level of ability they possess. Instructors can further facilitate learning by various motivational skills open to them. Further, instructors should be aware of how they address students: Respect for students should always be uppermost in mind. Awareness of specific rights and responsibilities pertaining to both instructors and students is essential for both parties. Diversity and multiculturalism should not only be recognized and appreciated but *celebrated.*

See p. 407 for answers.

Review Questions

1. True or False: Green's quotation uses the expression "possession of purpose" as a synonym for the word *motivation.*
2. List at least three responsibilities given in your university catalog of which you were not previously aware.
3. To which Hierarchical Domain do all the responsibilities refer?
4. Among the members of your group, list at least five factors dealing with student diversity that were not included in the box on page 126.
5. Among your group, discuss McKeachie's discussion regarding memory and the learning of new material. Write at least two statements arrived at by the members of your group.

References

1. Green TF. Acquisition of purpose. *In* Chickering AW, et al., eds. The Modern American College. San Francisco, Jossey-Bass Publishers, 1988, pp 543–555.
2. Undergraduate Bulletin, Wayne State University 1993–1995. Detroit, Michigan.
3. Clinical Laboratory Science Student Handbook, Wayne State University, Detroit, Michigan, 1995.
4. Davis BG. Reentry students. *In* Tools for Teaching. San Francisco, Jossey-Bass Publishers, 1993, pp 52–55.
5. McKeachie WJ. Personalizing education. *In* Teaching Tips. 7th ed. Lexington, Mass, D.C. Heath, 1978, pp 244–245.
6. Davis BG. Diversity and complexity in the classroom: considerations of race, ethnicity, and gender. *In* Tools for Teaching. San Francisco, Jossey-Bass Publishers, 1993, pp 39–51.
7. Davis BG. Motivating students. *In* Tools for Teaching. San Francisco, Jossey-Bass Publishers, 1993, pp 193–202.
8. Mager RF. Sources of influences. *In* Developing Attitude Toward Learning. Belmont, Calif, Fearon, 1968, pp 31–38.
9. McKeachie WJ. Learning and cognition in the college classroom. *In* Teaching Tips. 9th ed. Lexington, Mass, D.C. Heath, 1994, pp 279–295.

Suggested Reading

1. Bell G-R, Marshall E., Chekaluk E. Academic performance of mature-age and other students in a physiotherapy program. Journal of Allied Health 1991, 20 (2): 107–117.
2. Bernstein R. Dictatorship of Virtue. New York, Alfred A. Knopf, 1994.
3. Bowden R, Merritt R Jr. The Adult Learner Challenge: Instructionally and Administratively in Education. Vol 115, A3. Spring 1995, pp 426–432.
4. Brookfield SD. Developing Critical Thinkers. San Francisco, Jossey-Bass Publishers, 1988.
5. Davis BG. Tools for Teaching. San Francisco, Jossey-Bass Publishers, 1993.
6. Eble KE. The Craft of Teaching. 2nd ed. San Francisco, Jossey-Bass Publishers, 1990.
7. Endorf M, McNeff M. The adult learners: five types. Adult Learning 1991 (May): 20–25.
8. Johnson GR. First Steps to Excellence in

College Teaching. 2nd ed. Madison, Wisc, Magna Publications, 1990.
9. LeGrys VA, Beck SJ. Clinical Laboratory Education. San Mateo, Calif, Appleton & Lange, 1988.
10. Lowman J. Mastering the Techniques of Teaching. San Francisco, Calif, Jossey-Bass Publishers, 1984.
11. Mager RF. Developing Attitude Toward Learning. Belmont, Calif, Fearon, 1968.
12. McKeachie WJ. Teaching Tips. 9th ed. Lexington, Mass, D.C. Heath, 1994.
13. Queen J. Teaching tips. Vocational Education Journal. January 1995, 13, 14.
14. Student Handbook of your CLS Department.
15. The Teaching Professor. All issues.
16. University Undergraduate Catalog: Students' Rights and Responsibilities.
17. Webb RA, Weimer M. Classroom Communication. Madison, Wisc, Magna Publications, 1989.
18. Weimer M, Neff RA. Teaching College. Madison, Wisc, Magna Publications, 1990.
19. Zemke R, Zemke S. 30 things we know for sure about adult learners. Training 1961 (June): 117–120.

9

Education and the Law: Be Aware!

OBJECTIVES

Upon completion of this chapter, the reader should be able to:

- Identify federal statutes applicable to the various factors involved in the admission process of the university.
- Paraphrase policies within the university catalog that deal with Equality of Opportunity.
- Summarize the "Non-Discrimination for the Handicapped" policy found within the university catalog.
- List and describe the Academic Regulations: specifically, those policies that relate to admission, probation, student conduct, attendance, and students' rights.
- Locate policies within the student handbook dealing with Academic Dishonesty; list the topics included in this heading and the disciplinary action taken toward students not adhering to the policy.
- List at least five considerations included in the Buckley Amendment.
- Report on various mechanisms that constitute the Defense System provided for the undergraduate students within the university government.
- Research and report on the university lawyers and the types of cases involving students they tried and/or settled.
- Research the function and role of the ombudsman; identify the types of cases in which he/she has represented students.
- Keep in mind possible legal issues that are involved in writing a letter of recommendation; write such a letter for a student.

KEY WORDS

policies
regulations
laws
infringement
lawyers
ombudsman

Introduction

The content of this chapter deals with a very challenging but necessary task. It is one that is superimposed on the very *conscious* activity that engages both your mental and physical energy when you are involved in teaching. It demands that you familiarize yourself with the legalities involved in every facet of the educational process, from admission to dismissal policies, and all legal issues that come between, pertaining to both faculty and student behavior. As you begin to teach, you realize that you must become knowledgeable about the existence of policies and the consequences of their abuse: that your subconscious—your mind's eye—must be always on the alert regarding your own behavior and that of the students and *any* abuse committed against the laws of the university and/or the department.

Within every university catalog (bulletin) are found policies that deal with admission, admission standards, entry level GPA, adverse behavior, and dismissal. Further into the catalog, the various colleges and their departments are featured, again each describing their own specific policies. The mission statement of the university sets the tone regarding the admission of students to the university (Fig. 9–1).

> As a nationally ranked university, Wayne State holds high expectation for the educational achievements of the students and consequently maintains selective admission standards.[1]

The terminology used by the university to express *law* is *policy*. "Policies and regulations" *are* "law," and the individual abusing these laws is faced with specific consequences, the severity depending on the nature of each policy.

University law pertains and applies to both university faculty, staff, and students admitted to the university. Ignorance regarding the existence of the policy or the consequences incurred by their abuse is not admissible. It is a good practice in every department to require that students, upon admission to the program, read the "Student Handbook," which reviews both university and departmental policies, and to verify this by having them sign a form so stating. In other words, *Document! Document!*

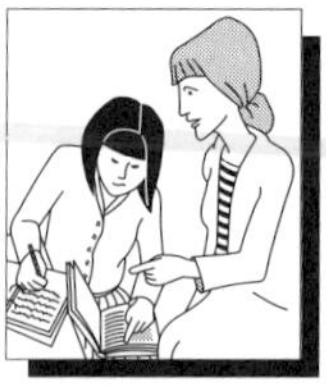

Activity I

1. Referring to the dictionary, define the words *policy* and *regulation*. Compare them to the definition of the word *law*.
2. Identify the domain with which this chapter deals (see Chapter 4). Comment.

Legal Issues Involving the Educator in Academia

PROGRAM DESCRIPTION: UNIVERSITY CATALOG

Faculty members submit updated descriptions of their program to the university to be printed in the catalog. It is the obligation of the faculty of each

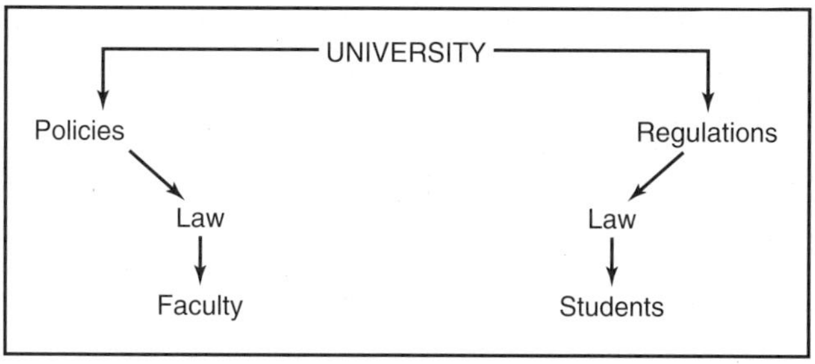

Figure 9–1 Academic law.

department to submit any changes in the curriculum dictated by their accrediting associations and agencies as these occur. If the department fails to communicate changes in its requirements to either advisors to undergraduate students or fails to update the university catalog, the student, by all rights, could claim to have been misled. *The student could then retain a lawyer.* (Catalogs are printed every other year; this is so stated within the text.)

ADMISSION POLICIES

Many legal actions have been brought against universities regarding admission policies: specifically against departments denying the student admission to their program. Nonadmission is based on the student's not having met specific criteria.

Given below are the results of several cases settled in court regarding admission standards and the policy generated by the settlement of each case.

1. *Federal jurisdiction precedes that of the state.*

> In formulating admission criteria, the federal constitution and federal statutory requirements, state statutory and constitutional requirements, and accreditation standards come into active interplay. It is important for the medical technologist to realize that if there is a conflict between the federal and state requirements, in general, the federal constitution requirements will prevail . . . it is against the 14th amendment's declaration that admissions standards, publications, solicitations, and the entire deliberative process will be measured.[2]

2. *Admission policies can be based on individualized assessments of an applicant's credentials and potentials for achievement.*

> Justice William O. Douglas stressed: Admissions process must be an individualized and particularized process which focuses on the *appropriate merits* as distinct from those of another applicant.[2]

3. *The court ruled that no individual could be denied admission to a program on the basis of race.*

> The interplay of the 14th amendment and Title VI formed the dynamic process by which the court enunciated its standard. Title VI of the Civil Rights Act of 1964 prohibits *discrimination on the basis of race* by any program or activity receiving federal financial assistance.[2]

4. *No individual can be denied admission to a program on the basis of a handicap.*

> In regards to nonadmission based on physical handicaps, in the case of South-

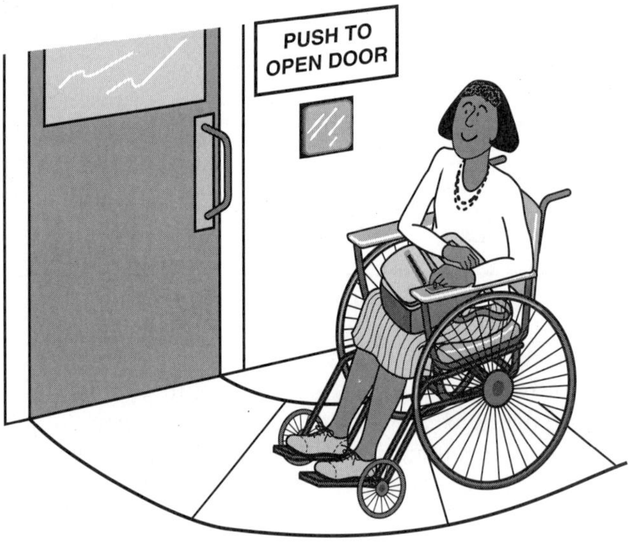

east Community College vs. Davis,[2] the language of section 504, the court found that physical handicaps are not in themselves a permissible ground on assuming inability to function in a particular medical, quasi-medical, or clinical context. Rather, an "otherwise qualified person" is one who is capable of fulfilling all the program's requirements *in spite of* the handicap.[2] Section 504 holds no requirement that an educational institution lower or adjust substantially its standards in order to accommodate a handicapped person. Rather, only "reasonable" accommodations must be made[2] (442 US 413 1979).

5. *The Admission Process must use the* ***criteria stated*** *in any printed material such as catalogs or brochures. Typical criteria utilized in the admission process are as follows*:

- A minimum cumulative and/or science grade point average (GPA)
- The completion of prerequisite courses
- An interview with the Admissions Committee
- Reference letters
- Test scores[3]

6. *Further described in the Introduction to the Allied Health Professions in the university catalog is the following*:

> Although academic achievement is important, personal qualities are considered of equal importance since the students selected will eventually be working as members of a team in the delivery of health care. Therefore, criteria for selection are also based on such qualities as maturity, motivation, knowledge of the profession, ability to communicate, personal integrity and empathy for others. Consequently, evaluations from faculty and advisers, as well as a personal interview, are given great weight in the selection of candidates by admission committees.[1]

By re-reading the preliminary pages in a university catalog, you will recognize the inclusion of the statute by every policy listed.

Activity 2

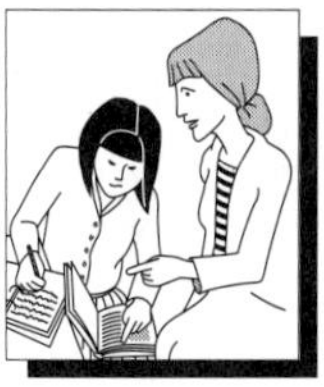

1. Referring to your university catalog, list other policies and the statute number that represent the legality of that policy.
2. A student seeking admission to the university reviewed a copy of his transcript. A number of his high school classes had been difficult and he had received some Ds. The student realized that these grades would greatly impede admission to the university, so he forged a transcript. This false transcript was indeed submitted to the university and upon inspection was immediately identified as such. What is the policy of the university (individual program) regarding forged transcripts? (Give the reference page in the Student Handbook.)

Grading and Evaluation of Students

Grading has already been discussed in Chapter 7 and constitutes "objective cognitive-based" data. The numbers translate to the academic ability of the student. Academic performance can be measured in the lecture setting and the student laboratory through quizzes and/or examinations, observation, and the performance of procedures.[3] This reinforces the earlier comment that grades should reflect the measurable performance of a student and that it be documented by both the instructor and the student.

Evaluating a student's professional performance is a more difficult task than the strictly objective-based academic review. The student's attitude and the manner in which laboratory assignments are carried out (including work habits, completeness of assignments, and even appearance) contribute to the factors evaluated in this category. As every lawyer and wise department chair will tell you, "*Document! Document!*" Every incident that involves adverse student behavior warrants documentation. Those consistent and noticeable traits that are not acceptable in a working site count against the student. As stated in the Wayne State University Catalog:

> Students must show diligence and are normally expected to complete the courses they elect. Irresponsible attendance is wasteful of both student and University resources. Those students who consistently receive excessive marks of "I" (incomplete) or "W" ("withdrawal") may be refused the privilege of further registration by the dean or the dean's designee of their school or college.[1]

Other examples of student type behavior to be documented would be lying or adverse behavior resulting in disruption of the class or laboratory. As earlier stated, grades deal with academic achievement; evaluations deal with student behavior. When such behavior is consistent, the faculty should meet with the student and point out that such deportment is incompatible with both the academic and the clinical laboratory workplace, and caution the student to modify his/her behavior pattern.

Disciplinary Action

The type of disciplinary action taken in response to adverse behavior can range from suspension to expulsion from the program. The nature of the behavior determines the severity of the disciplinary action. Before action can be taken, the department must have in place the policy by which the student is notified in writing as to unacceptable performance regarding the standards of the program (a meeting is advisable, but the written notice is essential as documentation) and notified a second time in writing of continual unacceptable performance regarding the standards of the program.

If the student continues to perform substandard, disciplinary action may be carried out. Institutions have the right to dismiss, suspend, or impose sanctions on students for behavioral misconduct and academic dishonesty. If there is an established procedure, it must be followed. Not following the procedure may be excused if the student waives his/her rights to them or if deviations do not disadvantage the student.[3]

Published academic and professional penalties at West Virginia University are as follows:

1. Reasons for Probation:
   - A grade of "D" in any course
   - Semester grade point average less than 2.0
   - Failure to adhere to dress code (after second warning)
   - Violation of safety practices (after second warning)
   - Failure to report illness or absence to Program office (after second warning)
2. Reasons for suspension:
   - Two or more "Ds" in any course
   - A grade of "F" in any course
   - Excessive absenteeism (greater than 10 consecutive school days)
   - Falsifying results
   - Violation of the Honor Code[3]

The various CLS programs are essentially similar in regard to legalities in that they are accredited by the same professional associations and agencies.

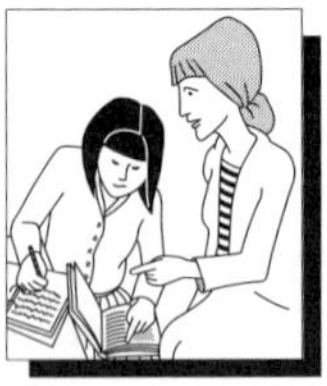

Activity 3

In your Student Handbook, find the disciplinary action taken against the following abuses by students:

1. During an examination, a student *allowed his eyes to roam* around the lecture room onto another student's paper. This is witnessed by the instructor. (Give the disciplinary action taken and the reference page in the Student Handbook.)
2. During a specific class, a student had been tardy 12 times over a 3-month period. (Give the disciplinary action taken and the reference page in the Student Handbook.)
3. A student, during the professional academic year, had failed to call in

when unable to attend class. (Give the disciplinary action and the reference page in the Student Handbook.)

4. A student enrolled in the CLS/MT program and finishing the academic year was preparing for final exams. He was confident regarding most classes, but one had been really difficult. During an exam, the student *looked* onto the exam paper of another student. At that very point, the proctor of the exam approached the student and cautioned the student to keep his eyes on his own booklet. (Give the disciplinary action for cheating and the reference page in the Student Handbook.)

Document! Document! Document!

Providing Letters of Recommendation

When a student approaches you to write a letter of recommendation, this implies that the student believes that you view him/her favorably and hopes for an honest evaluation. Sometimes, however, faculty members see (evaluate) students differently; perhaps not as positively as they see themselves. Whether you write an open-ended letter of recommendation or fill out a special recommendation form (that requests specific information) supplied by the asker, there are basic considerations that must be made before you begin composing the letter. Remember to be accurate and honest. Under the Family Educational Rights and Privacy Act of 1974, students have a right to see a copy of your recommendation unless they sign a waiver. Let the student know the general tone of what you are likely to write. He/she might not want to use you as a reference after all. Ask the student for a brief description of the job or the academic program he/she plans to enter to obtain a better perspective. If a good amount of time has passed, review the student's grades and any remarks you wrote, to refresh your memory.[4]

Udolf[5] suggests you will need to know at least the following points to write an effective letter of recommendation:

- To whom the recommendation is to be sent and when it is required to be submitted
- How long you have known the student and in what capacity, e.g., student, advisee, assistant, departmental assistant
- How well you know him/her
- What courses he/she took with you and his/her grades
- When he/she took these courses (so that you can check on the accuracy of his/her statements)
- What his/her grade point average is overall, and in his/her major
- What honorary societies he/she is a member of and prizes and awards received
- In what extracurricular activities he/she participated
- What his/her work experience is, if any

- What else he/she thinks you should know about him/her before writing your recommendation.

If this is an open-ended letter, a general statement regarding academic ability, demonstrated laboratory skills, personal traits, characteristics (especially those dealing with interpersonal relationships), ability to get along with others, even temperament, readiness to volunteer for various functions, written and communication skills, and special talents should be included. Information regarding making the dean's list and winning outstanding awards, and previous scholarships, will single students out. If this proves to be a negative letter, have supportive data for your statements regarding the student's low rank in the class and the performance of mediocre work (both in lecture and laboratory).[6]

Udolf notes that if you don't feel you can say anything positive about the student, then you should explain to the student what you would have to write and see if he/she prefers that you decline to write a recommendation.[5] Whatever you finally decide to include in your letter, identify the basis of your statements with documentation. Place a copy of the letter in the student's folder in the main office.

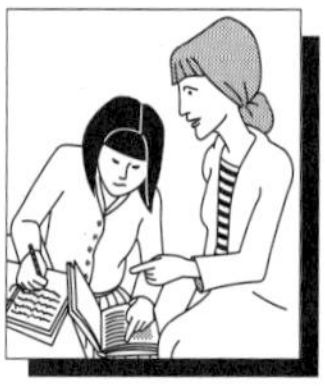

Activity 4

Discuss within your group at least five factors that you believe should be included in a letter of recommendation, whether the response would be positive/negative. List them by their importance.

Sexual Harassment

Illegal in the United States, sexual harassment is defined by university standards as unwelcome sexual advances, requests for favors, and other verbal or physical conduct of a sexual nature. The conditions include when:

- Submission to such conduct is made either explicitly or implicitly a term or condition of an individual's employment or education
- Submission to or rejection of such conduct by an individual is used as the basis for academic or employment decisions affecting that individual
- Such conduct has the purpose or effect of substantially interfering with an individual's academic or professional performance or creating an intimidating hostile or offensive employment, education, or living environment.[7]

When either faculty or student have been victimized by sexual harassment in the academic setting, an accurate report of the incident should be documented and filed with the proper authorities within the university for further investigation into the prosecution process.

Defense System: The University

Perhaps the strongest defense system the university possesses is the published documentation of its policies throughout the university catalog and in its

DEFENSE SYSTEM FOR UNIVERSITY
1. Printed policies
2. General counsel
3. State/Federal law

proceedings. Second, there exists the Office of General Counsel, through which the university lawyers primarily represent the president and the Board of Governors. Under appropriate circumstances, the Office of General Counsel will represent faculty and students.

On the departmental level, the stated and published policies are the strongest defense used by faculty against a student's claims. Those cases involving adverse behavior of the student rely heavily on the documentation of the incident; by nature, these cases are more difficult to settle. If students choose to sue a faculty member, they are entitled to do so but would have to independently retain a lawyer to represent their claim. The burden of proof lies on the student to provide adequate documentation as to the faculty's bias, prejudice, or ill will as the basis of the claim.

Defense System: The Student

Set in place are the specific mechanisms available to the student to plead a case for a variety of claims:

THE APPEAL PROCESS (GRADES)

Grounds for appeals involve the following reasons[8]:

- The application of nonacademic criteria in the grading process, as listed in the university's nondiscrimination and affirmative action statute: race, color, sex, national origin, religion, age, sexual orientation, marital status, or handicap
- Sexual harassment
- Evaluation of student work by criteria not directly reflective of performance relative to course requirements

DEFENSE SYSTEM FOR STUDENT
1. Printed policies
2. Appeal process
3. Hearing panel
4. Ombudsman
5. State/Federal law

The appeal procedure involves the student writing a letter stating why the disciplinary action taken should not have taken place. In most universities, the appeal process allows the student one year to appeal.[3] The student can appeal to the department chairperson. If the situation is not resolved at this level, the student can proceed to the dean of the college. Again, the burden of proof is on the student. This procedure reinforces the importance of each instructor informing students on the first day of class, via a class syllabus, the criteria used in determining the grades for the class. It is the instructor's prerogative to assign grades in accordance with his/her academic/professional judgment.[1]

THE HEARING PANEL

In cases that deal with students involved in cheating, a hearing panel will be formed according to the university's policies. Cheating is defined as academic dishonesty; plagiarism; unauthorized use of resources; falsifying, altering, or otherwise misrepresenting data or a signature; and obtaining or attempting to obtain or attempting to offer any unauthorized assistance in the performance of work or procedure for a course or other activity predicated upon or arising from student status in a particular professional program. The panel will consist of four faculty members and one student (not of the department in which the student is registered). The committee reviews the case, the charges made by the involved faculty member, and the documentation of evidence available. Serving at the dean's request, the committee makes its recommendation on what disciplinary action should be taken and submits its final report to the dean.

THE OMBUDSMAN

Within the structure of the university, there exists an official appointed (by the president) whose only function is to receive students' complaints and concerns involving abuses or "capricious acts" claimed to have been carried out by faculty, chairpersons, and staff members of the university. The ombudsman investigates these allegations in order to achieve a justifiable settlement. His/her office can investigate appeals and complaints and exercise independent judgment. Students may discuss with the ombudsman their concerns related to academic problems, problems related to admission, advising, degree requirements, discrimination, dishonesty, grades, harassment, records, registration and teaching; and on nonacademic problems relating to financial aid, housing, parking, payroll, tuition and fees.[1]

During orientation when the students receive their handbooks, the faculty make it a point to advise students as to the existence of the ombudsman and the location of his/her office. The ombudsman, after listening to the concerns of students, can offer advice to the students, perhaps facilitating communication between the student and the faculty member with whom the student is experiencing difficulty. Further, the ombudsman's office can investigate appeals and complaints. The office has no authority to change academic or administrative decisions, although it may be able to influence them.

THE FEDERAL LAW

Students may plead their case to the judicial system after the internal system within the university does not rule in their favor. In Lesser vs. Board of

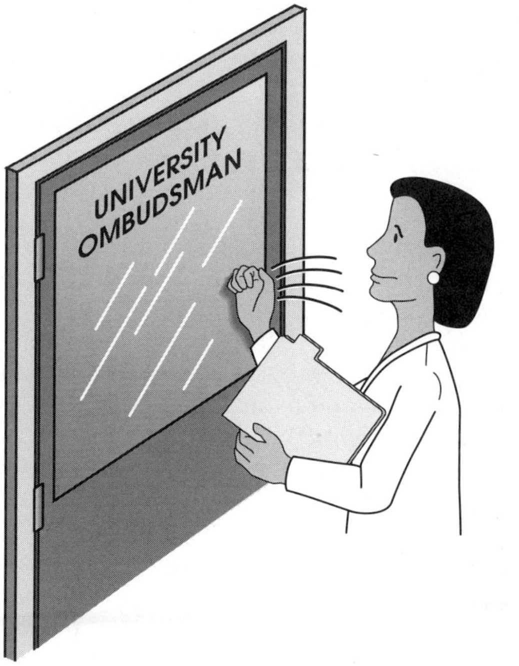

Education of N.Y. 18. A.D. 2d 388, 239 N.Y.S.2d 776 (1963), the student sued after being rejected based on the fact that his grade point was below the minimum. He argued that the college acted arbitrarily because it did not consider that he had been enrolled in a demanding high school honors program. The university ruling was *upheld.* The court stated that it should not intervene in situations relating to eligibility of applicants and determining standards.[3]

In another case, State ex rel Bartlett v Pantzer 158 Mont. 126, 489 P. 2d 375 (1971), the law school admission committee advised a student that he would be accepted if he completed a course. He received a "D" in this course. The law school claimed that a "D" was an acceptable but not satisfactory

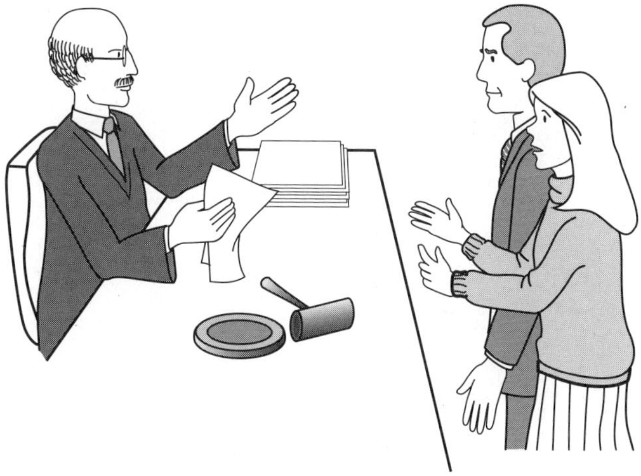

grade. He argued that the terms of a satisfactory grade were added after he had completed the course, and *the courts agreed.*[3]

THE BUCKLEY AMENDMENT (AMENDMENT TO THE FAMILY EDUCATIONAL RIGHTS AND PRIVACY ACT OF 1974)

This amendment was promulgated because of an abuse to a student's record. An instructor had written her opinion of a student in his record. She had labeled him "inadequate, retarded." Her impression was read by every teacher who thereafter consulted his record. Treatment of this student resulted in the student's parents' actions causing this amendment to be added.

The amendment provides protection for the right of privacy of parents, students, and guardians. The following is a right directed at the student as a result of the amendment: the right to amend educational records if he/she believes them to be inaccurate or misleading or to violate his/her privacy or other rights.[2]

As can be projected, the amendment has to clearly define the rights of the institution, the establishment of a hearing with the parties involved, and identification of the type of record included as "personally identifiable" that legally can be viewed by the student. As a result of the amendment, educational institutions must publish, at least annually, the following information[2]:

- The types of educational records and information contained that are directly related to the student and maintained by the institution
- The name and position of the official responsible for the maintenance of each type of record, the persons who have access to such records, and the purposes for which they have access
- The policies of the institution for reviewing and expunging of those records
- The procedures for a student to convene a hearing

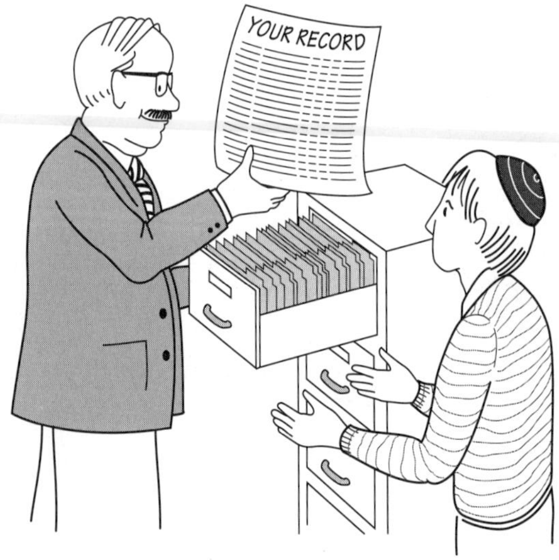

- The procedures for challenging the contents of specific educational records
- The cost, if any, that is to be charged to the student for producing copies
- The categories of information that the institution has designated as directory information
- Other rights and requirements set forth in the institution's policies.

Summary

This chapter emphasizes to both instructor and student that each has guaranteed rights, privileges, and obligations during the semester the student is enrolled in the instructor's class. If abuses take place by either party, policies exist to defend the one and discipline the other. The cases given touch on the more common types of infractions to existing policies.

The applicable law in its actual wording, together with its reference, has been quoted. This chapter stresses the importance of students and instructors becoming aware of policies, the rights of others, and the consequences they face when they abuse a law. Emphasis is placed on documenting all work, quizzes, exam papers, and course syllabi with specifics to guide students adequately through courses, dates, and so forth. The references given contain much explanation and background to the policies covered. Other policies regarding education and the law are explained.

Review Questions

1. What recourse do students have when they believe that one of their grades is not fair and should be changed?
2. Research this in the student handbook or your university bulletin and paraphrase the policy or procedure.
3. What do you consider to be "reasonable accommodations" that the university would have to provide for handicapped students?
4. Give at least four resources that the university provides for students to obtain legal assistance.
5. List at least three laws related to admission standards and the provisions of each.

See p. 408 for answers.

References

1. Wayne State University Undergraduate Bulletin 1993–1995.
2. Roller EL. Legal aspects of medical technology: education and clinical practice. American Journal Medical Technology 1982; 48(12):973–994.
3. Holter J. What Do I Do? ASCP Spring 1992 Teleconference Series: Legal Issues Involving Students. pp 1–16.
4. Davis BG. Writing letters for recommendation. *In* Tools for Teaching. San Francisco, Jossey-Bass Publishers, 1993, pp 407–412.
5. Udolf R. Interaction with students. *In* The College Instructor's Guide to Teaching in Academia. Chicago, Nelson-Hall, 1976, pp 25–36.
6. Davis BG. The first day of class. *In* Tools for Teaching. San Francisco, Jossey-Bass Publishers, 1993, pp 20–27.
7. McKeachie WJ. Ethical standards in teaching. *In* Welmer M, Neff RA, eds. Teaching College. Madison, Wisc, Magna Publications, 1990, pp 33–34.
8. Wayne State University, Clinical Laboratory Science Student Handbook. 1995.

Suggested Reading

1. Davis BG. Academic accommodations for students with disabilities. *In* Tools for Teaching. San Francisco, Jossey-Bass Publishers, 1993, pp 31–33.
2. Eble KE. Cheating, confrontations, and other situations. *In* The Craft of Teaching. 2nd ed. San Francisco, Jossey-Bass Publishers, 1990, pp 164–180.
3. Holter J. Legal issues involving students: "What Do I Do?" ASCP Spring Teleconference. Accompanying Handout for Subscribers. pp 1–16.
4. Lowman J. Evaluating student performance: testing and grading. *In* Mastering the Techniques of Teaching. San Francisco, Jossey-Bass Publishers, 1984, pp 184–209.
5. Roller EL. The law: legal aspects of medical technology: education and clinical practice. American Journal Medical Technology 1982; 48(12).
6. Strickland CG. Student's rights and the teacher's obligations in the classroom. *In* Weimer M, Neff RA, eds. Teaching College. Madison, Wisc, Magna Publications, 1990, pp 29–31.

10

Education in Clinical Laboratory Science: An Overview

OBJECTIVES

Upon completion of this chapter, the reader should be able to:

- Identify the contribution that the government, various associations, and agencies have made toward clinical laboratory education.
- Research articles from journals regarding the various professional associations.
- Describe the University-Based CLS Program and the role of Competency-Based Education in CLS.
- Define the term *goal.*
- Explain the relationship between "Competencies" and "Objectives."
- Recognize and identify the sequential steps of the Educational Process.

KEY WORDS

accreditation
certification
licensure
competency-based education

Introduction

All that you have experienced with the Educational Process was affected by myriad agencies and associations responding to the needs of health care at given times in history. Today's efforts remain consistent with those of the past: that is, to graduate competent laboratorians in the face of governmental regulations and policies that would threaten the quality of the educational program. It is important for all laboratorians to realize and know the contributions that each organization and agency has made to clinical laboratory education.

Allied Health Professions and CLS

AMERICAN SOCIETY OF ALLIED HEALTH PROFESSIONS (ASAHP): 1967

Whether you realized it or not, when you chose clinical laboratory science as your profession, you became a member of the Allied Health Professions (AHP),

ASSOCIATIONS AFFECTING CLINICAL LABORATORY SCIENCE EDUCATION

1928	ASCP	Professional and certifying association
1933	AMA	American Medical Association (established in 1847)
1933	ASCLS	Professional organization for CLS
1948	JCAHO	Accrediting agency for healthcare organizations
1967	Government	Allied Health Professions Personnel Training Act '67:CLIA '67
	CAHEA	Accrediting agency for allied health educational programs
	ASAHP	Professional support organization for all allied health professions
1973	NAACLS	Accrediting agency for CLS educational programs
1977	NCA	Certifying agency for CLS
1988	Government	CLIA '88
1992	Government	CLIAC
1994	CAAHEP	Replaces CAHEA as accrediting agency for allied health professions

Legend:
ASAHP = Association of Schools of Allied Health Professions
ASCP = American Society of Clinical Pathologists
ASCLS = American Society of Clinical Laboratory Science (previously American Society for Medical Technologists [ASMT])
CAHEA = Committee on Allied Health Education and Accreditation
CAAHEP = Commission on Accreditation of Allied Health Educational Programs
CLIA '67 = Clinical Laboratory Improvement Act
CLIA '88 = Clinical Laboratory Improvement Amendments
CLIAC = Clinical Laboratory Improvement Advisory Committee
JCAHO = Joint Commission on Accreditation for Healthcare Organizations
NAACLS = National Accrediting Agency for Clinical Laboratory Science
NCA = National Certifying Agency

a strong alliance of health-related professions that provide diagnostic and therapeutic assistance to members of the medical field in the treatment of their patients.

The Association of Schools of Allied Health Professions (ASAHP) was incorporated in 1967. It was known as the American Society of Health Professions in 1973, but with a change in its bylaws, it resumed its original title in 1991. The function of the Association was and remains the same: to provide interaction to academic institutions with established allied health educational programs and assist them in maintaining programs of excellence. It achieves its mission by providing leadership and representation for its members, fostering the development of new allied health programs, and publishing results from its involvement in educational research.

Today, ASAHP consists of members from universities, colleges, community colleges, professional associations, individual members, and other groups involved in some aspect of health care disciplines. ASAHP is not a regulatory organization, nor is membership mandatory. Individual membership numbers over 300, with various educational institutions and agencies close to 100. Its quarterly publication, *The Journal of Allied Health,* ranks with top journals in quality and formal presentation of subject. Articles dealing with interpretation and analysis of governmental regulations and their effect on allied health professions are often published in the journal. ASAHP's monthly publication, *Trends,* is a newsletter that provides notification of meetings, announcements of new members, governmental policies affecting AHP, accreditation, and so forth.

Relevance: The profession of Clinical Laboratory Science has been and continues its representation through membership in ASAHP.

Activity 1

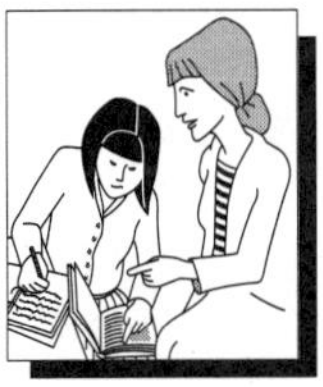

From the several Allied Health Journals provided, write a critique on several articles that relate to CLS.

The Government: 1967

In 1966, when demand for allied health professionals far exceeded the number of competent practitioners, the first act of Congress, through The Allied Health Professional Personnel Training Act of 1967, concentrated on upgrading the existing educational programs of allied health professions. It provided monies for clinical laboratory science to increase opportunities for training students entering the discipline. Focus was placed on the development of quality personnel. Students qualifying for other allied health professions were also supported. In addition, funds were directed toward the established training schools to enhance the quality of education.

This funding was administered by *grants* awarded to those institutions that implemented basic improvements of the curriculum together with the establishment of advanced clinical "traineeships."[1] In 1967, the Surgeon Gen-

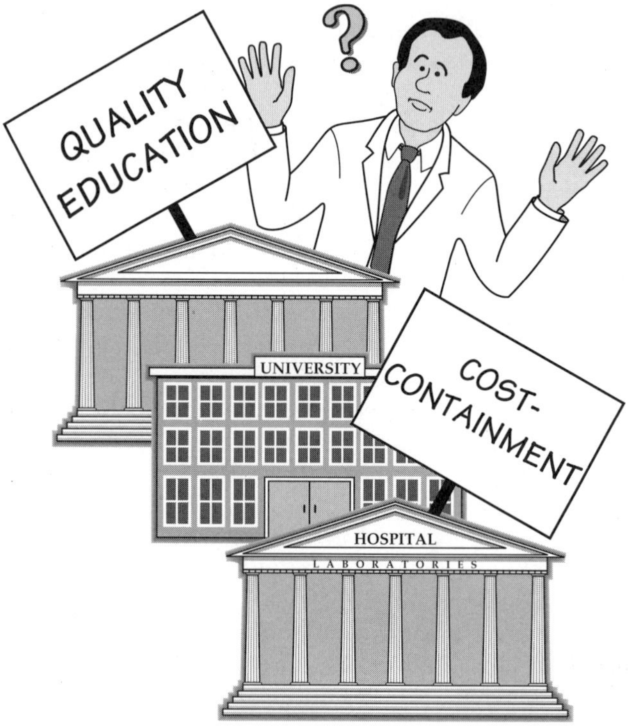

eral requested the Allied Health Professions Education subcommittee of the National Advisory Council to conduct the first comprehensive study on the allied health professions. The outcome of the study identified the need to increase the number of allied health educational programs. Also of significance was the designation of the university as the *primary site for all educational allied health programs.*"[1]

Relevance: The government, through the United States Department of Health and Human Services, continues to award grants to institutions submitting innovative programs dealing with such items as expansion, retention, curriculum, and new instructional models.

CLINICAL LABORATORY IMPROVEMENT ACT (CLIA) 1967

The passing of CLIA '67 not only implemented regulations dealing with laboratories engaged in interstate commerce but also defined *educational requirements* of laboratory personnel assuming "bench," supervisory, or managerial positions in the clinical laboratory. The law raised the standards and quality of the educational program, with the result of providing competent individuals for these positions.

1970s

During the late 1970s, the health workforce was estimated to be between 1.3 and 3 million. Consequently, the federal government turned its attention away from manpower production toward problems of maldistribution, coordination of resources, and cost containment. At the same time, allied health educators were coming to recognize the value of better planning for their educational programs and continued to assume leadership in this regard to avoid outside control by a governmental regulatory system.[1] The allied health professions continued to become stronger and independent as regards control by both the government and AMA.

1980s and 1990s

In 1988, the government introduced *CLIA '88* (Clinical Laboratory Improvement Amendments). CLIA '88 was the "birth child" of the government, a response to the media's coverage and reporting of misdiagnosed Pap smears and other inaccuracies in laboratory results. These incidences provided the government with two reasons to become involved in health care issues: to protect public health and welfare and to ensure the quality of services paid for by tax dollars.[2] The four main areas affected by CLIA's regulations were as follows:

- Test categories, performance standards, and laboratory certification
- Fees and applications
- Enforcement rules
- Accrediting bodies and state-exempt programs, effective for all sections.[3]

In 1992, a Clinical Laboratory Improved Advisory Committee (CLIAC) was established to advise and make recommendations on technical and scientific aspects of CLIA '88.[4] In 1994, CLS acquired representation on the committee. The recommendations made by the CLIAC subcommittee were approved by the full committee. The Department of Health and Human Services (DHHS) is to take that under advisement. Policies, acts, and amendments issued by the federal government supersede prior regulations established by professional agencies and associations.

THE AMERICAN MEDICAL ASSOCIATION, THE COMMITTEE ON ALLIED HEALTH EDUCATION AND ACCREDITATION, AND THE COMMISSION ON ACCREDITATION OF ALLIED HEALTH EDUCATIONAL PROGRAMS

The American Medical Association (AMA) has been involved in the formation and accreditation of the formal educational programs of all the professions since 1933. The AMA can be compared to a parent organization during the formative years of the various allied health professions. In 1966, the AMA established a Department of Allied Medical Professions and Services, out of which grew the Committee on Allied Health Education and Accreditation (CAHEA). CAHEA functioned in this capacity for three decades playing a major role in allied health accreditation.

In 1978, as new allied health professions were organized, CAHEA in collaboration with the AMA developed the *Essentials,* which dealt with the education of personnel together with initiating review procedures for various new emerging occupations. Eventually, the allied health professions made it known that they no longer needed to be controlled by AMA through CAHEA and that they desired to be accredited by an independent association. As a result, in the early 1990s, the AMA formed an advisory committee for the creation of a Commission on Accreditation of Allied Health Educational Programs (CAAHEP). CAAHEP emerged and was introduced in April 1994 as the new accreditation agency. CAHEA conducted its final meeting in May 1994 at which it transferred all records and similar materials to the new organization. The clinical laboratory science profession, with several other allied health professions, chose to be accredited by the National Accrediting Agency for Clinical Laboratories Sciences (NAACLS). Many of the AHPs continue to be accredited by CAAHEP.

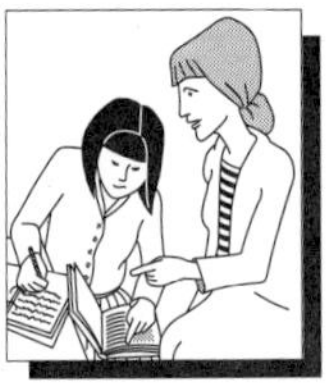

Activity 2

Referring to both professional journals—*Laboratory Medicine (Microscope in Washington)* and *Clinical Laboratory Science (Washington Beat)*—discuss with the members of your group what laws and/or policies the government has passed or is about to initiate that will affect the education of students enrolled in CLS programs. Summarize at least three that you agree are timely and important. Identify the nature of the involvement with CLS. Include your reference.

NATIONAL ACCREDITING AGENCY FOR CLINICAL LABORATORY SCIENCE

In 1973, the two professional organizations—American Society of Clinical Pathologists (ASCP) and American Society of Medical Technologists (ASMT), now American Society for Clinical Laboratory Sciences (ASCLS), which represent the clinical laboratory science profession—met to discuss the need to establish an independent agency with designated authority and control over program accreditation. The NAACLS was officially formed in 1973 and has been accepted by the CLS profession as its independent accrediting agency. So stated, each program must at least meet the minimum standards or exceed these standards in the quality of their educational program.

> Accreditation is a process of external peer review in which an agency grants public recognition to a program of study of an institution that meets established qualifications and educational standards.[5]

The accrediting process involves preparation of an extensive self-study in which the institution "examines itself." A team representing the accrediting agency visits the institution with the sole purpose of confirming adherence to the *Essentials.* Accreditation is then granted to those institutions fulfilling all requirements.

NAACLS has developed in its *Essentials,* the *Competencies,* which are broadly stated skills that must be mastered by all students enrolled in an accredited CLS program.

Relevance: Because NAACLS is an independent agency, CLS is no longer under the supervision of AMA.

Activity 3

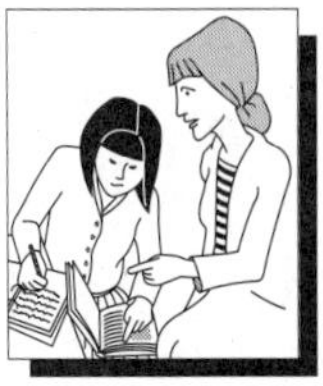

Ask the chairperson of the CLS department if you can borrow the "Self-Study." Examine the extensive documentation necessary to comply with NAACLS. Find the area dealing with student input. Summarize the impressions of your group of this work.

JOINT COMMISSION ON ACCREDITATION FOR HEALTHCARE ORGANIZATIONS (JCAHO)

JCAHO is a nongovernmental commission that was formalized in 1948 with authority of granting accreditation to hospitals that comply with its standards and regulations. Accreditation by JCAHO is not mandatory; however, hospitals comply with the standards in order to maintain quality care, to qualify for grants and Medicare reimbursements, and to gain status for their staff and educational programs.

Relevance: When hospitals are accredited, the *performance* of every allied health discipline is reviewed and included in the accreditation process.

Professional Organizations

AMERICAN SOCIETY OF CLINICAL LABORATORY SCIENCE (ASCLS), FORMERLY AMERICAN SOCIETY OF MEDICAL TECHNOLOGISTS

This professional organization, founded in 1933, is administered by clinical laboratory scientists *for* clinical laboratory scientists. The organization focuses on educational issues and those of a political nature affecting both quality of education and laboratory performance. Through its membership, it has won political alliance with many state legislatures, thus gaining representation on Capitol Hill.

The national organization has established 10 major regions consisting of clusters of states per region based on geographic proximity. There are also state organizations with further breakdown to districts representing a group of nearby cities. ASCLS is not a regulatory organization but states that its mission is as follows:

> . . . to promote the profession of clinical laboratory science and to provide beneficial services to those who practice it and to enable its members to provide quality service for all who practice it. To enable its members to provide quality service for all consumers, the society is committed to the continuous quest for excellence in all its activities.[6]

Relevance: ASCLS offers a reduced membership fee for students. It is important to become aware of the issues that both foster and threaten the high standards of the profession.

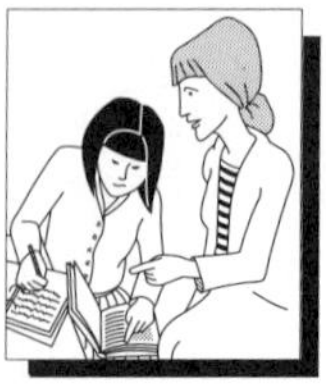

Activity 4

Have your group ask to view the ASCLS *Body of Knowledge* Manual. Summarize your impression of the contents.

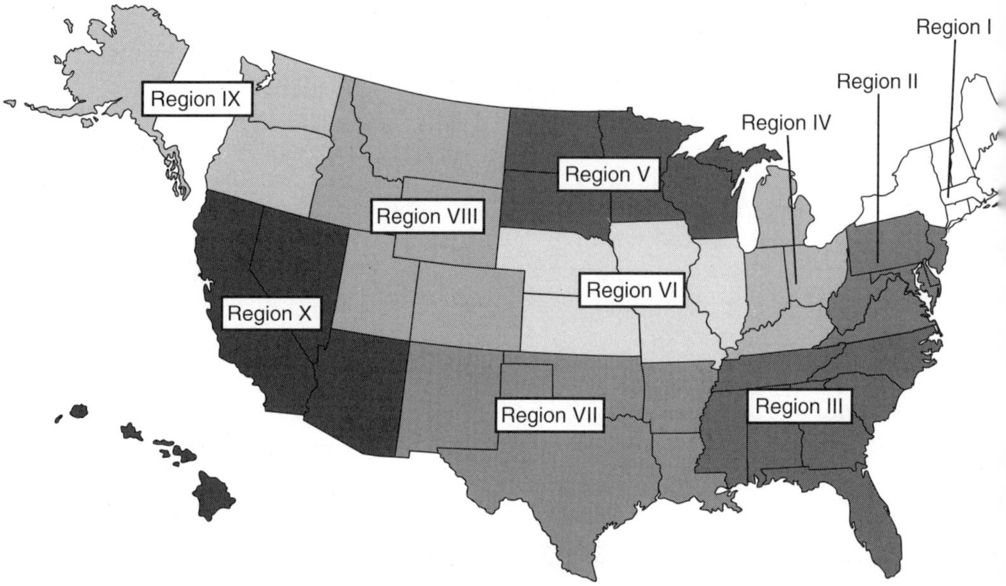

Region I	ME, VT, NH, MA, RI, NY, CT	**Region VI**	NE, IA, IL, KS, MO
Region II	PA, NJ, WV, VA, MD, DE, DC	**Region VII**	TX, OK, AR, LA, NM
Region III	TN, NC, SC, GA, AL, FL, MS, PR*	**Region VIII**	WY, MT, ID, UT, CO
Region IV	IN, OH, KY, MI	**Region IX**	AK, WA, OR
Region V	ND, SD, MN, WI	**Region X**	CA, NV, AZ, HI

* Puerto Rico not shown on map

Figure 10–1 Regions of ASCLS in the United States.

AMERICAN SOCIETY OF CLINICAL PATHOLOGISTS (ASCP)

Founded in 1928, ASCP is the oldest organization that is concerned with education and training of students, and through the administration of the registry examination it is the earliest known certifying agency in the country. The governance of ASCP consists of committees composed of pathologists and medical technologists whose concerns also deal with education, governmental policy-making involving laboratory issues, and certification of graduates from accredited programs.

It is one of two agencies that, through examination, certifies competent students graduating from an accredited educational program. The examination questions reflect Competencies established by its own organization.

Its format of examination is by computer, offered multiple times during the year at specific sites. Both ASCP and ASCLS have developed continuous educational programs offered throughout the year. Both organizations conduct annual conventions that feature experts on the various disciplines in the field of clinical laboratory science. Recent meetings have featured review sessions for students preparing to take the certifying examination.

Relevance: ASCP has been involved in providing quality education for CLS since its inception, either by providing the structure for the course work in the curriculum or in developing registry certification examinations.

NATIONAL CERTIFICATION AGENCY (NCA)

NCA was established in 1977 as an independent, nonprofit certifying agency. It administered its first certification exam in 1978 and continues to do so semiannually. It is also the first agency that established a national recertification program for practicing CL scientists either by re-examination or participation in acceptable educational activities and programs. Students should not be discriminated against by the potential employer in regard to the agency that granted their certification.

Relevance: NCA grants graduates of CLS accredited programs certification after successfully passing their examination confirming their competency.

LICENSURE

For clarification, licensure is a permit granted by a government body (California and New York issue licenses for laboratory personnel) to competent practicing laboratory scientists, which allows them to seek employment in that specific state. These states will issue a State Licensure Examination to both competent graduates of accredited programs living in state and out of state. Graduates who have not passed the examination cannot be hired into the laboratory system of that state. California now requires documentation of continuing education for those seeking annual renewal of their license.

Relevance: The various state professions through their state legal system established licensure to ensure quality of practice in their laboratory system.

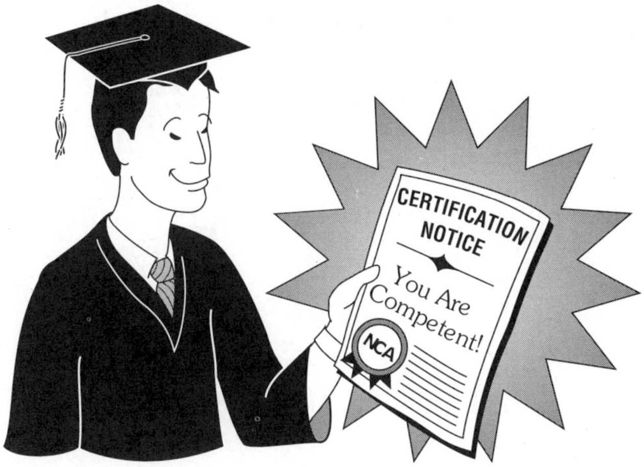

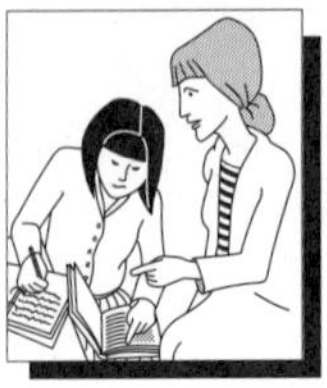

Activity 5

Do a search through the various professional laboratory journals and list those states that have licensure policies.

Activity 6

Compare several issues of *Laboratory Medicine* (ASCP) with *Clinical Laboratory Science* (ASCLS) as to their presentation of governmental issues that involve laboratory (both education and practice) concerns, continuing education, featured technical articles, and description of new procedures. As a student, how do these two journals relate to you? Summarize your findings.

REVIEW! ARE YOU CONFUSED? What should you remember regarding your CLS agencies? Let's see if this helps!

For Clinical Laboratory Science Programs

1. NAACLS	Accreditation of the educational program
2. JCAHO	Accreditation of the hospital performance
3. ASCP Board of Registry	Certification of qualified individuals

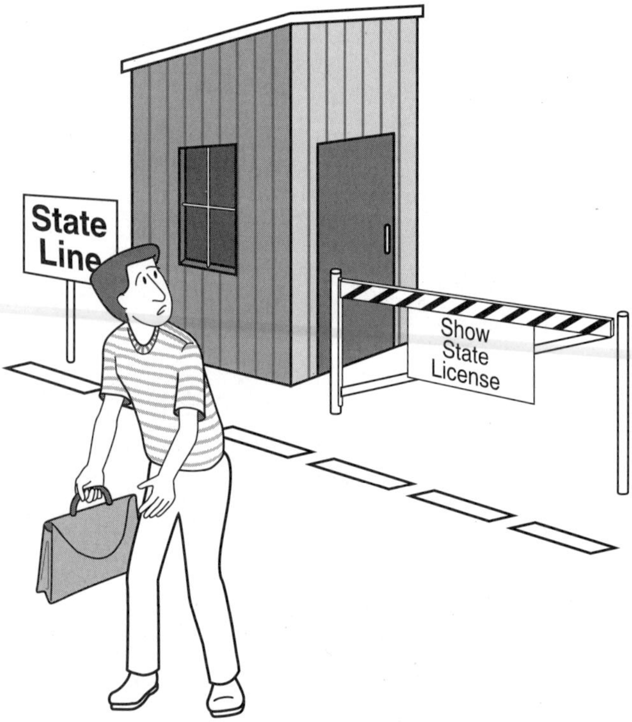

4. NCA Certification of individual students
5. ASCLS Professional program for CLS

Laboratorians may hold single or multiple certifications through ASCP, NCA, and other agencies.

Competency-Based Education (CBE)

DESCRIPTION

Historically, the educational system used in training potential clinical laboratory scientists has based its instruction on producing competent graduates. Before the title "Competency-Based Education" became popular, it was already being used in clinical laboratory training programs.

Educationally, CBE relates to certification granted by an external organization that recognizes students who have fulfilled all the requirements necessary to practice in the field and have achieved this by having been graduated from an accredited program and passed the certification examination.

Certification relates to *competency.* Practically, it describes an individual who has developed the ability to combine the realms of cognitive learning with the mastery of technical skills in generating accurate and reliable results in performing laboratory procedures (see Chapter 3.)

THE BASIS OF THE CLINICAL LABORATORY SCIENCE PROGRAM: THE COMPETENCIES

Within the *Guide to Accreditation,* published by NAACLS, is a description of the profession that lists competencies, constituting the required knowledge and skill every student enrolled in CLS programs must master. The competencies by nature are stated in broad terms; however, each competency designates a specific task. You observed in Chapter 3 that the competencies must be stated in such a way that students are given clear directions regarding the purpose of the procedure, the equipment, the reagents to be used, and the formula used for calculating the final red blood cell count.

The competencies are expressed in the Essentials and Guidelines of Accredited Educational Programs at the Baccalaureate Medical Technology Level (see Table 10–1). A recent graduate, when newly employed by a clinical laboratory, is required to demonstrate entry-level skills.

INSTRUCTION IN A COMPETENCY-BASED EDUCATIONAL PROGRAM

Establishing such a program involves many players and a highly organized flow system of successful instruction with one primary goal: to graduate competent students. An overview of the process is given in Figure 10–2.

GOALS

Goals, by definition, are ends toward which effort is directed. They are exterior to and exist outside the program. The long-range goal of the university (via

Table 10–1
COMPETENCY TO STATED OBJECTIVE

Competencies[7]	Stated Measurable Objectives
The students will be able to do the following: • Correctly perform a manual WBC count using the Unopette system • Establish procedures for collecting and processing biologic specimens for analysis • Perform analytic tests on body fluids, "cells," and products • Integrate and relate data generated by the various clinical laboratory departments while making judgments regarding possible discrepancies; confirm abnormal results; verify quality control procedures; and develop solutions to problems concerning the generation of laboratory data • Make judgments concerning results of quality control measures and institute proper procedure to maintain accuracy and precision • Establish and perform preventive and corrective maintenance of equipment and instruments as well as identify appropriate sources for repairs • Evaluate new techniques, instruments, and procedures in terms of their usefulness and practicality within the context of a given laboratory's personnel, equipment, space, and budgetary resources • Demonstrate professional conduct and interpersonal communication skills with patients, laboratory personnel, and other health care professionals and with the public • Recognize and act upon individual needs for continuing education as a function of growth and maintenance of professional competence • Lead supportive personnel and peers in their acquisition of knowledge, skills, and attitudes • Apply principles of management and supervision • Apply principles of educational methodology	The students will be able to do the following: • Correctly perform a manual WBC count by diluting the whole blood accurately using the specific vial and pipette, counting the WBCs in the designated area on the hemacytometer, and accurately calculating the final WBC $\times 10^9$/L within 10 min

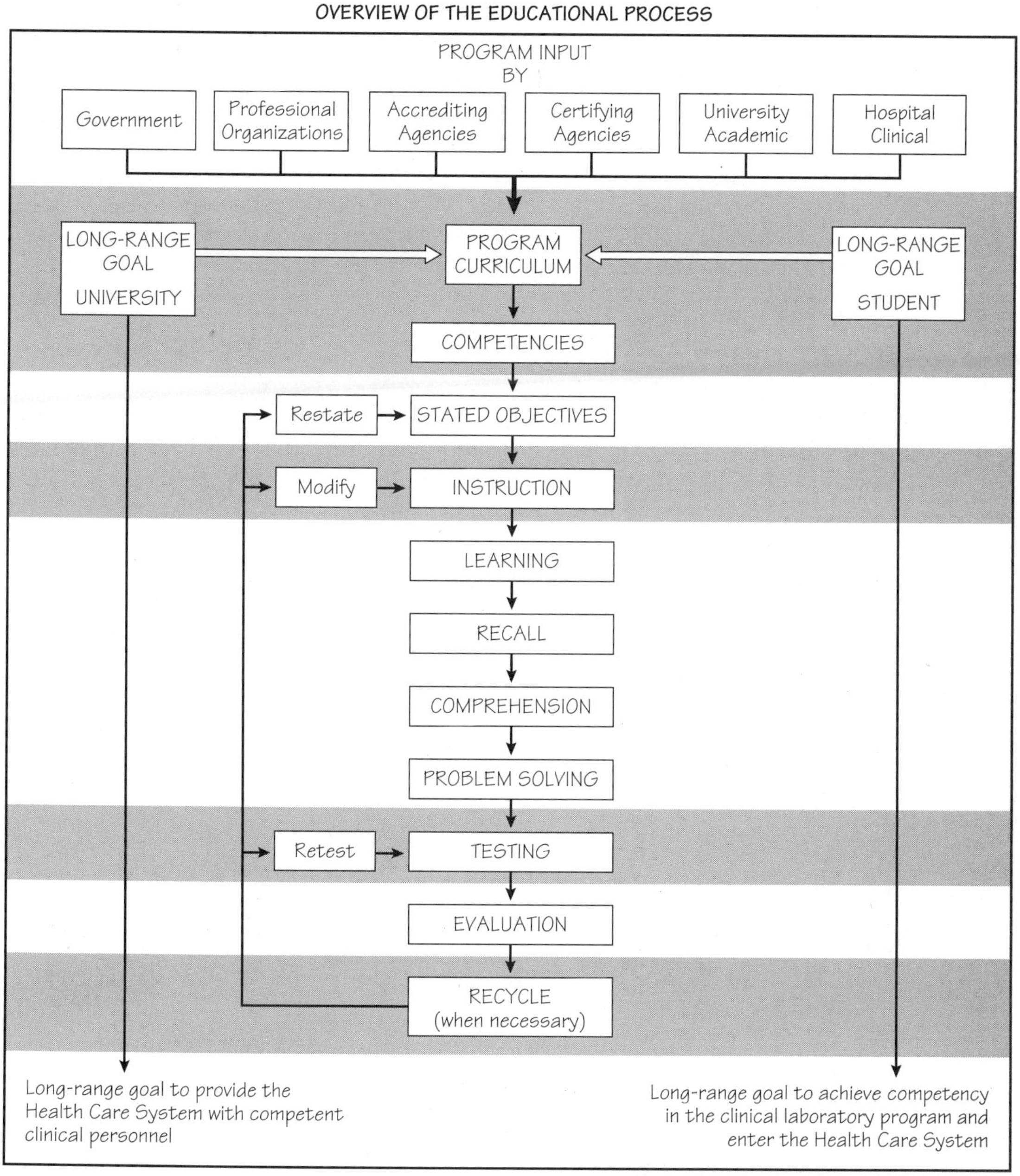

Figure 10–2 Overview of the Educational Process.

the CLS Department) is to provide the health care system with competent clinical laboratory scientists. The long-range goal of a student would be to graduate successfully from an accredited program in order to be hired into the health care system. Both reflect involvement in a multiyear time frame. Attaining this goal involves sustained effort and consistent performance in completing the curriculum.

Behavioral objectives (instructional for the teacher and measurable, observable, and behavioral for the student) translate the not-so-specific competencies into specific clear tasks and skills that must be measured. Criteria regarding amount of time in which the task must be performed, the degree of accuracy, and the conditions under which the task is to be performed are all specified. These objectives are found in the course syllabus of every lecture and laboratory session (see Chapter 3). The mode of instruction and testing are many and variable and have been discussed in previous chapters as well the process of evaluation.

Summary

Today, the curriculum of CLS programs throughout the nation bears the quality of education that reflects concerned input from the institutions that have contributed to its development. CLS and other allied health programs are now independently accredited by the organizations of their choice. The federal

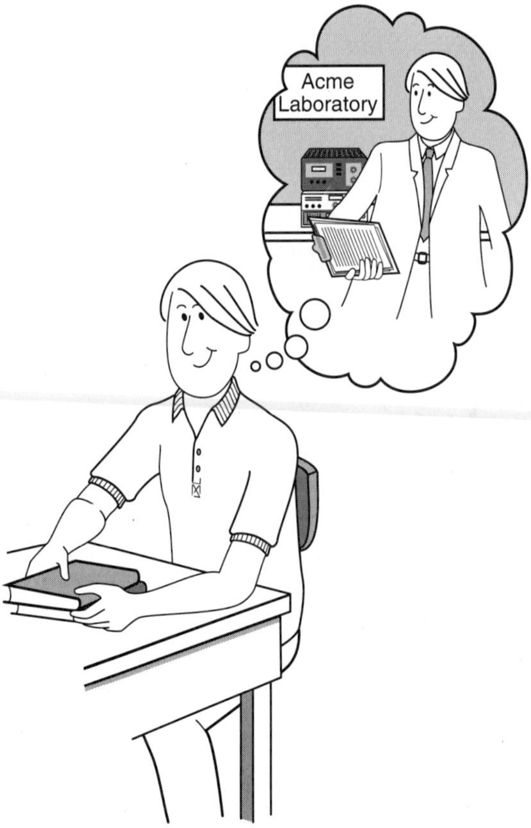

government continues to regulate various aspects of the laboratory. Its focus at present is on cost containment that involves targeting procedures by complexity and difficulty of performance. This allows lesser-trained laboratory personnel to perform less difficult procedures.

Students entering CLS today will participate in a competency-based educational process that will enable them to develop necessary skills and process necessary information to graduate as competent clinical scientists.

Review Questions

Encircle the letter that precedes your answer of choice for Multiple Choice, True/False. Write in Short Answers for the incomplete statements on the space provided.

1. The organization that grants accreditation to the hospital health-care services is
   a. ASCLS.
   b. NCA.
   c. NAACLS.
   d. ASCP.
   e. JCAHO.

2. A student who has finished the Academic and Hospital Programs will take an examination and become certified by ____________________ .

3. True/False: ASAHP is both a regulatory and educational organization for the allied health professions.

4. True/False: The government has precedence over any professional organization or agency dealing with the education of laboratory personnel and the practice of laboratory medicine.

See p. 408 for answers.

References

1. National Commission on Allied Health Education: The future of allied health education. *In* The Allied Health Concept in the Next Decade: New Meanings and Challenges. San Francisco, Jossey-Bass Publishers, 1980, pp 1–16.
2. Karni KR, Viskochie KR, Amos PA. Clinical Laboratory Management. A Guide for Clinical Laboratory Scientists. Boston, Little, Brown and Co, 1982, p 497.
3. Gore MJ. CLIA'S impact on the practice of clinical laboratory science. Clinical Laboratory Science 1992; 5(5):264–271.
4. ASCLS Today. 1994; 8(6):1–3.
5. LeGrys VA, Beck SJ. Clinical Laboratory Education. San Mateo, Calif, Appleton and Lange, 1988, pp 9–32.
6. American Society of Clinical Laboratory Sciences. Body of Knowledge: Content and Delineation of Tasks. ASCLS, Bethesda, 1981.
7. Guide to Accreditation of the National Accreditation Agency for Clinical Laboratory Science. Chicago, NAACLS, 1992.

Suggested Reading

1. Bucher WF, Brown JA. The impact of health care reform on the clinical laboratory. Medical Laboratory Observer 1994; Mar:30–36.
2. Clerc JM. An Introduction to Clinical Laboratory Science. St. Louis, Mosby-Year Book, 1992.
3. Fiorilla BJ, Maturen AJ. Statements of competency for practitioners. Clinical Laboratory Science 1981; 47(8):647–652.
4. Gore MJ. Health care reform: how it may reform clinical laboratories. The Washington Beat. Clinical Laboratory Science 1994; 7(2):72–77.
5. Green TF. Acquisition of purpose. *In* Chickering AWE, et al., eds. The Modern American College. San Francisco, Jossey-Bass Publishers, 1988, 543–555.
6. Heyman J. Microscope on Washington. Dramatic strides alleviate personnel shortages. ASCP Washington Office. Laboratory Medicine 1994; 25(6):359–360.
7. John M. CLIA '88 after year 1: no help to patients and a hindrance to labs. Medical Laboratory Observer 1994:20–26.
8. LeGrys VA, Beck SJ. Clinical Laboratory Education. San Mateo, Calif, Appleton and Lange, 1988.
9. Maclearn BL. Technical curriculum models: are they appropriate for the nursing profession. Journal of Advanced Nursing 1992; 17(7):871–876.
10. NAACLS Guide to Accreditation. Chicago, National Accrediting Agency for Clinical Laboratory Science Agency for Clinical Laboratories, Feb. 1992.
11. National Commission on Allied Health Education. The Future of Allied Health Education. San Francisco, Jossey-Bass Publishers, 1980.
12. O'Grady T, O'Brien A. A guide to competency-based orientation: develop your own program. Journal of Nursing Staff Development 1992; 8(3):128–133.
13. Saunders RL, Saunders DS. Consequences for teaching: student services and administration. *In* Chickering AW, et al., eds. The Modern American College. San Francisco, Jossey-Bass Publishers, 1988, 500–511.
14. Seibert ML. Establishing criteria for competency-based education. American Journal of Medical Technology 1979; 45(5): 368–371.
15. Washington Beat: ASMT awaits final verdict on CLIA '88. Clinical Laboratory Science 1992; 5(3):132–136.
16. Washington Beat. State licensure under attack in Florida and California. Clinical Laboratory Science 1994; 7(3).
17. Williams AL, Heath C. Reform and rationing: process lessons from the states. Clinical Laboratory Science 1994; 7(3): 136–140.

Management

Management, as both theory and practice, belongs in all businesses and activities regardless of their purpose. In laboratory science, pathology, and health care, the need for dynamic management strategies and applications has increased due to customer and legislative demands. Enhanced effectiveness and efficiencies are needed to control costs, improve quality, and streamline activities.

Laboratorians in training will find the management knowledge and skills they learn in their collegiate and clinical courses to be valuable when they begin their careers in laboratory settings. Some laboratorians currently working seek opportunities to learn more about management on their own and arrange activities for their own education. Additionally, the attitudes, attributes, traits, and effective behaviors laboratorians develop as professionals will place them in great demand as employees and prospective supervisors.

Various management functions—planning, organizing, directing, controlling, coordinating, and evaluating, plus financial and regulatory involvement—constitute many of the day-to-day responsibilities of supervisors and managers. With basic competence in these functions, laboratorians will be able to meet the challenges which all health care givers face.

11

An Overview: The Management Process and Managers

OBJECTIVES

Upon completion of this chapter, the reader should be able to:

- Explain one management concept in terms of its application to a laboratory environment and laboratory medicine.
- Briefly describe three management functions and relate each to a managerial role.
- Assess one's own leadership abilities according to the qualities presented.
- Discuss select situations and describe appropriate effective versus ineffective managing styles/behaviors.
- Describe personal traits that would enable new managers or supervisors to successfully undertake their responsibilities.
- Outline a self-training program to acquire knowledge of management concepts, develop leadership skills, augment one's own prevailing attitude, and distinguish effective attributes from ineffective ones.

KEY WORDS

management process
management functions
managing and leading styles
management responsibilities

Introduction

Health care has become competitive, and an organization must offer better services (or be perceived to offer better services) in order to attract and retain customers. Consumers of health care—patients, their families, physicians, and other health care givers—seek quality service and products for their diagnoses, therapies, and cures. Hospitals, health care organizations, and laboratories rely on personnel with expertise, knowledge, and skills to provide the quality that customers expect and demand. Health care administrations must ensure the smooth, effective flow of superior services to accomplish this goal. Managers and supervisors with education and experience will facilitate successful operations that support delivery of quality services.

These chapters will introduce laboratory science learners to the basic facets of management as a process and its functions, including supervision and leadership. The art and science of management span vast and complex disciplines; only the foundations of selected topics are presented here with the advice that aspiring managers and supervisors extend their education and experience. Career entry-level laboratorians who learn fundamental elements of management will better understand their roles as employees in health care and can perform their work for employers and customers more effectively.

Traditionally, laboratories existed in health care facilities and were managed according to consistent structures. Responsibilities were well defined, and authority was reflected through an established chain of command. Review the traditional organizational chart presented in Figure 11–1. In later chapters, innovative realignment and, occasionally, removal of authority lines are discussed. Becoming a manager may not be what you aspire to at this time, but people with strong science and medical education and interests in clinical and research laboratory work often find themselves supervising employees and managing laboratories.

The Management Process

Similar to the educational process, the management process is structured with sequential steps of logical thought and planned activities that culminate in achieving established goals. Key steps to the management process comprise several functions: planning, organizing, directing, controlling, coordinating, and evaluating. Each function supports the next and is intertwined from beginning to end. Regardless of the management level or position—chief executive officer (CEO) or assistant supervisor/team leader—responsibilities, in the simplest of terms, begin with determining the organization's goals, which are usually broad but reflect the organization's mission and values. Subsequently, specific and attainable departmental objectives are developed and communicated to all members. Next, methods are selected to accomplish the designated objectives. Finally, evaluation of the process and outcomes tie the operation together. The meld of activities contributes to the overall success of the organization's endeavors.

HISTORICAL PERSPECTIVE

The popularity of management today stems from emerging technologic, social, and cultural needs. Not unlike ancient times, products and services that serve

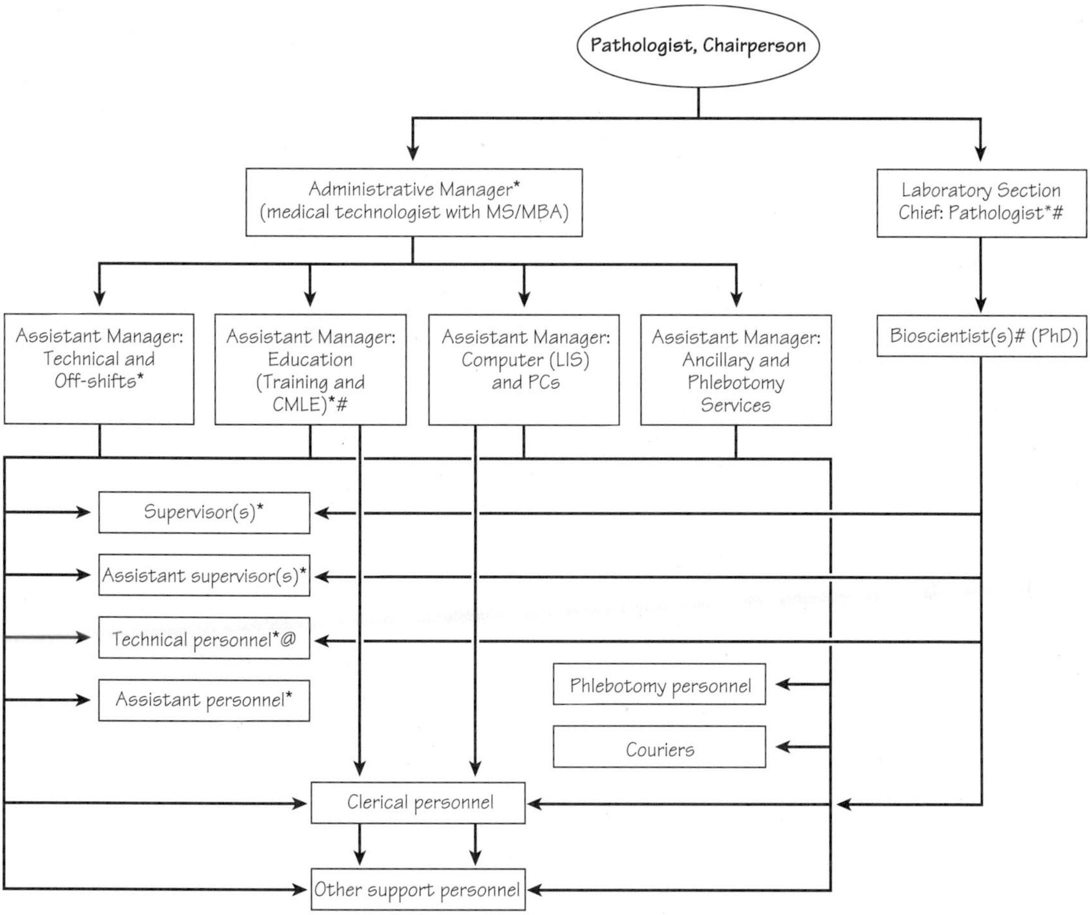

* Laboratory Sections: Chemistry, Hematology, Coagulation, Urinalysis/Body Fluids, Transfusion Medicine/Blood Bank, Microbiology, Immunology: others might be Molecular Pathology, Flow or Analytical Cytometry, Virology, or Anatomic Pathology-Histology, Cytology, Cytogenetics, and Electron Microscopy.

@ Technologists, technicians, plus other personnel, such as medical assistants, physicians, nurses, respiratory therapists, cardiovascular technologists, trained and certified or licensed to perform laboratory tests.

Additional areas of responsibility might include pathology residency, technologist, technician, and phlebotomy educational training programs.

Figure 11–1 Organization chart: Traditional large hospital laboratory.

a purpose—make life better and work easier, entertain, and save lives—are demanded. Peter Drucker's opinion is that "the best managers in history were those responsible for building the pyramids of Egypt."[1] They knew management but unfortunately didn't share their information. Throughout the history of the world, evidence exists that management was practiced. For example, in the early 1400s, the Arsenal of Venice, Italy, built ships and produced armaments with over 1000 workers. Accounting systems, planning, assembly-line techniques, interchangeable parts, inventory controls, and a formal system of personnel management were used.

Modern management evolved during the Industrial Revolution of the mid-eighteenth century in association with the factories in Great Britain. One hundred years later, the New World (North America) used steam power to fuel the demand for transportation and products as people moved west. This

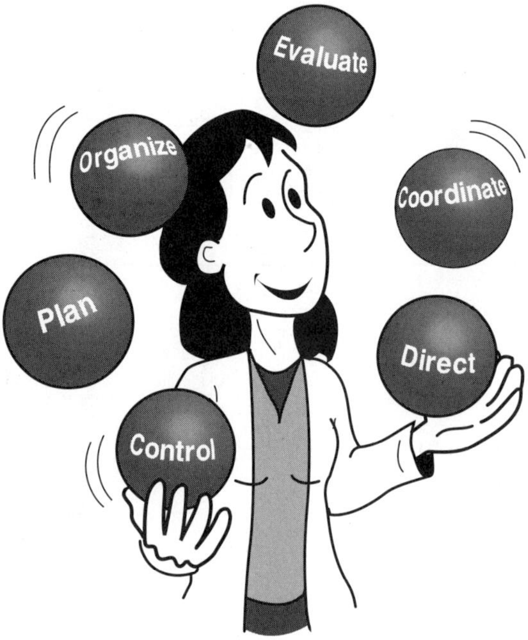

nation grew and prospered because of practical and hands-on systems requiring little theory or principles. Then, in 1881, college business courses were established at the University of Pennsylvania in Philadelphia by Joseph Wharton. Literature since late 1880s has marked the rapid development of management as a science, developing as engineering did.[2]

MANAGERIAL CONCEPTS

Profits, customer satisfaction (which includes employees), image and reputation, recognition, sense of fulfillment, and competition are all factors that drive managers to read, study, and change work processes. As a practical art, "*management* is the coordination of human and nonhuman resources toward the accomplishment of organizational goals."[3] How this coordination is accomplished by managers depends on their beliefs, knowledge, and style of managing. Drucker states: "Every achievement of management is the achievement of a manager. Every failure is the failure of the manager. People manage, rather than forces or facts."[4]

Scientific Management

Classic theories describe applications of the scientific method to management activities beginning in the early 1900s as manufacturing escalated and became highly specialized. Frederick Winslow Taylor, a mechanical engineer, advocated scientific principles to determine empirically, quantitatively, and qualitatively how to perform job tasks in order to improve efficiency instead of relying solely on common sense and intuition.[5] Taylor emphasized the specifics of jobs (tasks) along with development of individuals (behavior and relationships) for the greatest efficiency and productivity. Scientific management provided control over work with regulation of quantity and quality through analysis, prediction, and setting standards. Deviations from standards could be identified and corrected resulting in maximum efficiency. The logic of *efficiency* remains a key element in managerial behavior today, with many strategies refined and modified over several decades. (This is not likely to change as managers seek the perfect managing method.)

Management by Objectives

Early proponents of goal setting were Drucker[6] and Odiorne,[7] who espoused motivating employees to work harder and consequently improve their performance through mutual understanding of objectives. Objectives reflect goals set by an organization; thus, objectives can be used to measure the success of the organization and assess the contribution of each worker.

Management by objectives (MBO) is considered a proactive rather than a reactive style of managing, as goal setting (and writing specific objectives) occurs during planning but before operational implementation. The MBO process communicates to and requires involvement of employees. They want to know what they are to do and then how well they did it (their performance). Using objectives—that is, specific criteria or standards—as the measure or yardstick with which to compare their results becomes less biased than using arbitrary standards. Self-assessment can be accomplished before formal supervisor evaluation takes place. When employees know that they meet or exceed objectives, they feel good about their accomplishments. More importantly, they want their efforts and work to be recognized in terms of money, job challenges, praise, opportunities for growth, and awards.

Organizations apply MBO in various ways: to define employee jobs, to motivate employees, or to check work (performance) and modify it when necessary. After evaluations are complete, employees can be recognized for their contributions with monetary rewards, career development, and employee advancement. For maximal effectiveness, objectives must be clear, specific, attainable (although not necessarily easy), and agreed upon or accepted by employees. Other important aspects of successful MBO managing are as follows: (1) it encompasses everyone from top-to-bottom, (2) it requires commitment and involvement, (3) it is integrated into everyday operations and throughout all levels of activity, and (4) it is supported by sufficient resources for training personnel. A reasonable time frame for achieving objectives is usually 1½ to 2 years for concrete results to be observed, with the flexibility to alter programs when necessary.

Quality Management

Known by various titles such as quality improvement process (QIP), continuous quality improvement (CQI), and total quality management (TQM), quality systems advocate that employees are not the problem but should be recognized as part of the solution. Deming wrote that the job of management is not supervision, but leadership.[8] The decision to produce quality is a policy decision and involves more than just the worker doing quality work. Recognized founding fathers of quality management include W. Edwards Deming, Philip B. Crosby, Joseph M. Juran, Armand V. Feigenbaum, and Walter A. Shewhart. See Suggested Readings for more information.

Four consistent components surface in most prevalent quality programs, regardless of the author or the corporation: (1) statistical analysis, (2) training and education, (3) intervention, and (4) evaluation. Crucial to any improve-

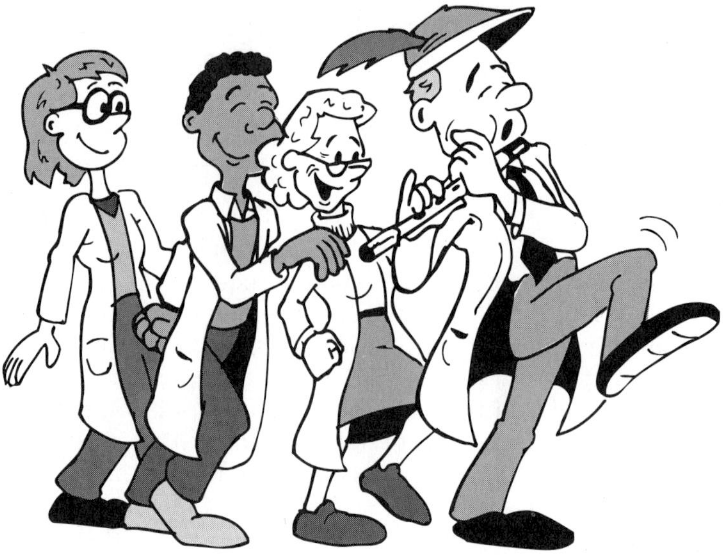

ment process is understanding (supported by statistics and facts and involvement of employees) the situation and the problems, developing solutions, and monitoring implementation to assess change (improvement). Technology, which is rapidly advancing with computers and information systems, communications, and data-base acquisition, will provide greater access to quantitative analysis of services allowing more scrutiny of data.

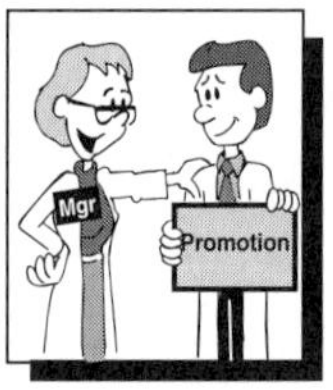

Activity 1: Quality Management Components

For this Activity, select one laboratory section: Chemistry, Hematology, Blood Bank, Microbiology, Immunology, Coagulation, or Body Fluids. Discuss the four common components of a quality management program that could be applied to improving operations in this laboratory section.

1. What does statistical analysis imply to you? What types of data are important to collect and study? Consider sources of data, amount of data that would be needed, and collection times.
2. What training and education should be developed for this laboratory section's employees regarding nontechnical issues and skills?
3. Think about intervention: that is, the applications or steps that might be necessary in this laboratory section to improve the work, environment, or processes.
4. Consider evaluation of steps, results (product), and quality management program as a whole.

See Activity Discussion 1 at the end of this chapter.

Note that a quality system works when everyone is involved and the commitment emanates from the highest person in the organization throughout all levels of personnel. Quality improvement activities can happen within a laboratory section or with a group of people who want to monitor and change their work for the better (quality improvement) and dedicate themselves to the quality philosophy. The maxim of quality is "You cannot manage what you cannot measure," according to Patrick Galvin, vice-president of corporate systems development, Federal Express.[9]

Activity 2: Management Concepts

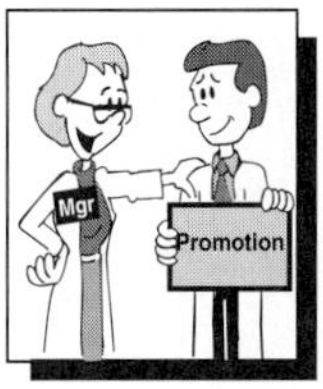

Select one management concept for this discussion. Write two to four objectives that you think appropriate for the operations of a hospital-based laboratory. Describe why you think the management concept you selected would best achieve the objectives.

Managerial Functions

Management functions identify what managers do: managing the "something" or operations to be done, the "somebodies" who perform the technical work, the "somehows" of the work getting done, and the "someplaces" where it occurs.

Six management functions represent the range of activities for most managers. Basic principles of each are presented individually in the following chapters but are intertwined to a great extent in application. These six functions incorporate myriad skills that support and enable managers or supervisors to do their work. In the clinical laboratory, technical skill competence, acquired through formal education and training, are essential for testing personnel. The ability to transfer concepts (abstract thinking) associated with technical skills enables new supervisors to succeed.

Planning requires conceptual or thinking skills. The planning function considers plan formats, essential components of a good plan, and implementation processes to be most effective. Planning, described in Chapter 12, addresses the primary skill of how one goes about accomplishing tasks. This section covers most of the 40% non–human-oriented supervisory work. The focus on people includes suggestions for team planning from authors who advocate quality systems.

The *organizing* function (see Chapter 13) covers interpersonal skill development definitions, categories, and explanations to prepare managers to better deal with people. The importance of developing oneself as well as employees as effective managers ranks high.

Directing, presented in Chapter 14, explains and reveals the ins and outs of four supervisor skills: communicating, motivating, delegating, and coaching. Theories of motivation consider reinforcement of behavior and needs of the individual. Getting to know employees reporting to you becomes an asset in determining what their needs are and what talents they may have.

Decision making and *problem solving* are considered as separate topics in Chapter 15: Controlling. Laboratorians acquire and develop good problem-solving skills performing analytical procedures. Some people demonstrate an aptitude for mechanics and work well with troublesome instruments; others have visual aptitudes and display expertise resolving cell morphology abnormalities identification. People with such strong technical skills can capably transfer their problem-solving conceptual abilities to supervision. Decision making spans most of the management functions, if not all. Sorting through information constitutes a professional and personal never-ending process to reach action or conclusion.

Coordinating (see Chapter 16), *evaluating* (see Chapter 19), and *complying with (external) rules and regulations* (see Chapter 17) relate to long-term programs requiring committees, task forces, employee involvement, and applying strategies to achieve objectives.

Financial acumen—the ability to find ways of saving money, increasing income, and better spending of money—has taken on a very high priority for health care administrators and managers (see Chapter 18). Competition and regulations drive managers to seek quick cost controls, and, occasionally, they forfeit quality because of these short-term fixes. Methods that are statistically founded and involve the organization as a whole have been reported to be much more productive. Employees frequently assist in seeking ways of identifying costs that can easily be controlled.

These functions keep most managers quite busy. Handling multiple tasks simultaneously requires a good calendar, reminder notes, vision, and help from well-trained, competent employees.

Managerial Roles

Managers and supervisors fill the mid-level tier of authority in traditional operations. Two federal acts describing supervisor work are shown in the boxed areas. Managers ensure that the right job gets done and supervisors make sure the job gets done right. Historically, managers learned their jobs as they worked: being told by owners, learning from the "elders," and "trial and error."

Knowing managerial roles and methods, plus personally developing managing skills along with identifying resources, become extremely beneficial for managers and supervisors in fulfilling their obligations. Examples of valuable skills for both managers and supervisors are identified in the third boxed area. Abilities such as efficiency and effectiveness in performing tasks rank equally high. Learning about theories, successes and failures of others, standards, and processes takes place through reading (primarily), listening to others, and personal experience (trial and error).

One role assumed by managers is that of agents or representatives of the organization, its owners and (higher) authorities (board of directors or

NATIONAL LABOR RELATIONS ACT

The National Labor Relations Act, Section 2(11) states:

The term *supervisor* means any individual having authority in the interests of the employer to hire, transfer, suspend, lay off, recall, promote, discharge, assign, reward or discipline other employees, or responsibility to direct them or to adjust their grievances or effectively to recommend such action if in connection with the foregoing, the exercise of such authority is not of a merely routine or clerical nature, but requires the use of independent judgment.

FAIR LABOR STANDARDS ACT

The Fair Labor Standards Act defines a supervisor as any employee "employed in a bona fide administrative capacity":

a. Whose primary duty consists of either:
   1. The performance of office or nonmanual work directly related to management policies or general business operations of his employer or his employer's customers or . . . and

b. Who customarily and regularly exercises discretion and independent judgment, and

c. 1. Who regularly and directly assists a proprietor of an employee employed in a bona fide executive or administrative capacity, or
   2. Who performs under only general supervision work along specialized or technical lines requiring special training, experience or knowledge or
   3. Who executes under only general supervision special assignments and tasks, and

d. Who does not devote more than 20%, or in the case of an employee of a retail or service establishment who does not devote as much as 40%, of his hours worked in the work week to activities which are not directly and closely related to the performance of the work described in paragraphs (a) through (c) above.

administrators). Selection as the representative—that is, appointment to the position—reflects that a manager has the abilities, knowledge, skill, and interest to perform managerial functions and duties. A manager is charged with responsibility and authority to implement strategies that will achieve the mission and goals of the organization.

Another role that managers fulfill relates to providing resources that enable employees to do their jobs. As primary resource persons, managers communicate to, with, and from employees (to administrators and owners); they provide materials, supplies, and finances; they nurture, advise, and admonish as needed.

MANAGING

For mutual understanding, in this book the term *manager* refers to the description of what a person does rather than the title a person is given. Traditionally,

SUPERVISOR SKILLS: ESSENTIAL COMPETENCIES FOR EFFECTIVE SUPERVISION

1. Accomplish tasks: planning
2. Accomplish tasks: time management
3. Interpersonal skills with customers: patients and physicians
4. Interpersonal skills with employees, coworkers, and superiors
5. Communicate
6. Motivate
7. Delegate
8. Make decisions
9. Solve problems

technologists and technicians have advanced up a career ladder from technical jobs to supervisory responsibilities. Then they might move up into administrative levels (as entry-level managers) with less emphasis directly on managing and supervising people and products (results) and more on process and regulations. In Figure 11–2, time spent differences are shown of the skills used by top-level managers, middle-level managers, and first-line supervisors. Technical skills performed predominately (approximately 48%) by first-line supervisors deal with the operation. Their ability to manage methods, processes, procedures, and techniques serves to meet organizational objectives concerning product (laboratory services). Human skills performed appear consistent for all three levels of managers (approximately 43%) and concern working effectively with (managing of) people. Conceptual skills relate to one's thinking ability to generate ideas, ponder abstract concepts, perceive the organization as a whole relative to the mission statement and goals, and acknowledge how decisions made in one area have impact on other areas. This skill predominates (approximately 48%) for top-level managers.[10]

LEADING

What can a leader do? A leader can generate energy and enthusiasm among workers. Optimistic and positive outlooks become contagious. Often, leaders are not committed to the organization's goals but find satisfaction in getting others to do work. Leadership is generally defined as the art of getting things done through people. Leaders are persuasive, approachable, emotionally appealing, trustworthy, and communicative. They cultivate a high caliber of followers, promote competence, offer fulfillment of people's needs, and induce a sense of commitment. Most leaders love their work and the people they reach. They portend the future, enticing others to follow. Tom Peters describes how "bad" characteristics of leaders inspire strong followings. He implies that President Clinton is manipulative in "preaching inclusion . . . orchestrating every context to present the desired message." One can be dictatorial about one's vision, although "compromise is necessary to build consensus for action." Peters also states that the best leaders are avid students of power, concentrating on the competition and "the contest."[11]

Leaders are drawn to emulate the people we'd like to become. Of all

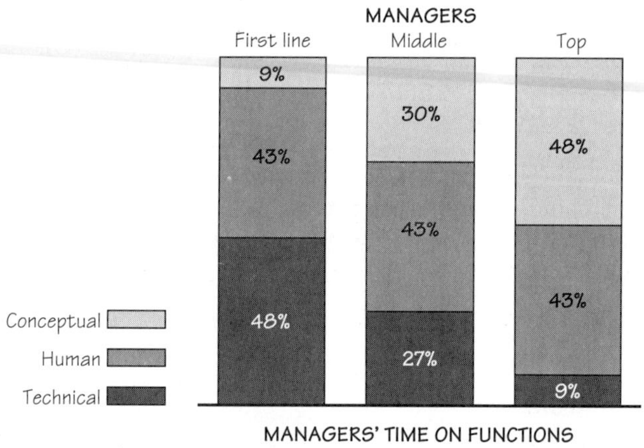

Figure 11–2 Three management levels: Time on functions.

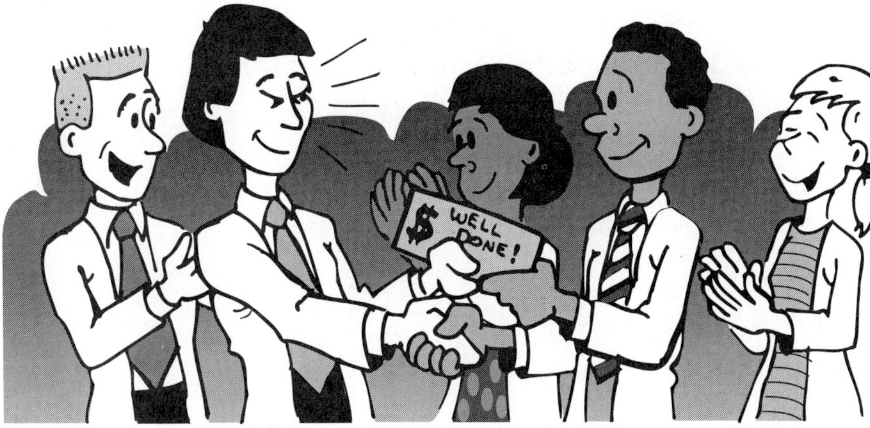

characteristics that managers admire and respect, credibility tops their lists. Research indicates that with creditability, leaders inspire pride, team spirit, sense of association and attachment, and a sense of ownership in the organization.[12]

Known as an outstanding manager and leader in laboratory medicine, Bettina Martin wrote and talked during her lifetime about her experiences in a large university teaching hospital laboratory. She gave practical advice to supervisors on how they should behave. She explained that how supervisors act and think is based on (their) studies, experiences, beliefs in what is right (their values), and the specific modalities with which they feel comfortable. Through her extensive writing and speaking, Martin mentored hundreds of laboratory professionals with her teaching, coaching, and pulling. She encouraged risk-taking with no fear of failure. Her ideas advocated that taking risks diminishes the comfortable feelings that come from following long-established patterns handed down by (our) predecessor and superiors. She noted that performing out of rote (habit) or retaining policies because "we've always done it this way" isn't valid. Being comfortable isn't always best, especially when creativity, innovation, enthusiasm, and improvement are squelched. See the Suggested Readings list for some of her writings.

Activity 3: Getting Into Leadership

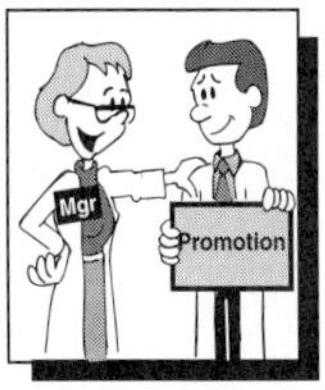

Circle the number you feel most accurately reflects the amount of each leadership quality you possess.

	None	Minimum	Average	High	Maximum
Honesty	1	2	3	4	5
Enthusiasm	1	2	3	4	5
Energy	1	2	3	4	5
Give compliments	1	2	3	4	5
Sincerity	1	2	3	4	5
Creativity	1	2	3	4	5
Like myself	1	2	3	4	5

Continued on following page

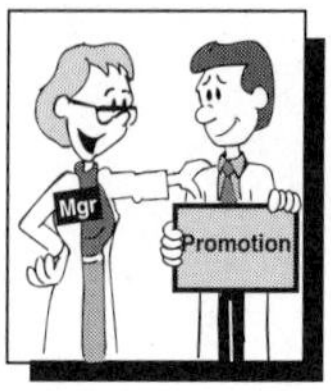

Activity 3: Getting Into Leadership *Continued*

	None	Minimum	Average	High	Maximum
Like others	1	2	3	4	5
Love what I do	1	2	3	4	5
Believe in others' worth	1	2	3	4	5
Give others center of attention	1	2	3	4	5
Competent	1	2	3	4	5
Inspirational	1	2	3	4	5
See big picture (global)	1	2	3	4	5
Trustworthy	1	2	3	4	5
Sense of humor	1	2	3	4	5
Show appreciation of others	1	2	3	4	5
Clear expectations of others	1	2	3	4	5
Friendly	1	2	3	4	5
Change-oriented	1	2	3	4	5
Total Scores	_____	_____	_____	_____	_____

Add all total scores for your overall score = __________.

Following is the key to interpreting your score.

100	=	run for President of the United States or of a laboratory professional society
90 or greater	=	start your own company
80 or greater	=	seek a laboratory manager position
70 or greater	=	organize the accreditation inspection of the lab
60 or greater	=	organize a fund-raiser
50 or greater	=	organize National Medical Laboratory Week events
Less than 50	=	You're OK; be happy being on the team!

Note: This exercise was simply created for learners embarking on their first professional position and is not based on designated research. Any similarity to other validated surveys is purely coincidental.

Styles of Managing and Leading

By inference, style describes the way something is said or done as distinguished from its substance. Developing one's own management or leadership style may occur as a result of (1) observation of other managers (your boss or mentor), (2) work assignments and experience (functions), and (3) education. Often style appears easy if one also possesses intuition and luck.

Most clinical laboratories traditionally function under the "boss aspect": that is, someone is responsible for, plans, and directs others. Even though futuristic models for laboratories involve robotics and automation, people will continue to perform many tasks and use a variety of skills that machines and computers have yet to completely mimic. Someone is needed to manage personnel, some of whom may not be employees but rather temporary, contingent, consulting, or transitional workers.

Managing styles for hospital and health care administrators and managers changed significantly when health care reform became a national issue. Competition drove them to focus, truly and sincerely, on patients as customers. Directing this focus outward brought about marketing and customer satisfaction programs.

Managers who observe and assess internal assets, including employees, facilities, and processes, use a "managing by wandering around" (MBWA) style.[13] This style conveys the message that (hospital) administrators and middle managers do know what's going on. They tune into quality and efficiency issues quickly and prevent troublesome incidents from occurring. They keenly desire to maintain a competitive edge by implementing changes as needed. And it works!

Manager styles depend quite a bit on the individual. In the boxed area below, descriptors of a variety of styles of "good" managers are presented; these are desirable styles. The more successful supervisors adapt to situations, their boss, employees, professional growth, and external influences, and continue to do so. Evidently, supervisors responsible for larger numbers or a more heterogeneous mix of people are required to adapt more readily. In the next boxed area, several examples of undesirable styles of managers who most people wouldn't want to work for (or become) are described. Several of these styles apply to leadership also. Remember: a "can do" attitude affects competence, knowledge, and skills. A "want to" attitude demonstrates commitment and motivation. Combine both attitudes for success!

Catching onto management trends often signals low self-confidence or

DESIRABLE MANAGING STYLES

- Respectful: Explains orders. Requests input regarding work. Describes behavior rather than personality. Works together on long-term expectations. Is a committed partner. Recognizes and respects everyone's own space. Avoids interrupting. Seeks all facts before reprimand or criticism is given.
- Supportive: Establishes and develops working environment. Desires all to achieve organizational goals. Values employees' input. Recognizes contributions. Implements others' ideas to increase work productivity. Listens. Praises. Employs democratic philosophy.
- Consultative: Accepts opinions and input from employees. Acknowledges usefulness of employees' ideas and suggestions. Coaches and advises readily. Retains decision making as own responsibility.
- Participative: Utilizes team approach sharing responsibility and authority equally between managers and employees. Desires that all will own the idea or decision. Provides guidance and general oversight. Provides acceptable working conditions. Seeks equal contribution of resources from all employees.

UNDESIRABLE MANAGING STYLES
• Paternalistic: Father figure, "I know what's best!" Creates dependency; relationships good as long as getting own way. Asks for input and opinions only to be nice.
• Maternalistic: Mother figure, "Here's a batch of cookies 'cause I know you tried. I'll do your work." Often thinks employees are incapable. Needs to be needed.
• Autocratic or authoritarian: Thinks there is only one opinion and one way. Possesses unilateral power. Believes must be present for work to be done and done right. Lacks tolerance for initiative. Strong and powerful.
• Chauvinistic: Same gender most often. Locked into self. Unaccepting of others' race, place, education, or even sports played.
• Quick fix-it-upper: Believes one solution will solve all problems. Considers latest fad to be best.
• Accommodating: Very friendly and approving. Does what is wanted by others when they're looking. Attitude of "If it isn't broke, it don't need fixin'."
• KISSer: Attitude of "keep it simple, sweetie." Thinks problems have simple, easy solutions. Avoids complexities.

minimal ability. Some managers also seek generic strategies or think a single approach will solve a whole problem. They search for a panacea: a magic cure. Supervisors who do this need to get educated and take into consideration the experiences they and others have had to create their most effective and personal manager style. Watch for future styles to be derived from ethics and from using computerization (looking for quickies, again).

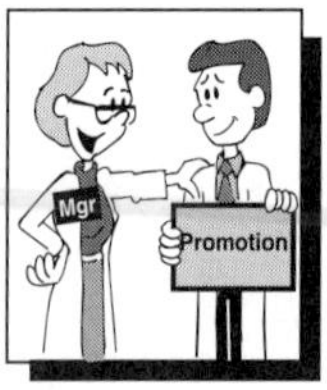

Activity 4: Managing Styles

1. Match the best suited "style/behavior" to each of the following situations. Fill in the blanks with the letter depicting the style/behavior.

SITUATION	STYLE/BEHAVIOR
___ Give a compliment on good work done. It's good news.	a. Bargain, explain relevance, establish mutual objectives.
___ Give a reprimand for an error made. It's bad news.	b. Outline in clear and straightforward manner, be available to answer questions.
___ Delegate a five-step assignment for the first time to a new employee.	c. Relaxed, friendly, enthusiastic.
___ Give assistance in planning and action in implementing a CMLE program.	d. Diplomatic, serious, concerned.

2. Identify three laboratory-related situations. Discuss two or more styles/behaviors for each situation and select which one could be most effective. Explain your reasons for ranking each style/behavior.

Strategies

Consider certain strategies to determine how you should behave or react. Matching your behavior to the situation, circumstances, or people involved for favorable outcomes may influence how you establish your expertise. Learning to accurately judge which manner of style will be most effective in obtaining results (productivity and quality) takes a bit of intuition and luck, with a hefty dose of experience. Many outstanding managers adapt their style to one that fulfills a particular need.

Another strategy is self-assessment. Are you comfortable with the style you've developed for yourself? Do you think you're effective, especially in delivering fair and consistent treatment of others? As your personal style is developed over time and by trial and error, ask colleagues, bosses, and employees to provide you with essential feedback. Build your confidence and techniques. It is more important to be respected than liked.

Often, fresh viewpoints and alternative experiences, when cultivated, beget cost savings, efficiency in performance, and improved services to customers. Supervisors who manage by allowing and supporting suggestions create an atmosphere in which employees will strive to contribute. Supervisors look good to their bosses when employees assist supervisors and each other in significant achievement of organization objectives.

Personal Traits

Many positive and effective traits are included either implicitly, indirectly, or specifically in supervisor job responsibilities and performance standards. Rankings will be high for successful and effective managers. You will have certain choices based on your own personality, beliefs, and work ethic. Should you be personal or impersonal, forceful or passive, warm or cool, flippant or serious, colorful or beige?

Personal style, such as a supervisor's method of operating, innate and honed by experience, influences how he/she manages. Just as likely, employees' style influences their reception to being managed. The supervisor who gets employees to follow directions by asking, but has to ask more than once, might be thought of as a conscientious supervisor by some or a nag by others. The supervisor who usually delegates special assignments to one or two employees might be considered knowledgeable of his/her employees' abilities to get the job done by some, or showing favoritism by others.

Activity 5: Supervisor Behaviors: Good Versus Poor

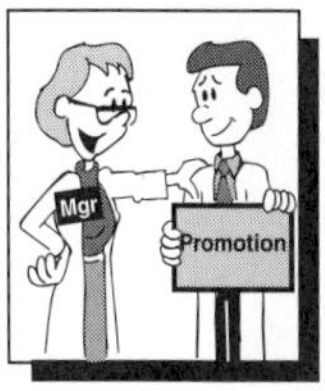

Think of yourself as an employee (or group) in each of the following situations listed on page 182. For each behavior, write a brief statement about why you think it's good *or* why you think it's poor; explain why you like or dislike the behavior; and write a short description suggesting more appropriate behavior by the supervisor.

Supervisor's behavior

1. Follows policies with no exception.
2. Keeps office door open, but chairs are cluttered with papers and test kits.
3. Stands when you enter office.
4. Is always late for meetings.
5. Plays practical jokes during work time—only on subordinates.
6. Does not allow anyone to go to coffee break unless the work is completely done.
7. Does not allow personal time, even though personal time is authorized by Human Resources, because of the heavy workload.
8. Does not ask (or allow) anyone to participate in laboratory committees, such as safety, National Medical Laboratory Week, continuing medical laboratory education (CLME).
9. Approves all vacation time requests based on seniority.

Job Responsibilities and Competencies

Owners and administrators select managers and supervisors to do the job based on abilities and attributes: those special talents or gifts that would distinguish you as the right (most effective) supervisor on the job. Abilities needed are the KSAAs: knowledge, skill, attitude, and attributes. But what is the job? A list of major job responsibilities appears in Appendix 11–A.

Many experts estimate that the time spent by a supervisor on dealing with people is 60%! The corollary is that supervisors spend 40% of their time on the professional and technical aspects of their work. In Figure 11–3, average times spent on certain tasks are shown.

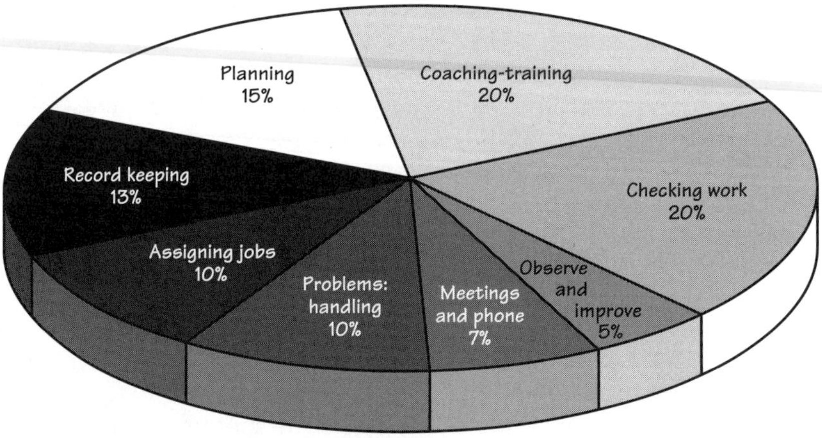

Figure 11–3 Supervisor's time on tasks.

Activity 6: Job Responsibility Weights and Time on Skills

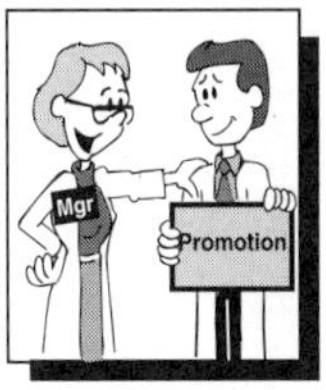

Review the list of job responsibilities in Appendix 11–A and time spent on particular skills (tasks) in Figure 11–3.

1. Estimate the approximate hours per week (40 hours) and per month (40 hours/week × 4.3 weeks = ~172 hours/month) that this supervisor would spend on each of the eight job responsibilities and performance standards (PS). Keep in mind that certain responsibilities are cyclical: budgets are reviewed and justified usually 4 months before the end of the fiscal year; actual accreditation inspection preparation is heaviest 2 to 3 months before actual visit, and mock or internal inspections might be mid-cycle or at regular intervals.
2. Do you think there are any missing or inappropriately weighted job responsibilities?
3. Describe which performance standards (see Appendix 11–B) would be measured by quantitative means (using numbers: statistics, percentage increase in volume, dollars saved) and which would be determined by qualitative or subjective means (compliments or criticisms: 1 to 5 ranking of descriptive statements on surveys by employees).

Training and Transition

One of the most important tasks an effective administrator assumes is to uncover managerial potential in employees. Some managers have become known for preparing their replacements. This is especially true in organizations that support a promote-from-within policy: laboratory directors and administrators are constantly attentive to those prospective candidates for advancement.

Begin building your own KSAA foundation: knowledge, skills, attitudes and attributes. Seek a mentor or role model from among your professional colleagues: internal or external. Look for the doers, and study their strategies and tactics. Act on recommendations from those persons you can trust. Acquire tools for communicating one-on-one and in groups. Control situations by adhering to planned agendas. Be active instead of reactive: anticipate situations and consequences. Develop your own list of objectives and promote its importance regularly. For example, you might want to increase on-site continuing education opportunities.

In fact, no ideal formula exists to educate up-and-coming supervisors, nor are there rules about the who, what, when, and how of supervision. There are, however, explicit principles. Several authors provide a succinct directive that graduates of management programs in health services must be superbly prepared professional managers thoroughly grounded in the concepts, theories, skills, tools, and techniques of the (management) discipline. They add that successful management of health care will be dependent on a multitude of factors including (1) strategic and financial planning, (2) refined management skills, (3) predictive market analysis, and (4) computerized decision support systems.[14]

DO IT YOURSELF OR GET A MENTOR

Design your own "self-training" program; get yourself ready and in position for a supervising job. Read, watch videos, take classes, attend seminars. Ask and accept assignments that will enable you to develop skills other than technical. Assignments might be method and equipment evaluations that require following certain specifications and objectivity. If you've identified a problem, offer solutions. Think about changes in work (for example, workflow or equipment) that will save money by reducing costs or increasing revenue. Go beyond your workplace; get involved locally, statewide, and nationally.

Become a volunteer with charitable or professional organizations to develop skills and leadership abilities that will transfer to career growth. You can embark on this direction by joining a society, attending educational and social functions, and offering your time to work on activities. Raise your hand, sign up, or call when volunteers are sought. Look for notices in societal newsletters and invitations from officers.

Observe the laboratory professionals who lead, and watch for those who will share their knowledge and experiences. Ask for their opinions and advice. Offer your energy and time for projects that they are managing. Take their suggestions seriously to improve what you do and how you do it.

MOVING UP

Are you beginning to think like a supervisor? Can you think of ways that your contributions would improve selected situations or specific results? As a technical generalist or specialist, the category of knowledge and skills you used will not be needed (as much if at all beyond minimally) as a supervisor. You can transfer abilities employed in your technical (scientific) work to management: planning, prioritizing, organizing, quality assessment, problem solving, decision making, to name a few. Be aware that your employees and colleagues will think of you differently! You are now a *boss*! You will develop a different perspective on the work to be done and how it will be done. Your values and motivation will shift from "let's get the work done and go to coffee" to "how can we accomplish this work more efficiently?" Friendships among former coworkers might diminish or become strained because of your new position.

Certain characteristics, such as perfectionism, can be detrimental to the success of a supervisor: every detail *must* be absolutely right no matter what the cost or how much time it takes. Being task-oriented rather than attentive to people and having a preference to work from a habitual format instead of using creative thinking can also be detrimental. Technical employees plan short-term instead of long-term projects and focus on a single issue rather than seeing the big picture (global perspective; they think in black-and-white of procedures rather than the gray of managing people) and are often more practical than visionary.

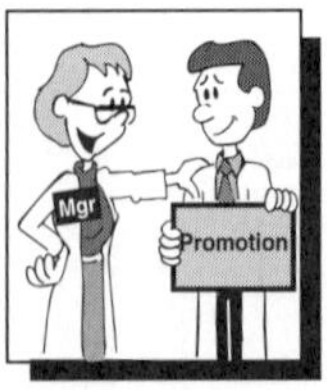

Activity 7: A Self-Training Program to Become an Effective Manager

From the topics presented in this chapter, you have now learned about many aspects of managing, leading, and managerial functions. Given your responses in the previous exercises, list the most important information (knowledge), skills, attitudes, and attributes you would want to acquire and enhance for yourself. Develop a plan for your own training program; include specific activities that would best suit your learning style and management needs.

Summary

In general, individuals are selected to fill manager positions because of evidence of sound technical knowledge that includes problem-solving skills, team contributions, managerial potential, and personal traits compatible with the organization and bosses. Aspiring managers and supervisors formulate their readiness to assume managerial functions and responsibilities by attending seminars or classes and seeking mentors. Successful organizations depend on their managers to have vision and to identify forces in economic and political arenas that can influence and affect health care, laboratories, and the laboratory medicine professions.

As a learner, it is important that you gain knowledge of management theories, competencies, expectations, concepts, and activities as a basis of management, even if you look at becoming a supervisor as a far-away goal. Acquire skills initially with minor tasks in the workplace or in professional or community organizations. Appropriate attitudes and attributes round out the desirable characteristics of "good" supervisors and can be sincerely demonstrated only when valued and incorporated into one's personal and professional philosophy. Enhancing your image to others depends on your self-awareness. Learn to judge accurately and for yourself those management principles that will prove to be most effective and valuable assets for you as a manager.

Activity Discussion 1: Quality Management Components

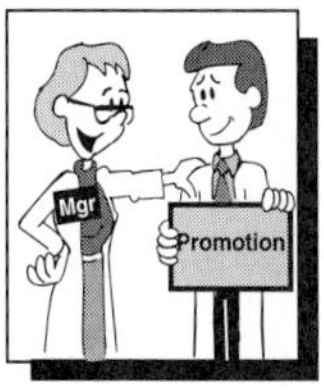

1. Laboratory managers want to know number of tests performed per day (of the week), time of day, and cost of performing that test: labor, equipment and supplies, turnaround times (TAT) from ordering to reporting results, or discarded reagents due to expiration.

2. These issues consist of how to be a member of a committee or a task force; act in a consensus group; facilitate a meeting; communicate with higher-level management, especially on technical issues; design an employee recognition program; become a viable member of a work team; or use appropriate problem-solving methods. People orientation and contact skills can be learned through activities and planned interactions. For many workers in industry, training focuses on how they could use their minds instead of doing physical work; for laboratory technical employees, including phlebotomists, training might focus on how they could use their qualitative and thinking abilities (affective or valuing) instead of quantitative or rote (cognitive or knowledge) and physical (psychomotor or manual) skills. Training within an organization will teach tools of the quality system and how to use them; communication will occur in the same language (vocabulary).

3. Did you think of trouble-shooting an instrument or solving a problem with unacceptable quality control? Interventions can range from simple, such as turning off lights when leaving a room to conserve energy and save money, to complex, such as altering philosophies in management (changing from traditional authoritarian to worker-ownership or teams).
4. Did you think only of products or did you think about people also? Consider periodic feedback and discussions with employees about their performance rather than simply using annual performance appraisals. Also consider comparing two or more instruments or methods and evaluating against predetermined criteria to select one best suited to your needs. Other areas where evaluation would be beneficial are review of a work-flow process to determine efficiency, or clinical assessment of effectiveness of test results in determining a specified diagnosis. Again, training in designing appropriate evaluation tools and protocol precedes actually doing an evaluation process.

Review Questions

Directions: Circle the one best answer.

1. Most laboratories have a management-employee structure that establishes the guidelines for official chain-of-command (responsibility) and communication. What is this structure called?
   a. Administrative outline.
   b. Directory of laboratory personnel.
   c. Organizational chart.
   d. Table of organization.
   e. Policy and procedure table.
2. When "management by objectives" is used, evaluation of employees focuses on what premise?
   a. Number of tasks performed per month.
   b. Attitudes displayed.
   c. Knowledge of test procedures.
   d. Results accomplished.
   e. Personality.
3. What percentage of time do supervisors spend on people-oriented activities?
   a. less than 10%
   b. 20%
   c. 40%
   d. 60%
   e. 80%
4. Which of the following management concepts employs statistical analysis as the basis for achieving better results?
   a. Management by objectives.
   b. Quality systems.
   c. Scientific method.

5. Given a situation in which an employee wants to go to breaks with you and talk about other employees, which tactic would be most likely to get your message across of "No gossip allowed!"
   a. Avoid going to breaks with that person.
   b. Be direct: tell the person you'd rather not discuss others.
   c. Include others at breaks.
   d. Listen, but then tell your boss.
   e. Only go to breaks at the end of the month.
6. In your opinion, which of the following personal traits would be most helpful to a new manager/supervisor?
   a. Perfectionism.
   b. Creative thinking.
   c. People orientation.
   d. Ability to figure out costs.
   e. Perceptiveness.

See p. 409 for answers.

References

1. Duncan WJ. Great Ideas in Management. San Francisco, Jossey-Bass Publishers, 1989, p 3.
2. Travers ME, McClatchey KD. Laboratory Management in Clinical Laboratory Medicine. Baltimore, Williams & Wilkins, 1994, p 5.
3. Duncan WJ. Great Ideas in Management. San Francisco, Jossey-Bass Publishers, 1989, p 12.
4. Drucker PF. Managing for Results. New York, Harper & Row, 1964, pp 1–50.
5. Taylor FW. Principles of Scientific Management. New York, Harper & Bros, 1911.
6. Drucker PF. The Practice of Management. New York, Harper & Row, 1982.
7. Odiorne GS. Management by Objectives. New York, Pitman, 1965.
8. Deming WE. Out of the Crisis. 2nd ed. Cambridge, MIT Center for Advanced Engineering Study, 1986, p 5.
9. Dobyns L, Crawford-Mason C. Quality or Else: The Revolution in World Business. Boston, Houghton Mifflin Company, 1991, p 270.
10. Katz RL. Skills of the effective administrator. *In* People: Managing Your Most Important Asset. Boston, Harvard Business Review 1988, pp 45–57.
11. Peters T, Waterman RH. In Search of Excellence. New York, Harper & Row, 1988.
12. Kouzes JM, Posner BZ. The credibility factor. Clinical Laboratory Management Review 1994; 8(4): 340–355.
13. Peters T. A case for being 'bad.' Peters on excellence. CAP Today 1993; 7(8): 70.
14. Reddick WT. Simulation: A complementary method for teaching health services strategic management. Philadelphia, SCAMC, Inc., 1990, p 308.

Suggested Reading

1. Bass B. Bass and Stogdill's Handbook of Leadership. New York, The Free Press, 1990.
2. Covey SR. The 7 Habits of Highly Effective People. New York, Simon & Schuster, 1989.
3. Fryer B. Managing technology: When you're bit of a techie. Working Woman 1995; Oct., pp 24–25, 98.
4. Levey S, Hill J, Cyphert S, Levey LI. Viewpoint: A prescription for leadership excellence. Clinical Laboratory Management Review 1993; 7(3): 269–274.
5. Martin BG. The CLMA Guide to Managing a Clinical Laboratory. Malvern, PA, Clinical Laboratory Management Association, 1991.
6. Martin BG. Changing roles, changing goals: team development in a competitive environment. Clinical Laboratory Management Review 1993; 7(3): 260–262.
7. Martin BG. Credibility, decisiveness and flexibility. Management Briefs 1993; January: 12.
8. Martin BG. Safe passage through an uncharted territory. Clinical Laboratory Management Review 1991; 5(4): 316–317.
9. Martin BG. Live your life—now! Clinical-Laboratory Management Review 1992; 6(5): 470–472.

10. Scherkenbach WW. The Deming Route to Quality and Productivity: Road Maps and Roadblocks. Washington, DC, CeePress Books, 1986.
11. Special article on Bettina G. Martin. Teamwork, credibility, uncharted waters and life. Advance/Laboratory 1993; 2(5): 35–42.
12. Umiker WO. How to build supervisors' management skills. Medical Laboratory Observer 1993; 25(7): 61–63.
13. Walton M. Deming Management at Work. New York, Pedigree, 1990.

APPENDIX **II–A**

Supervisor Major Job Responsibilities (MJR)* and Weights (WT = 100)

MJR		WT
#1	Supervise and coordinate daily activities of the assigned laboratory section to provide high-quality, uninterrupted services.	25
#2	Supervise and evaluate professional, technical, clerical, and other support personnel assigned to perform duties in designated laboratory section.	35
#3	Serve as a laboratory resource professional to the department (laboratory) and medical staffs.	10
#4	Assist in preparing operating and capital budgets. Strive to maintain cost effectiveness.	5
#5	Work with the pathologist in charge of the laboratory section to maintain complete, accurate, and up-to-date procedure manuals.	5
#6	Monitor evaluations on new test methods, equipment, and instruments. Evaluate new products.	5
#7	Demonstrate effective interpersonal skills to work productively with others inter- and intradepartmentally.	10
#8	Perform other tasks/special projects as assigned or required.	5

*Punctuality, attendance, and compliance with safety and regulations are additional expectations noted elsewhere, as they are not included as job responsibilities.

APPENDIX **II–B**

Performance Standards (PS) for Supervisor Major Job Responsibilities (MJR)

MJR	PS	
#1	PS-1	Monitor that staff are appropriately scheduled to complete work assignments.
	PS-2	Maintain, monitor, and evaluate quality control results, instrument maintenance, proficiency testing, and other quality assurance measures.
	PS-3	Maintain an adequate inventory of supplies.
#2	PS-1	Instruct staff on methods and procedures.
	PS-2	Verify orientation, training, and education of personnel for ability to perform work assignments.
	PS-3	Review work for quality and timeliness. Verify abnormal results.
	PS-4	Participate in interviewing, hiring, evaluating, counseling, and terminating of assigned laboratory section employees following hospital policies and procedures.
#3	PS-1	Provide advice and guidance to the department (laboratory) staff on technical and procedural matters.
	PS-2	Effectively confer with medical staff to resolve problems or special concerns.
	PS-3	Demonstrate effective analytical and problem-solving skills.
#4	PS-1	Effectively complete the budget(s) in an accurate and timely manner.
	PS-2	Maintain and provide the necessary related records to complete and support budget requests.
	PS-3	Demonstrate effective analytical and problem-solving skills.
#5	PS-1	Write, revise, and update procedures in standardized format as needed. Review annually.
	PS-2	Ensure that employees are aware of current information and work requirements.

#6	PS-1	Effectively coordinate, evaluate, and discuss findings with the pathologist in charge of laboratory section, technical staff, and vendors.
	PS-2	Keep abreast of current technologies and trends in laboratory testing.
#7	PS-1	Encourage and promote a harmonious work environment.
	PS-2	Communicate effectively with persons of varying educational, experiential, and cultural backgrounds.
	PS-3	Remain alert to laboratory section morale, conveying pertinent issues to the pathologist in charge of the laboratory section and/or the department manager.
#8	PS-1	Participate in monthly open-communication laboratory section meetings.
	PS-2	Work closely with associated hospital and medical departments.
	PS-3	Ensure that laboratory section personnel adhere to safety—both laboratory and hospital policies.
	PS-4	Ensure that laboratory section personnel adhere to general policies from both laboratory and hospital expectations.
	PS-5	Ensure that the laboratory section is in continual compliance with regulatory agency guidelines.
	PS-6	Maintain progressive professional growth. Support professional growth and career development of laboratory section personnel.

12

Planning: The First Management Function

OBJECTIVES

Upon completion of this chapter, the reader should be able to:

- Compare and contrast at least three types of plans, and provide an example of how each type might be used in a clinical laboratory.
- Explain the rules for planning and managing assignments and describe the steps of these two processes.
- Develop a Gantt chart or similar diagram listing five to 10 activities and timelines for implementing a new laboratory procedure or a selected project.
- Prioritize supervisory tasks according to importance and estimate times to accomplish each task.
- Determine which "time robbers" impact on assignments; describe switching them to "time grabbers."

KEY WORDS

planning
plans
goals
objectives
prioritize
time management

Introduction

Most people have and use plans, probably more for personal use than for business activities, until they are placed in leadership or managerial roles. Plans serve multiple purposes; the most remarkable would be to attain goals and, in today's fast-paced world, execute several plans simultaneously. Therefore, when developing plans, several considerations must be addressed. What is to be accomplished, that is, the ultimate *goal* (of the plan)? What *objectives* are necessary to attain the goal? What *research* has been conducted or *information* gathered that indicates the need for a plan? What *timeframe* is required to formulate and implement the plan? What *steps* should be taken to initiate and *implement* the plan? And what additional *resources* or *people* might be needed to fulfill the plan? Thinking about these questions provides a head start in the process of *planning.*

Mackenzie, author of *The Time Trap,* wrote "Nothing is easier than being busy and nothing more difficult than being effective." He continued on to describe that with *planning* (some) assurance exists that your efforts "will be in the right direction."[1]

Planning: the First Management Function

Plans are defined as advanced decisions with rational predetermination about what is to be done, figuring how to go about doing it (both the plan and the assignment), developing a list of "to-dos," and then putting the plan into action. The "figuring out" part depends on analyzing information from past activities and determining the effects of those activities. The "to do" part is called *setting objectives.* "Putting into action" becomes the implementation part, which requires designated strategies. Differences exist between company plans and personal plans, but the process of planning prevails for both. Certain elements within each can be compared, differing perhaps only in scope and volume.

The Nature of the Planning Process

Business plans prepare employees to do activities to accomplish work. These plans address needs for resources, time, and budget to achieve the intention(s) of the company. Business plans integrate assignments from a variety of departments and systems. Supervisors have a major responsibility to inform employees of what their work and its purpose are, how to perform it through specific processes, and what the expectations are of them in the workplace, that is, their behavior.

Driving forces from outside of an organization often propel the planning process. Certain external forces consist of reduced revenues from payers, loss of available resources, competitors offering better or preferred services, and changes in deadlines. Internal forces (those occurring from within the company) may come from the board (of directors or trustees) with a new mission, desired improvement in products or services, a shift from manual to auto-

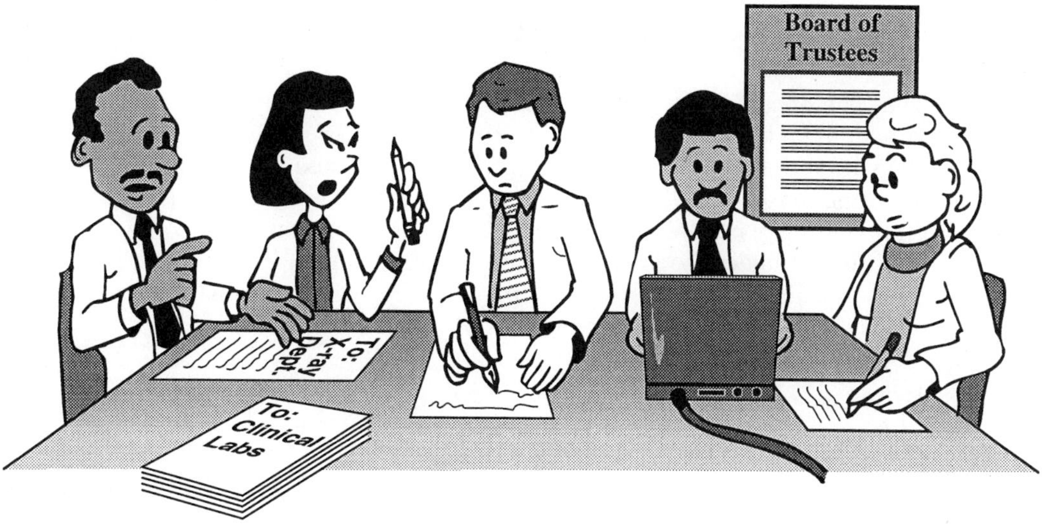

mated production, or changes in priorities. For health care organizations, the *external force* to improve services and control costs is happening through innovative strategies primarily known as *managed care.* The highest level of administrators through all of the hierarchical levels of personnel must react by changing the manner of their day-to-day business because much of it is simply not acceptable anymore. This is because the present system is not cost effective. Correcting this problem requires detailed assessments and a variety of significant plans that address multiple facets of the total operation. Other chapters in this book will address restructuring services and staffing.

Uncertainty surrounding expected outcomes can be offset only when risks and unknowns are calculated. A laboratory manager may desire an economic gain or profit. He/she will plan changes in operations to increase efficiency, anticipating reduced costs and increased revenues. Assessing the impact that planned activities and changes will bring *before* final implementation allows alternatives to be considered and assumptions to be validated. Brainstorming and analyzing the "if this is done, then this should happen" process reduces errors and prevents mistakes.

Plans evolve over time in complexity and effectiveness. Large companies often maintain minimal short-term plans along with significant broad-based all-encompassing plans. At any given time, a laboratory manager might have several plans in progress: ones that embrace two to three steps to achieve minor or immediate goals and others with multiple phases to achieve major goals. It may become necessary to act quickly in order to resolve significant issues. There may be no time to sit down with others and think about what to do. Under these circumstances, intuition (gut feelings) and experience take precedence over planning, especially when the outcome is crucial. Extensive investment of time, talent, and energy on unimportant or petty topics would not be wise.

No plan exists forever as originally developed if the organization faces rapid growth or struggles to survive, or if the group has served its purpose. Good plans offer flexibility and can be modified as needed. More important, preparing employees through participative planning enables change to be accepted and plans implemented.

The Components of Planning

Once the necessity of taking action to achieve some outcome has been determined, the means that will produce this outcome must be identified. Declaring one's intentions to act initiates the planning process. The first component of planning involves needs assessment or surveys to establish a rationale for the plan. Setting *goals* defines the desired results or outcomes. Specific objectives identify the logical sequence of actions with designated time frames or deadlines. Securing approval for the plan and modifying it as needed precede implementation.

GOALS

Achieving a goal becomes an end point toward which management directs its efforts. Setting a goal implies that an ongoing business, hospital, laboratory, or school seeks something different, something new, correction of problems, or improvements.

Goals also serve to motivate employees, control destinies of organizations, and add challenge to mundane and staid operations. A sense of achievement develops from attaining goals. Goals enable people to adopt a results-orientation by working smarter, not harder. Stress is relieved through accomplishments. Good supervisors set three goals for themselves: to be effective, to be efficient, and to be systematic.[2]

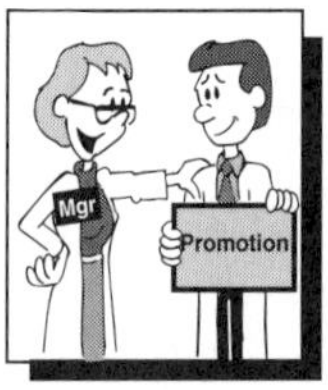

Activity 1: Writing Goals

Goals "work" best when written. Write two goals related to your studies or career.

Write two goals individually or with your group based on an *ASSIGNMENT* identified by your instructor or created by yourself or your group.

OBJECTIVES

Effective demeanor is associated with achieving objectives. Objectives serve as guides to what is desired to be accomplished; several may be used to support a goal. Objectives are statements that describe the mechanism by which the goal is to be achieved. Similar to educational objectives in format, they differ in structure in that learning objectives deal only with guiding students in mastery of information, skill, or behavior. Managerial objectives relate to any focus of business. Not only is the organization affected by the attainment of a goal and corresponding objectives or failure to attain, but also it is affected by outcomes: its product, employees, and customers.

Objectives are "directives" that clearly describe how a goal will be achieved. These statements address specific details and relate to a relatively shorter time frame than goals. The approach to writing good, usable objectives follows the acronym *SMAART: S*pecific, limited to one idea, focused on a

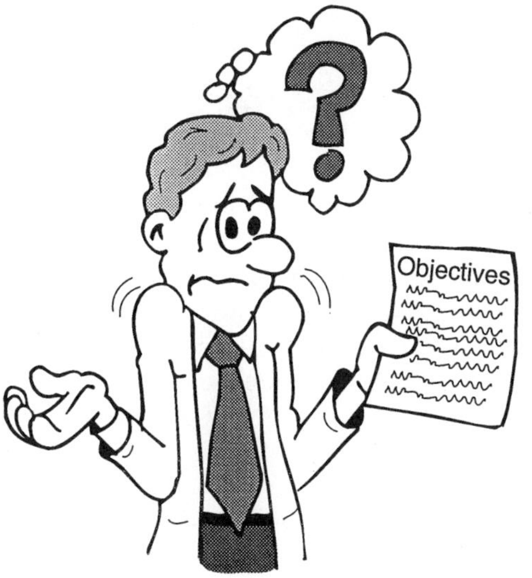

single target. *M*easurable, quantitative or qualitative as compared with predetermined criteria or existing standard. *A*chievable, feasible, and can associate with activities of similar constituents or comparable means; supported by availability of resources, talent, and finances; assumptions, obstacles and contingencies have been addressed and tested. *A*greed upon objectives have been approved in writing among the group members or by those who will evaluate the achievements. *R*ealistic, worthwhile to the individuals, the organization, or customers; makes sense; has practical value. *T*ime-bound, has predetermined dates for completion; deadlines required by driving forces must be met.

Writing objectives is not easy. Experience gained from writing objectives for the Education section of this book should help. The same rules apply to managerial objectives. It is suggested that when first writing objectives associated with business plans, keep them simple, direct, and succinct. Identify sensible timeframes and dates. Eventually, objectives should be written with details and complexities. The "how-tos" of writing objectives imitate the ABCDs: "*A*" describes the audience, the employees who will be doing the work; "*B*" describes the behavior, what they will be do, and is the verb (remember that this verb must represent a measurable action); "*C*" relates to the criterion or criteria, what is expected to be accomplished by the action performed: (it becomes the statement of the expected outcome); and "*D*" describes the degree expressing when, how much, to what amount the action is to achieve (measurable outcomes). Clarity rates of the utmost importance for understanding by all involved parties. If complete definitions or descriptions within objectives are lacking, the employees may not know how to proceed or how to perform all the steps.

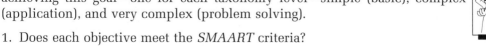

Activity 2: Writing Objectives

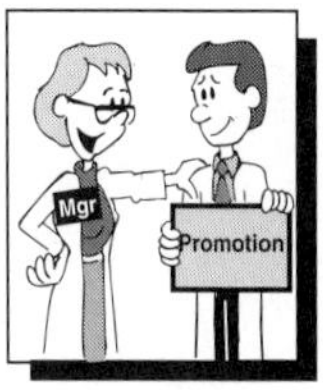

Select one of the GOALS written in ACTIVITY 1. Write three objectives for achieving this goal—one for each taxonomy level—simple (basic), complex (application), and very complex (problem solving).

1. Does each objective meet the *SMAART* criteria?

2. Does each objective contain the ABCDs?
3. Is each objective clearly understood by others outside of your group?

It is important to remove misconceptions about plans. *All* of the following statements are *not* true: Planning can be accomplished only by the most important person in an organization (the boss does the planning and tells employees what to do). The best, most effective plans are quick and easy to develop. Plans should be rigid, constant, and long-lasting. If planning is not in the employees' job descriptions, they do not have to be involved. What is *true* is that employees really are necessary elements in the planning process *if* the plan is to be successful. Even if their input is minimal or happens at one stage only, employees should have a say about how their work will be incorporated into the whole scheme of the organization.

Types of Plans

Plans may be *limited* in that they are confined to an immediate group, area, or department; laboratorians use a limited plan for a 1- to 3-hour continuing education presentation. Conversely, plans can be *comprehensive* and extend beyond a department or institution, even to encompass several organizations of similar mission and activity: for example multiple health care facilities working together on a major community project such as Children's Miracle Network. *Short-range* plans represent designated and restricted intervals; they are specifically related to current services involving 1- or 1- to 2-year periods. Upgrading five personal computers within the laboratory reflects plans of this type. *Long-range* plans extend for 3 to 5 years and occasionally 10 or 25 years, depending on the project, need, goals, and resources. These plans might include constructing a new building or renovating an existing one or expanding services to cover multiple malignant diseases. Many managers look at the "Yr 2015" in a speculative frame of reference but identify projects that will affect work into this time element.

Incremental planning refers to an internal process that specifically examines survival or growth of activities from confined times. Recruitment and retention programs, representing incremental plans, may be implemented in several stages. *Strategic* planning looks at what is to be done and how to do it in relation to the institution's mission and value statements, goals, and forecasts of where the organization wants to be, financially or proximally (for example, statewide or worldwide goals for complexity of operation). Strategic planning is extensive and situational: that is, looking at myriad activities from an external viewpoint. Strategic planning frequently employed by businesses and professional (volunteer) groups uses the "*TWOS*" process during which members identify *T*hreats, *W*eaknesses, *O*pportunities, and *S*trengths associated with the group. From these lists, priorities are determined and plans for future action are developed. Such strategic plans might delineate activities to promote strengths and overcome weaknesses in order to achieve certain goals such as growth of membership, increasing public awareness, or collaboration (networking). This process is often referred to as the "SWOT" or "WOTS" analysis.

Activity 3: Plan Types for Laboratory Events

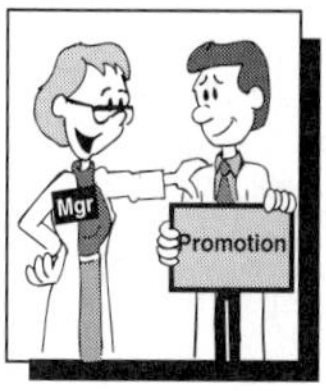

Discuss in groups, with the assistance of clinical instructors or others, various assignments and activities that might involve employees in a clinical laboratory for each of these six types of plans.

Good strategic planners picture a "vision" in their minds. This can happen when individuals comprehend the long-term improvements sought for an organization's growth and profitability (or survival). These people induce employees and others outside the organization to embrace the vision. They ask probing questions that make other people think about what they are doing. Strategic planners establish direction and entice others onto the path. They initiate action with others who will also make a lasting impact on the organization and outcomes. These people are totally honest with themselves and others, never pretending to be what they're not. They recognize and accept their strengths and weaknesses and seek out others to complement their team. They also recognize those characteristics of the organization that promote and enhance strengths; they set about to solve problems and diminish weaknesses.

THE PROCESS OF PLANNING

Rarely during any planning process will one individual develop a plan and carry it out alone. Whether a work group or team, a continuing education program committee, or a problem-solving task force, individuals are either appointed or elected. Often members are recruited or selected for their special talents or abilities. Certain responsibilities pertain to the leader and other responsibilities to the members, but all should acknowledge these responsibilities before agreeing to participate.

Leaders' Responsibilities

Leaders direct group activities. Important attributes that enable a leader to readily facilitate the planning process are (1) the ability to promote discussion without judgment among the members through listening and interpreting skills; (2) competence in logical, rational, and persuasive techniques; (3) an appreciation of the value of members' time as evidenced by prioritizing important items; (4) the ability to select materials and resources for group meetings as well as for members to use during the planning process; (5) the ability to integrate multiple pieces of information, systems, goals, and functions and assess the impact on other people and work units; and (6) conscientious attention to results that will produce improvements rather than acceptance of status quo or traditions.

Leaders are known for their ability to visualize the "big picture," in which outcomes appear very real to them. They may lack an orientation to details and must rely on others to think and discuss the specific, minute details of plans. Leaders nurture the group through the planning process because their strengths are in convincing and in encouraging members. Sticking to the task becomes the responsibility of all members under the guidance of the leader.

Group Members' Responsibilities

Members of the planning group need to accept coordination and integration from the leader. They should expect to spend time on brainstorming by using their imagination and experience. Most important, they need to desire common outcomes. Possessing the following key abilities enables members of the group to better assist in implementing plans: they should be able to identify real priorities; be flexible and adaptable; apply the scientific method by reviewing records, data, and reports; avoid guessing or making assumptions; take responsibility for their own actions and recognize responsibility and authority of others. They should be curious and ask questions about the status of situations, how the work is being done, and what it is that workers like about doing it. They should involve colleagues and employees in planning processes at appropriate stages and be willing to seek help from experts for their knowledge of content or planning abilities; and they should have the courage to criticize plans (pending or current) when appropriate. The scientific method helps to enhance imagination, creativity, and boldness during any planning process once the situation and associated information is known.

RULES FOR PLANNING AND MANAGING ASSIGNMENTS

Randolph and Pozner[3] created a clever process for planning assignments or projects, titled *GO CARTS.* The acronym representing these elements, similar to the mnemonics used as educational learning tools, help teach the planning process for any assignment. First, set a clear ***g***oal, then add more detail by determining ***o***bjectives. Next, establish ***c***heckpoints, ***a***ctivities, ***r***elationships, and ***t***ime as the means of delineating which things are to be done, in what order things will be done, and the monitors that will be used to track progress. They advised mapping out a ***s***chedule by drawing a chart, diagram, or a

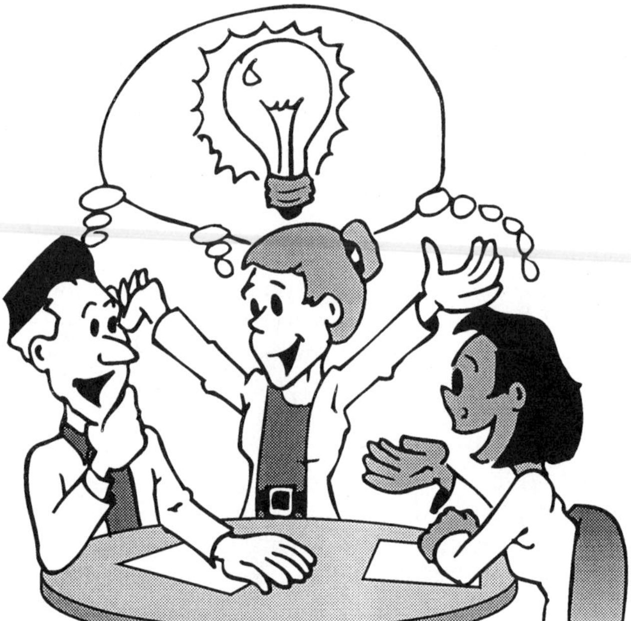

picture to portray the total scheme. They also recommended "rules" for utilization of the plan. Following their previous analogy, *DRIVER* became the acronym for the steps of this management method. Group member must be ***d***irected through communication, motivation and involvement, must ***r***einforce their commitment by getting people excited, and must ***i***nform others continually in order to reduce and remove communication barriers. This requires active listening skills. Continue to ***v***italize people by building agreements, and assist them in working through conflicts and disagreements. ***E***mpower group members; lack of authority to get people on track is a problem that requires a leader's finesse. Acknowledge that when people believe that they make a difference, productivity improves. Group (team) members want honesty, confidence, direction, and inspiration from leaders. Commitment and compliance follow. Finally, becoming ***r***isk-takers encourages and generates creativity and promotes competitiveness (the desire to be first and best among others outside the organization).

Policies, procedures, methods, and rules concerned with efficiency in reaching objectives must be included in the plan. These materials, usually available from the organization's human resource department, might be supplemented by specific departmental ones. Details within these support materials constitute a clear diagram of *who* will do the actions, *what* is to be done, *when* it is to be done, *how,* and *where.* These provide distinctive resources to determine criteria and standards. NOTE: *Why* an action should be undertaken is inherent in the goal statement.

For managers and supervisors, scientists, and technologists, details of activities and times from plans can be presented using various charts and diagrams. These tools become valuable again after implementation of a plan as means for collecting statistical information during the evaluation phase. Gantt charts indicate specific activities and the time frame/deadlines for accomplishing each one (Fig. 12–1). Flow charts depict the plan as separate components from the start to completion. This helps demonstrate the relationship of one component to another (Fig. 12–2). Program evaluation review techniques (PERT) are best used when more than one milestone is scheduled for the same time. The critical path method (CPM) provides a visual aid to spot checkpoints, determine relationships among activities, and estimate appropriate times. A critical path is defined as the chain of events and the total time required for completion of an assignment. Computer software programs easily facilitate these drawings.

Prioritizing Plans

Advantages can be gained for people who prioritize. Using a system and creating labels helps to distinguish assignments accordingly: "High" means it is critical, goal-related, must be done today, or is urgent. "Medium" categorizes it as important, goal-related, must be done soon or can be delegated. "Low" implies that it would be nice to get it done, may or may not be goal-related, can wait, and has no significant time pressure, "No" does not relate to a goal but someone thought that the thing should be done anyway or thought it would be fun to do.

Assignments of greatest importance usually require more resources and time. Involvement on the part of the leader and other people will also be more extensive. Satisfaction derived from completion may be diminished because of this heavy investment. Sometimes the least important assignments, which

OBJECTIVES	J	F	M	A	M	J	J	A	S	O	N	D
1. Student Recruitment Master Notebook												
a. Brochure (revised)		▲		□								
b. Handouts for Career Days (to include middle schools)			△	▲				□				
Inquiry Response Cards			△		▲	■		□				
c. Outlines for Presentations (update old/create new ones)	▲				□							
2. Selection/Acquisition/Creation of Audio-Visual Materials				O	N	G	O	I	N	G		
3. Inquiry Log Monitor (to be evaluated; revised?)				△	▲	■	□					
4. Recruitment Team of Hospital Employees				O	N	G	O	I	N	G		
5. Career Day Participation/Class Presentation	*	*	*	□				△				
6. Press Release/Media Coverage (news ad)		▲	■					△	□			
7. Tours of Hospitals/Departments		*	*	*	■				△			

* Event occurred: Details in Student Recruitment Notebook
△ Planned start date
▲ Actual start date
□ Planned completion
■ Actual completion

Figure 12–1 Gantt chart.

are the easiest and most pleasant, generate a stronger sense of accomplishment when they are done.

New supervisors ask, "Are there any foolproof ways to manage competing priorities effectively without sacrificing quality?" The following steps are helpful: (1) Determine responsibilities and interests; (2) reassess and reprioritize items based on their relevance to objectives: put first things first; (3) select the "vital few" rather than the "trivial many" situations that need attention; (4) seek others to help, particularly with urgent activities; (5) extend deadlines for those important items that are not on a critical timeline; (6) delegate activities of medium priority; (7) eliminate activities that are unimportant or ones that you've labeled as low priority; and (8) seek new, different, or advanced resources to use such as computers and software.

Supervisors should learn to say "No" and not feel guilty. Decide what *must* be done and what is *desired* to be done and say no to all the rest. No exceptions can be made for those assignments either *delegated* by one's bosses (or the company president) or *influenced* by the potential impact involving a significant amount of money.

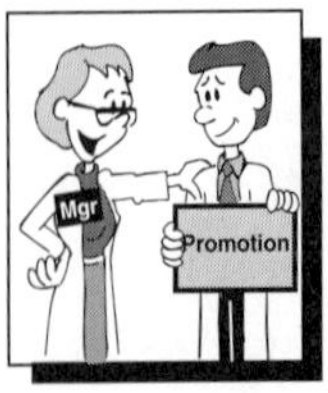

Activity 4: Prioritizing Supervisory Tasks

Jane, the supervisor of hematology, has a "to do" list on her desk. The day is Monday, the first workday of the month. Label each of the following assignments, #1–15, pp 203–204, according to priorities: High, Medium, Low, or No. Identify whether or not the task could be delegated, and, if yes, indicate to whom. Estimate when, during the month, each item should be completed.

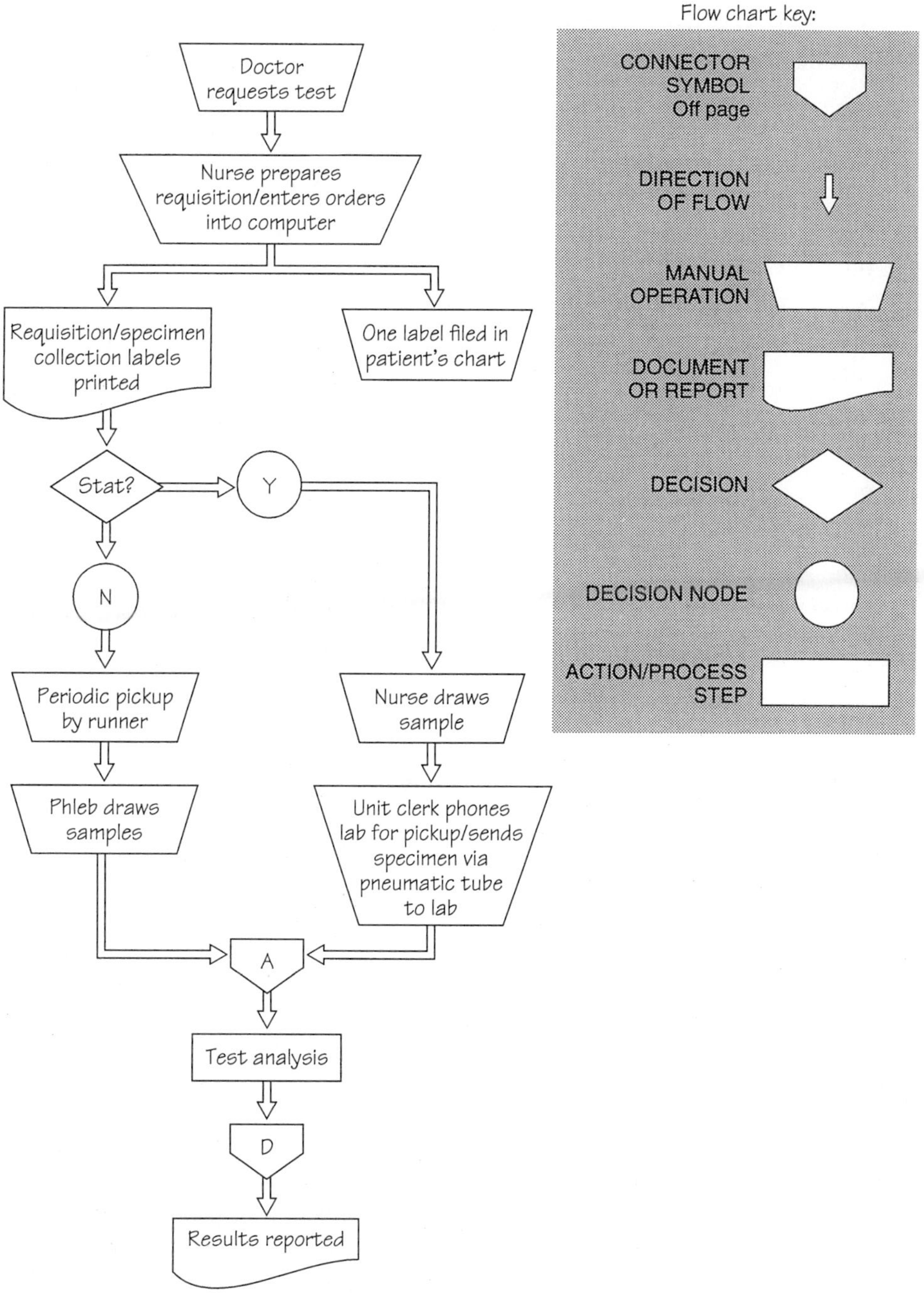

Figure 12–2 Flow diagram with legend for symbols.

---

1. Review daily problem log.
2. Upgrade Coulter STKR analyzer software with technical representative (2 hours).
3. Stainers: inventory supplies and reagents. Move hazardous chemicals to new "Boom Room."
4. Confirm Emergency Center-lab meeting Thursday AM. Review phone log

Continued on following page

and draft TAT list for ECs most frequently ordered tests. Any recommendations from hematology personnel?

5. Performance appraisals due this month: Tom, Nancy, and Clare.
6. Identify how 10% can be saved in costs for next quarter. Confer with lab section chief and submit in writing to lab director and manager.
7. Phone MDA company regarding factor assay problem on new coagulation instrument.
8. Write and e-mail new policy for reporting differentials without band percents or absolute numbers. (Get all necessary approvals and signatures!)
9. Review service contracts before the 10th: meet with lab-section pathologist and lab manager.
10. Read e-mail and check phone messages and messages from administrative secretary.
11. 2:30 PM meeting with manager of reference lab business and afternoon shift supervisor.
12. Continue to develop inventory worksheets on new computer program.
13. Finish technical training checklists, computer (new technologist and technician start Monday).
14. Prepare new lecture, the 18th, for students on cytochemical stains used to confirm leukemias.
15. Need new competence assessment materials of peripheral blood and bone marrow slides on acute leukemias (prefer lymphocytic).

BARRIERS TO SUCCESSFUL PLANNING

When some people are asked to plan ahead, they feel loss of freedom because they like to decide on the "spur of the moment" what they will do. They resist conforming to set guides. Some people feel loss of control if others have provided ideas. They must "own" the idea. Some people need instant gratification from here-and-now action. Others prefer acting to thinking.

Barriers flourish because of personal preferences. Emphasis tends to be placed on day-to-day operations. People think in terms of the here-and-now (the present). People like structure with certainty and predictability. Most individuals in laboratory professions, who are strong in sciences, prefer conservative methods, make decisions cautiously, and avoid taking risks.

Factors or assumptions that would have impact on plans might concern resources, personnel, finances, and methods. Key decisions should be based on identified assumptions that are supported by hard data rather than those only perceived to be facts. One should investigate and test assumptions by means of a questionnaire to people who will be affected, a mini-activity, a pilot test, or a trial run. Look for implications using concrete and validated data to check assumptions. Assume that the environment or key variables can change rather than remain static. Expect unknown or unpredictable events to occur during implementation of the plan. Consider how these situations will

DANGEROUS ASSUMPTIONS FOR LABORATORY PLANNERS

1. Customers will seek our laboratory services because we think we are good.
2. Customers will use our laboratory services because our services are medically superior.
3. Customers will agree with our perception that our laboratory services are "great."
4. Our laboratory services will sell themselves: word of mouth.
5. Physicians and nursing homes will send their patients and their specimens to our laboratory rather than continue to use their present laboratories.
6. We can provide new tests and results on time and on budget.
7. We will have no trouble attracting the right staff.
8. We can isolate our laboratory services from competition.
9. We will be able to charge price according to quality while gaining shares rapidly.
10. The rest of the hospital (company) will gladly support this plan and provide help as needed.

Adapted and reprinted by permission of Harvard Business Review. From McGrath RG, MacMillan IC. Discovery driven planning. Harvard Business Review 1995; 73(4): 44–54.

be handled. Evaluate the ability of the organization (its people) to implement the plan even when assumptions have been tested. In the boxed area, 10 implicit (unquestionable) assumptions are described that, if believed, could be dangerous unless tested.[4] The planning process should address whether or not each statement is valid. Without proof of these assumptions or supporting facts, pending plans may require alteration before and even during implementation.

Constraints or restrictions known as the "triple threat" have been recognized: poor planning, procrastination, and personal disorganization. The checklist in Table 12–1 can be used to ensure that a plan contains essential elements.

Managers and supervisors, leaders, and successful planners provide for contingencies when possible. This means that these planners are prepared with alternatives, additional resources, and other choices. Experts might also be identified to be called on to assist when necessary. Reserve finances should be created. Most of all, when plans go awry, keep calm and maintain a level head.

AIDS TO SUCCESSFUL PLANNING

Certain aids will cultivate acceptance of a plan: (1) inform the lab director and manager during the process and secure their approval and support; (2) verify that it is complete, well integrated, and comprehensive; (3) present it at the most appropriate time after thorough preparation; (4) include the implementation process; and (5) keep it flexible, changeable, and durable as long as needed.

Additional aids that might help include keeping plans up-to-date, scheduling *and* handling most important tasks first according to peak work times (or when best executed), and dividing large assignments for ease of handling (referred to as the "Swiss cheese" technique). Avoid doing easy, fun, small

Table 12–1
PLANNING CHECKLIST

Activity	Date Due	Date Done
1. Analyze present situation. *Where am I/are we now?*		
a. What needs improvement?		
b. What would I/we like to improve?		
2. Write objectives. *What do I/we want to do?*		
a. Relevant to a clear set goal?		
b. SMAART?		
3. Consider and test assumptions.		
a. What conditions might come about during implementation?		
b. What can I/we do about any unexpected events that occur?		
4. Decide on policies, procedures, rules, and actions to achieve objectives. *How will the plan be carried out?*		
a. Which ones already exist?		
b. Which ones need to be developed?		
5. Identify resources needed to achieve objectives.		
a. *Who and what?*		
b. Budget		
6. Identify alternative ways to achieve objectives.		
a. Other resources: people, finances, materials, methods.		
7. What will be oversight, control, or monitor procedures?		
8. What will be the evaluation process?		

items first. Save calendars of what has been accomplished. Departmental records often require all medical and administrative personnel to present their previous month's activities at the monthly department business meeting. One's own personal work records will be useful when seeking a raise, updating a resumé if seeking a new position or promotion, or even providing justification to maintain a current position.

A reverse hierarchy that often becomes more effective requires getting all employees involved from the bottom up and selecting representatives as "key" people. What these representatives have to say frequently carries more weight than comments from the president of the organization. When a major plan involves redesigning the work flow, input prior to finalization and inclusion of front-line employees' ideas will promote acceptance later on. "Key" people also have the authority to approve or reject a plan. Employees who can support or interfere with the plan must be identified; this includes employees affected by the plan. Communicate to people at all levels and in all jobs as much as possible, and don't overlook those people involved only peripherally. Other important strategies include developing formal communication channels such as "a telephone tree." Neutralize opposing influencers. Use a variety of strategies to increase supporters of the plan.

Time Management

Management expert Peter Drucker noted, "Time is the scarcest resource and unless it is managed nothing else can be managed."[5] Webster's definition of time indicates getting things done: "The period during which action or process continues." Estimate how much time managers and supervisors you've worked for in the past spent on each task; write down percentages. Consider the work that technologists and technicians perform. Technical personnel have little input into how they spend their time because their work is driven by testing system from volumes, procedures, instruments, and many external factors. Managers and supervisors, similarly, have designated work but often theirs is more self- (or higher-authority) imposed rather than system imposed. Refer to Figure 11–3 in Chapter 11 and review management tasks and time spent on each. The impact of systems on control of work rises significantly when systems are inadequate or heavily burdened. Invest planning time on significant assignments or ones of major impact and reflect on past experience, where you have been, and the services provided in the past that are still needed, no longer needed, or replaced by new services. Schedule time to probe and analyze multiple aspects of past plans related to current needs, and then align factors that will be most influential in the plan. Determine a hypothesis and arrange to test it. Communication among group members must be arranged. Supplementary conferences might be necessary with employees and authorities to negotiate the plans and component activities.

Projecting timelines on a graph or Gantt chart helps to ascertain feasibility of deadlines and due dates. Experts on time cite Parkinson's Laws: (1) Work expands to fill the time available; and (2) people tend to devote time and effort to tasks in inverse relation to their importance. On the basis of this, how can the estimated time be controlled or even reduced for an assignment? Leaders and managers can impose time limits on schedules and agendas for the purpose of devoting designed time to issues and activities in accordance with their relative importance and value.

Consequences associated with acceptance or denial by any person involved in the implementation of the plan and who might be affected by results can cause havoc with implementation. Major plans often take more time than initially anticipated in order to secure agreement. Allowances within plans that provide for additional time may be indirectly considered at the onset of planning.

TIME ROBBERS

So how do managers and employees get more time in a workday? The answer is to identify, control, and eliminate or curtail specific incidents, events, and situations that take away time. These factors prevent people from completing their work, meeting deadlines, and doing their best. Look realistically at what is to be done, what is desired, and the system and processes for accomplishing the work. Managers advise, "Work smarter, not harder."

Supervisors watch their habits and work schedules as well as their employees. What functions as time controls for supervisors might also apply for their employees. The primary responsibility of all employees is that work productivity should achieve the organization's purpose.

Managers and supervisors often team up to work on solving problems that plague the laboratory. The Pareto Time Principle (Fig. 12–3) illustrates that unless problems are identified according to their significance, workers could spend 80% of their time on unimportant issues, which only account for 20% of all the problems![1] Identifying which problems are significant and which are not becomes very important, because time, energy, and resources should be allocated where the impact will be the greatest. This 80:20 ratio relates to many common management practices: 20% of items in inventory

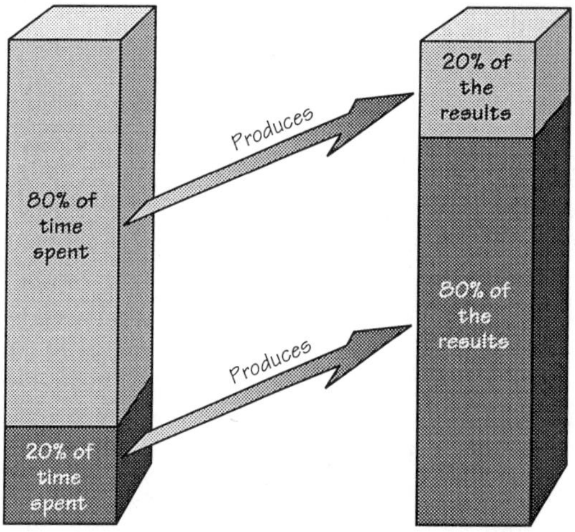

Figure 12–3 Pareto chart.

account for 80% of the total value. Obviously, it is better to apply 80% of one's time to generate 80% worth of results or other value.

Certain obligations will always consume time: one's bosses, phone calls, reading, visitors, regular or "standing" meetings, mail, and even commuting. It is possible to control some of these obligations efficiently with planning and commitment. Table 12–2 details more "time robbers" gathered from several reports.[6, 7]

Procrastination interferes with assignment success. People who procrastinate have characteristics that are different from those people who are more efficient. Group members or employees are considered perfectionists if they must do it right all the time or not at all, or rarely accept any lesser outcome. Leaders and managers must be tough and demanding on "perfectionists" to keep them on schedule. Other people dislike unpleasant tasks and avoid them. Still others lack self-confidence to perform difficult tasks and often cannot decide where to begin.

TIME GRABBERS

Many supervisors and employees go astray despite their good intentions. Consider what would more effectively enable people to manage their time. Revitalized commitment to and renewed interest in the project must be generated, especially when deadlines are near. Review priorities previously determined and assess their status. Certain questions demand answers related to continuing the assignment. Is there a better time to do this? Is there a better person (or other people) to do this? Is there a better way to do this?

Consider selectively adding new responsibilities only when ones that are no longer appropriate for the employee can be eliminated.[7] Stipulations can be imposed on how new assignments will be done and the amount of time that should be devoted to them. Negotiation should include willingness along with any constraints for completing the assignment, expressed without sending a negative message.

Managers and supervisors often consider other means to accomplish their work. They seek help, delegate work, develop teams, empower employees, and only go it alone when *a single person* is required to do the task. Another technique, when inundated with assignments and deadlines, requires manag-

Table 12–2

TIME ROBBERS (Managers, supervisors, and employees may be affected by these factors or attributes)

1. Inadequate Management Skills

Poor crisis management skills
Disorganized: cluttered workplace, poor filing system
Attempts too much; ineffectively delegates
Lacks self-confidence: I've never done this before, how can I do it now?
Style is so different; questions if it will be OK
Cannot delegate: "If I don't do it, it won't get done." *or* "If I don't do it, it won't get done right."
Unnecessary meetings
Poor listening skills
Can't set priorities

2. Insufficient Training or Education

Unfamiliar with organization's mission and goals
Gives unclear or too few instructions
Makes mistakes and doesn't know how to detect or correct
No definite deadlines; unrealistic time estimates

3. Interferences

Too long or unnecessary telephone calls
Reads junk mail
Drop-in visitors
"Bureaucratic red tape"

4. Decision Making Capabilities

Unable to make choices
Unable to reach conclusion or finalize
Detail versus global oriented
Unable to attain consensus
Perfectionist

5. Insufficient or Outdated Resources

Insufficient finances
Lacks information: Policies, procedures, rules, references, regulations, standards
Unavailable personnel: Office, technical, upper management, other support
Unavailable or inadequate equipment: Computer, office supplies, technical instruments

6. Lack of Self-Discipline

Procrastinates: "I'll do it later."
Likes to talk, socialize, eat, watch TV, play
Prefers to do something else: Clean office or house, cook gourmet dinner
Daydreamer

7. Not Healthy

Lacks sleep
Needs eyeglasses or hearing aid
Stressed
Fearful of failure, change, loss of control
Inadequate work setting and patterns (ergonomics): Lighting, instrument and equipment set-up, space for doing work, floor or chair
Poor diet
Gets little or no exercise

8. Right-Brained

Aptitude for other types of work
Low concentration for detailed tasks
Performs rituals: Daily routine, traditional
Worries about things far off in the future
Lacks sense of humor
Always late
Doesn't reward

ers to alternate major activities with minor ones. This will boost one's sense of accomplishment.

Computer technology provides excellent means of conserving time, especially with routine assignments and reports. Word processing software enables people to develop forms and templates to use repeatedly with the "merge" feature. Other time-saving features include reducing multiple forms to as few as possible, deleting extraneous information and implementing the daily turnaround times (TAT), weekly quality control, monthly incident and quality assurance reports, and yearly census of tests forms.

Unexpected situations often occur for managers and supervisors. For the surprise visitor or phone call, briefly explain time limitations and counter by offering a certain amount of time either then or later. Social visits should not be permitted when unannounced, during peak work times, during crucial situations, when other appointments or commitments are scheduled, and for prolonged times. Similar guidelines should extend to employees who may be performing STAT or difficult procedures during which interruptions might be devastating. For everyone in the department, other guidelines could handle most unexpected situations gracefully: make an appointment, assign a receptionist to screen visitors or phone calls, explain the work constraints and when time would permit conversation, and institute departmental policies. If time does permit the meeting, moving to a neutral area, such as the cafeteria or lounge, allows the employee to leave as needed. Supervisors have suggested other tips for handling unexpected visitors: (1) stand when the person enters the office and remain standing rather than sitting: it's polite but inhibits lengthy conversations; (2) use an egg timer and after 3 minutes, if more time is needed to complete the conversation, suggest an appointment at a mutually convenient time; (3) invite the visitor to walk along when going to a scheduled meeting; and (4) greet visitors in an open area of the laboratory or lobby or at the reception desk rather than in an office.[6]

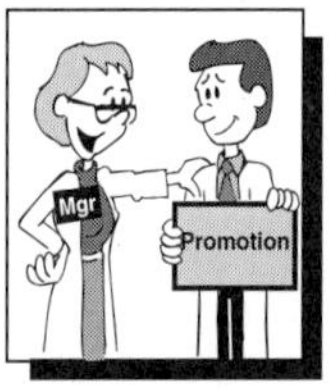

Activity 5: Changing Time Robbers Into Time Grabbers

Review Table 12–2, Time Robbers. Divide the topics among several individuals or groups. Complete all steps in this activity.

1. Describe why the "robbers" are so disruptive to the production of effective work. Discuss among your group how to avoid them.
2. List the ones that have interfered with your completing homework this term as a recent assignment. Identify tactics to control the specific ones working against you.
3. Designate a specific time, such as National Medical Laboratory Week, and hold a contest on ways to deal with time grabbers for the "most original," "most improved," and "most valuable," among the students and personnel in the building, within the program, or between classmates and instructors. Secure sponsor(s) and award prizes such as clocks, day-planners, personal calendar computer programs, or other time-management aids.

Identifying one's peak performance period of the day and setting aside this as "quiet time" facilitates time management. Depending on the job, an hour or two might be needed. An isolated block of time allows accomplishing three times as much work. This also applies when performing critical tasks. Identifying other times for mail works well to alleviate stress of concentrating hard on critical tasks. Handle mail, or any other paper, according to the acronym *TASK:* ***T***oss it out when in doubt. ***A***ct on it; only allow a piece of paper to cross your desk once. ***S***end it on if it relates to someone else's work. ***K***eep it: (a) handle within 3 minutes; (b) prioritize, categorize, and file if high or medium importance (delegate low-priority papers). Make "action" files in your system of "To Do," "To Call," "To Read" and date to take care at 1 week and at 2 to 4 weeks. Make 12 "tickler" files in your system for January through December.

Clean work spaces help work productivity. Accounting for 90% of what's on a desk is a reminder of things to be done and work items stored so they won't be forgotten, overlooked, or lost. Every 8 minutes one of these items becomes a distraction from work, which amounts to more than 40 hours. Suggestions are to schedule a "De-Stress Desk Day," and create holding files for correspondence, reading, projects to do and date, and miscellaneous. Sort through all paperwork and discard it, delegate it, do it now, or "decide when" it needs to be done. Review the "decide when" items to put them in the appropriate tickler file and record them on the calendar. At the end of the workday, clean and clear the workspace or desk. For technologists and technicians, safety requirements in the laboratory, such as wiping off counters with fresh bleach, storing reagents, and so forth, are normal; this trait also serves busy and productive supervisors as well.

High-profile, prolific authors advocate time management in terms of "me" management. Covey writes that his personal philosophy is to organize and execute around priorities.[8] People today tackle the challenge of managing themselves, according to Covey, by preserving and enhancing relationships and on accomplishing results."[8] "Not getting smarter is getting dumber," advises Peters.[5] He notes that instability in the workplace produces the desire to spend more time in situations that provide stability: the community, family, neighbors, church religious community, and special interest groups. At work, managers, supervisors, and their employees want an efficient and effective environment for maximum productivity.

EFFECTIVE TIME MANAGEMENT

Groups meet regularly to discuss planning, implement assignments, and evaluate progress and achievement of active assignments. When meeting, they follow an agenda with time allocations. All group members are kept involved and on track with their delegated or chosen activities. Activities divided according to members' abilities or experience limits learning new skills by novice members. Training members who lack knowledge, skills, and abilities to contribute their share is important. Replace members if their time and energy wanes. Allow members to work at their own pace, but tighten the control when deadlines become close. Murphy's Law states: "Everything takes longer than it takes." Tolerate some leeway if extra time is needed. Ask experts for advice and opinions. Seek approval of authorities when appropriate.

Many managers and planning advisors recommend visualizing the finished "product" and reversing the mental process for successful planning. This method often catches erroneous assumptions and conclusions. Use resources generously. Don't overlook ancillary materials, especially if they weren't available initially. Seek tools such as computers and software to facilitate the momentum of the assignment. (More than likely these items will last and have usefulness long after completion of the assignment.) Include rewards or some type of recognition for members and affected employees when milestones, even small ones, are accomplished. Allow opportunity for fun, and get some enjoyment from the hard work. Admit mistakes readily, and correct them in order to prevent serious mistakes. Expecting more from others than what one is willing to give sends a negative message about the importance of the assignment. When the assignment is finished and evaluations are critiqued, everyone should be thanked for involvement and contributions. No matter how the assignment turns out, each member should note what he/she learned from the experience.

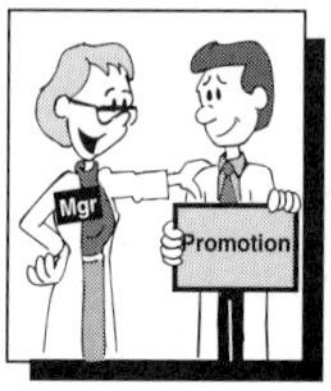

Activity 6: Crisis Assistance

An employee comes to you seeking your help with a particularly difficult project. You have learned that this person agreed to handle it several weeks ago and that the medical director is expecting the employee to present information tomorrow. What should you do?

See Activity Discussion 1 at the end of this chapter.

Summary

Planning is a straightforward process derived from the desires to fulfill the organization's goals. Planning includes constructing and setting objectives, outlining strategies, and distributing responsibilities. These directives describe activities that, when fulfilled, assist in achieving goals.

Various types of plans are based on length, depth, breadth, and scope of assignments. Rules for *planning* and *managing* assignments adhere to the acronym *GO CARTS DRIVER:* *g*oals, *o*bjectives, *c*heckpoints, *a*ctivites, *r*elationships, *t*ime, *d*irect, *r*einforce, *i*nform, *v*italize, *e*mpower, and *r*isk-taking.

Objectives represent the principal element and measurements for achieving goals. Complete objectives include the audience, the behavior (verb), criterion or activity, and degree. Employees should know what is expected of them regarding their work, how they should do it, when it should be done, and how they (and others) can determine their accomplishments. Planning requires time, resources, talent, and energy of the people involved. Diagrams and charts enable visualizing results.

When many assignments converge on one's desk, prioritizing and categorizing determine order and handling: some need to be done as soon as possible (ASAP), some next week, some with lots of help, some by someone else, and others not at all. Time management techniques can apply to improve personal, professional, and work situations.

Planning leads to accomplishments, which in turn produce results. The process and the outcome affect fulfilling organizational goals. Managers and employees also benefit from effective planning through involvement, their contributions, and satisfaction of doing good work.

Activity Discussion 1: Crisis Assistant

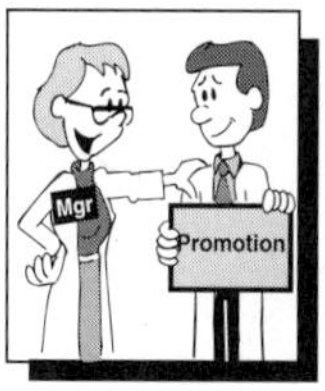

An employee comes to you seeking your help with a particularly difficult project. You have learned that this person agreed to handle the task several weeks ago and that the medical director is expecting the employee to present information tomorrow. State several responses you might give the employee. Which one would be the most appropriate? Consider these choices for your response:

1. "Yes, I'll help." (It will make YOU look good.)
2. "I'll do it for you." (If YOU drop everything else and take over the project, you'll do it better.)
3. "Here's my offer: Let's get together for an hour—no more than two—this afternoon. What about 2 o'clock?" (Cooperative but not taking over.)
4. "I suggest you approach the medical director and ask for a time extension." (Not willing to help at all.)
5. "I don't want to get involved at all." (It's better to let this person learn from this and suffer any consequences.)

Preferred response should be: "I would be happy to give you some advice on this project (resolve this issue or the problem). I believe that it is your responsibility and am confident that you can take care of it. If you still need my help, I can free up an hour, but I'll only be available after 3 o'clock."

Review Questions

For the multiple choice questions, circle the one best answer. For the short answer questions, write a brief response.

1. The primary reason to plan is to
   a. obtain the commitment of your employees to their work.
   b. ensure that your luck will hold.
   c. concentrate on the determined objectives.
   d. implement assignments that use less time and resources.
   e. meet organization annual review criteria.
2. Which is the best protocol to use for testing assumptions?
   a. Apply the Pareto Principle.
   b. Develop a Gantt chart.
   c. Prioritize the assumptions.
   d. Use the Scientific Method.
   e. Match to objectives.
3. What are the four rules for planning assignments?
   a. Identify TWOS.
   b. Establish CART.
   c. Use the Pareto Principle.
   d. Develop PERT.
4. Given the five characteristics of good objectives, define each and cite an example for each characteristic.

5. Given a list of activities, describe how you would go about prioritizing according to importance.
6. Given a list of "time robbers" from your instructor, and describe how you would control for each and switch each to "time grabbers."

See p. 409 for answers.

References

1. Mackenzie RA. The Time Trap: Managing Your Way Out. New York, AMACOM, A Division of American Management Association, 1972.
2. Merck WR: "Maxim"izing time. Clinical Laboratory Management Review 1995; 9(3): 226–230.
3. Randolph WA, Posner BZ. Effective Project Planning and Management: Getting the Job Done. Englewood Cliffs, NJ, Prentice-Hall, 1988.
4. McGrath RG, MacMillan IC. Discovery driven planning. Harvard Business Review 1995; 73(4): 44–54.
5. Peters T. Peters on excellence. Column in CAP Today. Northfield, IL, College of American Pathologists, October 1994, p 90.
6. Frings CS. Increasing Productivity Through Effective Time Management. (Seminar Book) Birmingham, Chris Frings & Associates, 1995.
7. Van Auken P. Seven pesky time management traps. Clinical Laboratory Management Review 1995; 9(1): 49–52.
8. Covey SR. The 7 Habits of Highly Effective People. New York, Simon & Schuster, 1989.

Suggested Reading

1. Alexander R. Commonsense Time Management. New York, AMACOM, 1994.
2. Blanchard K, Johnson S. The One-Minute Manager. New York, William Morrow and Co. Inc., 1982.
3. Davidson J. What fills your days and why? Clinical Laboratory Management Review 1993; 7(3): 237–242.
4. Fogg CD. Team-Based Strategic Planning. New York, AMACOM, 1994.
5. Lewis JP. Fundamentals of Project Management. New York, AMACOM, 1995.
6. Reeves PN. Strategic planning revisited. Clinical Laboratory Management Review 1994; 8(6): 549–554.
7. Zorn E. Getting your act together. Notre Dame Magazine 1993; Autumn: 26–29.

13

Organizing: The Second Management Function

OBJECTIVES

Upon completion of this chapter, the reader should be able to:

- Describe the process of organization and correlate associated duties.
- Given an example of a laboratory staff by title and brief job description, determine an appropriate organizational structure including responsibilities and accountability.
- Define *reengineering* as applied to the clinical laboratory.
- Discuss ways for improving work operations and work patterns.
- Define *ergonomics* and describe three examples of appropriate applications in the clinical laboratory.
- Select one topic presented in the materials management section, and prepare recommendations for improving the selection and acquisition process.

KEY WORDS

organization
work sequence
work site and facilities
reengineering
ergonomics
material management

Introduction

Recently, a new medical technology graduate accepted a position in a newly created molecular virology research laboratory. Space for this laboratory became available following a relocation of clinical microbiology-virology laboratories. The graduate faced a room filled only with counters and cabinets. No equipment, instruments, reagents or manuals were to be found in the room. The virology laboratory director supplied her with two pieces of information to use in organizing the lab: a list of the research tests prioritized in order of implementation and an accompanying literature review for each test. Fortunately, this new technologist possessed two favorable attributes: common sense and organization skills.

How would you proceed? It is hoped that the information presented throughout this chapter, which provides you with suggestions, ideas and activities, will enable you to use your own common sense and organizational skills if you ever find yourself in a similar situation.

Organization

The skill of *organizing* does not mean that *you* do all the work. According to Snyder and Senhauser, organizing means that you, as the manager, should develop a structure to facilitate the coordination of resources to achieve completion of long- and short-range plans.[1] Organizing consists of building a framework in which one portion is supported by another, and these are both supported by a third, and so on. Organizing provides the plan through which the work required to realize objectives (of the institution) can be accomplished. A manager becomes responsible for the work getting done through either a formal or informal structure. The relationship among what work is to be done, the person responsible for doing it, and the workplace environment must be determined. This relationship exists on a threefold foundation: *authority,* which allows the manager to direct others to do the work; *responsibility,* which refers to the work, tasks, and activities the employee has been assigned to do; and *accountability,* which obligates the people involved to successfully fulfill their assignments. Job descriptions support those holding authority in a legal sense, but employees accepting the work must convey a willingness to report to that authority.

Laboratories are highly organized and efficient operations. Laboratorians possess keen skills of organization, a methodical approach, and the ability to analyze minute details. They must transfer their excellent analytical abilities to integration, cooperation, computerization beyond data storage and retrieval, and facilitation with other medical and health care givers.

ORGANIZATIONAL DUTIES

Managers inaugurate the organizing function with major activities; see boxed area. Managers classify tasks as major and minor, then align each into sections or units according to similarity of analysis (functional departmentalization), physiology (product departmentalization), or geography (laboratory services closer to the patient). The workplace requires appropriate physical structuring.

MANAGERS' DUTIES FOR ORGANIZING WORK

Duties performed by managers within the organizing function produce work results such as:

1. Alignment of major tasks versus minor ones
2. Workplace physical structure
3. Job descriptions with delineation of authority, responsibility, and accountability
4. Communication, coordination, and reporting systems
5. Staffing to get the tasks done and personnel to do the tasks
6. Policy and operation manuals (standard operating procedures—SOPs), guides, and handbooks
7. Table of organization
8. Informal network of relationships
9. Functional committees, task forces, and special interest groups
10. Flexible framework

Managers will guide personnel with job descriptions delineating authority, responsibility, and accountability. They should establish systems for communication, coordination (teams), and reporting (chain of command for accountability). Other activities that require significant attention include determining staffing needs and staff selection. Policy and operation manuals (standard operating procedures: SOPs), guides, and handbooks must be prepared and produced. Employees must be informed of these materials and become familiar with the contents, especially those dealing with expected behavior and conduct, areas of responsibility, and duties. Confirmation of authority should be addressed. The official organization of personnel and titles should be documented with authority and chain of command, or teams should be delineated. This is also called an *Accountability Chart.* Supporting groups composed of committees, task forces, and special interest groups with designated functions are described and a list of members included (by title or position and name of the individual).

Organizing involves framework, obligations, and workforce: the where, the what, and the who. It is a method to carry out the plans developed based on the principle of division of work. Additionally, flexibility of the framework or alternate operational guides should be developed to support crises, stressful situations such as lack of staff or reduced workload resulting in lay-offs or reduced work time, or rapid growth of workload by volume or test expansion. Unifying the right workforce with the right workplace enhances the achievement of the organization's goals.

Activity 1: Organizing a Laboratory

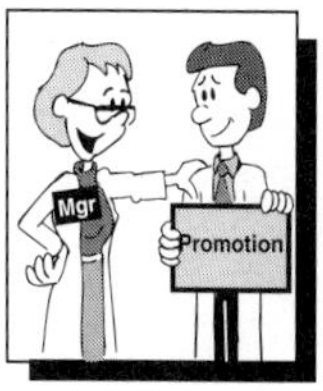

Select a specific laboratory section. Outline a framework for its operation; identify tasks and several tests. Describe important policies and manuals that a manager might want to acquire or develop first. Discuss a manager's obligations for chain of command, authority, responsibility, and communication.

Many books, articles, stories, and other resources are readily accessible that assist managers in "getting centered," "getting started," "organizing" and "reorganizing."[2]

Authority and Responsibility

"Invested authority" establishes the right to direct, invoke compliance, and allocate resources by one person. *Responsibility* defines the obligation to execute tasks and work. *Power,* often confused with *authority,* describes the ability to influence behavior. A basic principle of parity of authority and responsibility means that no one should be given responsibility without the authority to perform it. In this situation, authority refers to making commitments, using resources, and taking necessary actions. Both authority and responsibility must be commensurate in order for the individual to fulfill his assignment.

Authority from any of three sources conveys certain rights. "Legitimate authority" delineated in job descriptions can be exerted downward through all layers of management and employees. In the "acceptance theory of authority," employees respond to communication through a memo, but they must understand the communication, be convinced it is consistent with the mission of the organization, find it compatible with their personal interests, and comply with it. For the manager who is the single boss of employees, the "unity of command" authority theory gives legitimacy because of clarified lines of authority and reduces problems of conflicting orders from more than one boss.[3] Authority or influence over employees depends on the manager's style: autocratic (employees are told what work to do, when, and how), paternalistic (the manager helps and instructs the employee to do the work), or collateral (together manager and employee figure out who will do the work). The collateral style of managing occasionally backfires if the manager is perceived as a WIMP (Woe Is Me Person) because he/she does not take the responsibility but

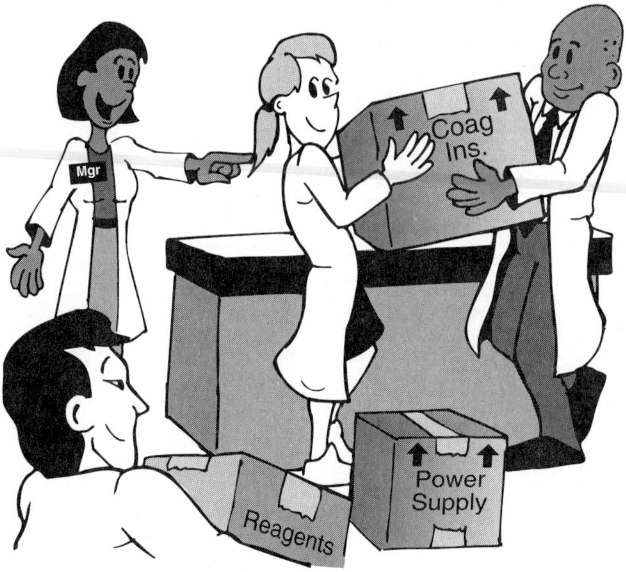

TEST CATEGORIZATION CRITERIA

- Requested as routine, urgent, STAT, or special
- Volume high or rare
- Analyte easy or difficult to detect and measure
- Assay qualitative or quantitative
- Methodology simple or complex
- Procedure manual, semiautomated, or automated
- Method availability*
- Instrumentation availability*
- Time of day specimens received
- Day of week specimens received
- Specimen type, preservative and amount: whole blood, serum, plasma, other body fluid
- Patient type based on diagnosis

*For example, in a large hospital clinical laboratory, 5 methods are utilized on 14 different instruments.

needs help from the employees in finding a solution. Employees can grab control and the solution still may not work.[4]

IDENTIFICATION OF TASKS AND TESTS

The customers determine job functions, tasks, and tests to be performed in a laboratory. The patient type (based on diagnosis), the patient's location at the time of specimen collection (inpatient, outpatient but at the hospital, outpatient but elsewhere such as doctor's office, nursing home, or at work or school), and the kind of specimens must be classified and counted. This essential information must be analyzed regularly to determine the total laboratory operation beginning with what will be done.

Test categorization depends on several factors; see boxed area. For most tests, turnaround times have been established in order to meet patient care requirements; this is also referred to as *patient-test management.* Tolerance by clinicians to prescribe therapy based on laboratory results affects turnaround times and the laboratory administration's decisions about whether or not the laboratory will perform the test in-house or send the specimens to a reference laboratory. The manager must address the reasons tests are performed and reported according to clinical (patient) schedules and requirements for other diagnostic procedures, therapies, or discharge.

Because of the multiple factors influencing decisions regarding tests, managers and employees devote much of their efforts and attention and spend hours to achieve optimal laboratory services delivery. Therefore, identification of tasks and tests cannot be fully accomplished until a careful analysis of data is completed.

TASK SEQUENCE, PLACE, AND TIME

Once job functions and tasks have been identified, the tests to be performed must be prioritized and assigned in a logical sequence, set up in specified laboratory sections, at designated workstations or modular cell units, and scheduled at appropriate times. Different strategies can be utilized to group tests, job functions, and tasks:

1. Similarity of analysis, called the *principle of functional departmentalization:* for example, all tests performed using radioimmunoassay methodologies are performed in one modular cell unit within one laboratory section.
2. Specimen type or pathophysiology, called *product departmentalization:* for example, body fluids other than blood are all processed and analyzed at several workstations within one laboratory section; hematologic studies or bacteriological studies are all performed in their respective laboratory sections regardless of specimen type.
3. Minimizing distances between site of analysis and patient: for example, open heart surgical suite laboratory; presurgical testing (PST) laboratory for electrolytes, CBC, and urine; point-of-care testing (POCT) at nursing units or at patients' bedside.

Additional data analysis requires calculating when peak testing times occur during the day and identifying which days of the week peak operations occur. A visual computerized display enables managers and employees to justify testing. Another time factor to be addressed is how long it takes to perform the procedure, taking into consideration method, instrumentation, and testing site.

Managers may be surprised about the information generated. There may be times when work volume is so low and routine that the staff languishes in boredom and other times when work volume is so high and crucial that staff members sweat through their frustrations. Managers need to develop plans and alternative solutions for these diverse circumstances. Traditional "we've always done endocrine testing on Monday and Wednesday mornings" routines may have to be changed. Just because the laboratory has not run chemistry profiles at 2000 hours (8:00 PM) before does not mean that the task will never be done at this particular time. Acquiring customers who want (and expect) their results on specimens collected late morning or early evening by early the next morning directs the laboratory to alter its "traditional" framework.

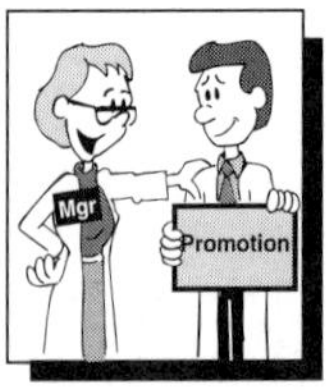

Activity 2: Test Sequence, Place, and Time

Use the same laboratory information from ACTIVITY 1: section, tasks and tests. Describe how you would organize the operations according to when tests should be done by priority, site of testing, and time of day/day of week.

TEST PERFORMANCE

Many preestablished criteria constitute the selection of methodologies and instrumentation to be used. Method evaluation procedures and instrument comparison protocols are well established and published (see Suggested Readings). Overall considerations are customer based as described previously, laboratory personnel and others handling specimens and performing tests under the auspices of the laboratory administration, and from financial reasons.[5] Each laboratory administration determines the best methods and instruments for its own operation rather than relying on manufacturer's information or input from other laboratories.

IDENTIFICATION OF EMPLOYEES

Task analysis offers managers valuable insight into the knowledge, skill, and ability levels required for acceptable performance. Separation of tasks into preanalytical, analytical, and postanalytical phases presents opportunities to develop new roles for clerical personnel, laboratory aides, technicians, technologists, and scientists. This might occur in a physical separation of rooms, work cells, or workstations. Many individuals can transfer their theoretical knowledge and skills from one discipline to another when similarities and limitations are well defined and clearly stated, even for the simplest activity. Employees can gain the needed self-confidence and skills after practice and competence assessment. The qualities that are difficult to teach are integrity, accepting and acting with responsibility, and follow-through. This is where coaching works best.

Again, review a task-analysis worksheet. Assess the work based on several factors similar to those described previously: (1) volume (tests of greater numbers rank high, those of fewer numbers performed in a day or week rank low); (2) numbers of results in normal versus abnormal ranges and how many require further investigation for verification before final report; (3) procedure variation from common and simple to unusual and complex; and (4) customer source of specimens whether from college students or insurance company physicals with a limited range of tests regularly requested or from pediatric oncology patients who need special tests derived from morphologic abnormalities. External forces to contain or reduce labor costs also affect personnel decisions.

Training before hire does not always guarantee personnel competence during employment. Managers should accommodate employees with further training as needed to review procedures and (any new) details. Regularly scheduled training sessions, in-services, and continuing education programs help personnel maintain confidence, retain manipulation dexterity, and control sources of error.

All these factors influence the most appropriate level of education and training necessary for personnel to achieve the objectives and commitments for laboratory services and the organizational mission. Personnel handling and processing specimens must be identified: testing personnel, laboratory assistants, clerical personnel, aides, and others. Personnel performing test procedures and reporting results must be considered: medical technologist/clinical laboratory scientist, medical laboratory technician/clinical laboratory technician, nurse, patient care technician, or even physician (occasionally an emergency center resident).

Reengineering: Ways of Working

Needs, issues, advancements in technology and science, and obsolescence precipitate change—the redoing of what has already been done to fulfill the needs you have today. What once worked well may not do so now. Accept

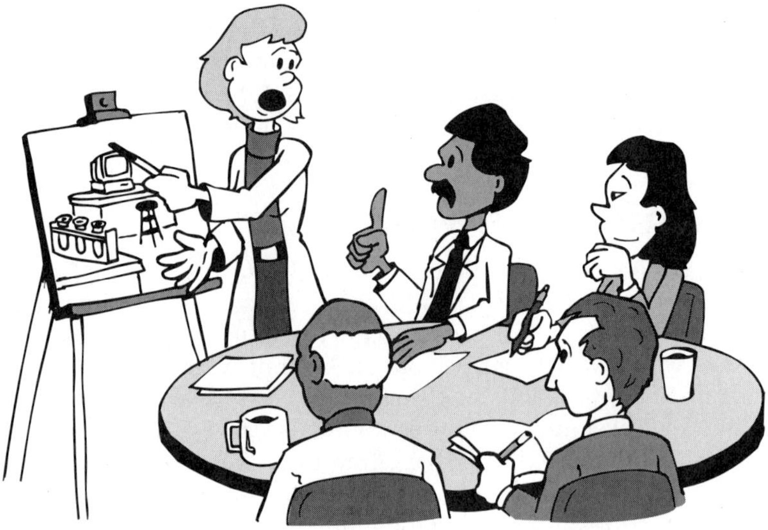

the fact that growth, change, and innovation are essential to keeping your customers (even if they also don't think new is better). Management theorists and practitioners advocate rethinking, creative thinking, experimenting, and validating to achieve new and more clearly defined goals.

Reengineering is defined as "the fundamental rethinking and radical redesign of business processes to achieve dramatic improvements in critical, contemporary measures of performance such as cost, quality, service and speed."[6] Laboratory managers explained that the driving forces for reengineering their laboratories came from developing a set of shared values as two hospitals as one system developed vision and mission statements (Johnson); developing a "fit" of the laboratory into the total health care picture (Lang); and hospitals, pathologists, and staff involvement in integration (Wilson).[7] By involving administrators, staff, and facilitators (consultants), all three managers invested much time discussing and teaching correlations of the big picture of values with a process. They advocated questioning why something is done. They planned to develop and "encourage and support teams toward a common goal . . . and manage staffing changes."[7] They described the "luxury of a phased-in approach," with no loss of staff (several FTEs were shifted to newly created positions), and requiring only several months for the designing process. Johnson reported the following benefits: (1) expanded space; (2) dramatically reduced turnaround time; (3) fewer staff (members) needed to perform clinical testing; (4) medical technologists serving in new information and outreach management duties; (5) expanded staff roles, allowing cross-training and diversity, supervisory roles; (6) reduced utilization; (7) reduced rates of error; and (8) improved clinical outcomes in documented cases with medical technologist interaction at point of care.[7]

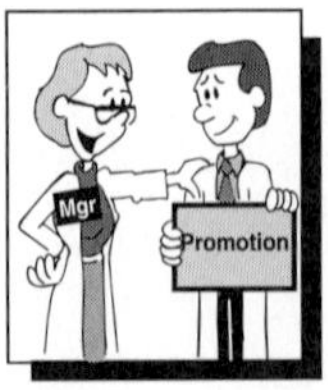

Activity 3: Reengineering Activities: Impact and Value

Discuss each of the eight benefits Johnson reported. What actions do you think were implemented to achieve these benefits? What impact do you think each benefit had on the services and personnel of this laboratory?

Ideas selected for implementation are usually scheduled in phases and assessed immediately. Certain ideas may be tried and discarded or changed, including instrument analyzers or workstation/modular cell arrangement. Work reassignment and staffing mix changes requiring extensive training dictate a thoroughly thought-out plan. All actions to be taken are best accepted and ensured of success if discussed and developed with the laboratory personnel involved. Individuals performing tasks to be changed bring knowledge and solutions when they participate in the decision-making process.

Johnson and colleagues determined the success of the activities implemented by consistently using measurement indicators to provide the data for evaluation. A simple diagram, Figure 13–1, depicts the thought process for resolving a real situation in which the objective was to improve patient services within a general laboratory setting. Actions taken and the evaluation tools used are shown. Could the desired objective be achieved by this plan?

Activity 4: Turnaround Time Improvement

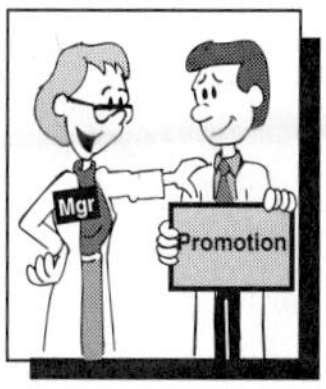

After reviewing Figure 13–1, discuss what value might be attained by achieving the objective. Why do you think fasting blood sugar testing and result reporting are problematic? Discuss implementation strategies of the five actions. Look over the collection of data and statistical evaluation information. What steps would have to be taken to obtain this information? How does not achieving this objective impact on the patient?

See Activity Discussion 1 at the end of this chapter.

In fact, Johnson also reported that more than 100 activities are (still) monitored, one specifically for real-time review of turnaround time on a twice-daily basis.[7]

Reengineering may appear easy and successful. It exacts extraordinary effort from all persons at all levels of the organization. It is a process that demands exceptional management of individuals, resources, and time. Without psychological and political commitment, resistance to change can sabotage the outcome, producing failure. Suggestions generated from more than 100 companies that experienced reengineering projects warrant study:

> . . . communication must be effective, continual, varied, and two-way to reach the diversity of employees . . . commitment must be visible from leaders and top-level managers and . . . expectations must be reinforced through key measurements of managers and employees alike.[8]

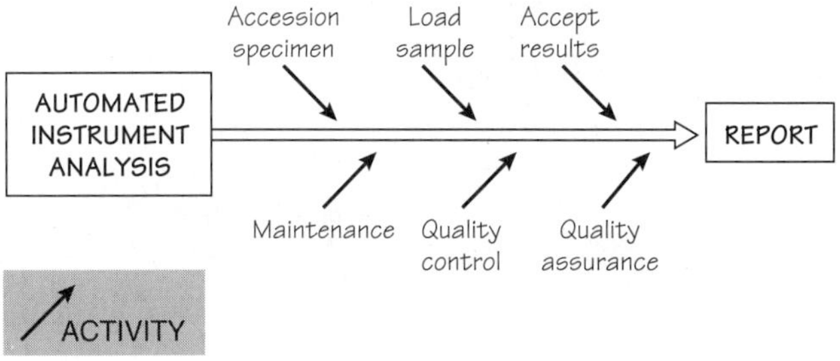

Figure 13–1 Automated specimen analysis.

Methods of Work Performance

Individuals performing tasks often rely on support materials such as basic office supplies, procedure manuals, equipment such as ventilation hoods and computers with appropriate software and programs, and other materials such as counters, drawers, stools, and floor pads. In the laboratory, most work requires special equipment. Examples are safety devices, instruments/analyzers, and specifically designated reagents. Certain functions and tasks pose dilemmas for managers seeking to expand or improve operations, increase safety protection, and reduce tedious repetitive tasks. Increasingly, managers are incorporating automated devices, such as computers and robotics, that are built-in or connected or interfaced with instruments and analyzers. These devices perform redundant manual steps and save labor. Reengineering is proving to facilitate task performance and cost control.

Robotics

Mechanical devices performing tasks usually carried out by personnel offer more benefits by increasing productivity, reducing accidents and injuries, and, in many cases, enhancing reliability. Advantages to using roboticized devices and automated systems stem from improved technology in the mechanics and devices themselves and developments in computer hardware and software. Independently, mobile robots purposefully meander through corridors in hospitals and laboratories, going in and out of rooms, using elevators and carrying information, specimens, meals for patients, and equipment. Routine and repetitive tasks have been programmed into the computer of these devices. (Remember R2D2 in *Star Wars?*)

Further benefits have emerged as workers no longer handle hazardous specimens and reagents: increased volumes can be managed by one facility

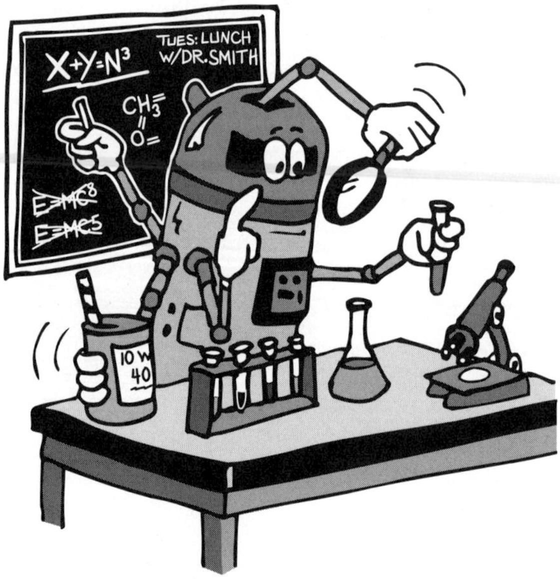

and fewer personnel are needed to perform mundane, repetitive tasks. All these factors affect finances favorably. Still, constraints exist that slow down complete implementation of robotics and automation: technology (converting other business manufacturing technology to health care applications), feasibility, cost, and education of people.

Activity 5: Automation and Robotics

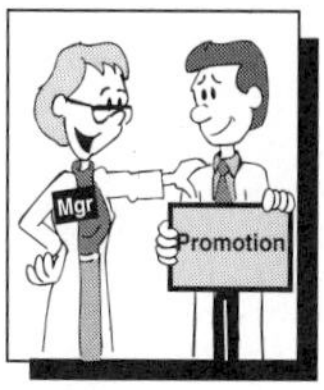

1. Write a brief description of three to five mechanical devices that you have seen and/or used recently at work, for entertainment, in offices, stores, restaurants, or anywhere else.
2. Summarize why you think each device is beneficial.

ERGONOMICS

Environment, composed of physical materials and items, determines the comfort and concentration level maintained by an individual. *Ergonomics,* the Greek word for "the laws of work," describes the science of designing workstations and equipment that are compatible with the human anatomy.

In everyday situations, people encounter hindrances in performing simple activities. Observe: a left-handed person using a pair of scissors designed for right-handed persons, a short person or child washing dishes at a standard height kitchen sink, a professional basketball player stooping down to get through the doorway.

An obvious situation requiring attention to ergonomics is the workstation. The diagram depicted in Figure 13–2 shows the most appropriate measure-

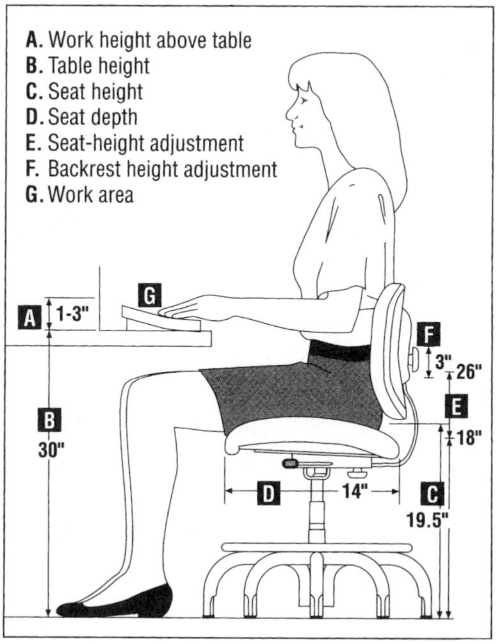

Figure 13–2 Relation of seat height to work level. This diagram has been modified from an advertisement to include printed information included elsewhere in the Biofit brochure. (Courtesy of Biofit Engineered Seating, Waterville, OH.)

ments for a person seated at a standard table height workstation.[9] This company states that "comfort and efficiency of a seated worker depend a great deal upon the relation of the seat height to the work level . . . with an adjustable variation upward or downward to fit the size and body type of the worker."[9] The distance from the floor to the worker's fingers should be at a height between 30 inches and 38 inches, and the chair have a seat adjustment between 18 inches and 26 inches.

Additional concerns address musculoskeletal disorders and illness influenced by environment and biological factors. Environmental factors include demands on the body that exceed working strength and endurance such as heavy lifting, constant twisting, and repeated motions such as pipetting or data entry. Biological factors are the physical characteristics of the worker including size, endurance, range of motion, and strength. If the worker cannot satisfactorily meet the job requirements at any given time, an injury can occur. Injuries known as *cumulative trauma disorders* affect tissues, nerves, tendons, tendon sheaths, and muscles. Six tendon injuries are tendinitis, tenosynovitis, DeQuervain's disease, trigger finger, Raynaud's syndrome, and carpal tunnel syndrome (CTS). Back disorders result from poor posture, lifting too heavy or big items, lifting improperly, and falls. Although laboratories are usually temperature controlled, attention must be paid to handling frozen or hot materials properly. Even if the laboratory is comfortable, hallways and other areas may be hot and humid, causing depletion of energy and fatigue.[10]

Often, work environments are initially accepted by employees without attention to possible discomfort or distress. Noises, especially if loud or constant, can be irritating but over a period of time are adjusted to without complaint. Background or low-level (white) noise, such as music, sounds from instruments, and even talking, can produce subtle irritations causing the worker to be unconsciously distracted. Lighting that creates glare or causes heat, is too strong or too weak, is not directed properly to the work area, or causes reflections or distortions requires attention also. Resulting headaches, fatigue, and personality changes are signals that the work environment is unhealthy. Complaints about room temperature frequently appear on seminar evaluation forms because uncomfortable settings may impair attention span.

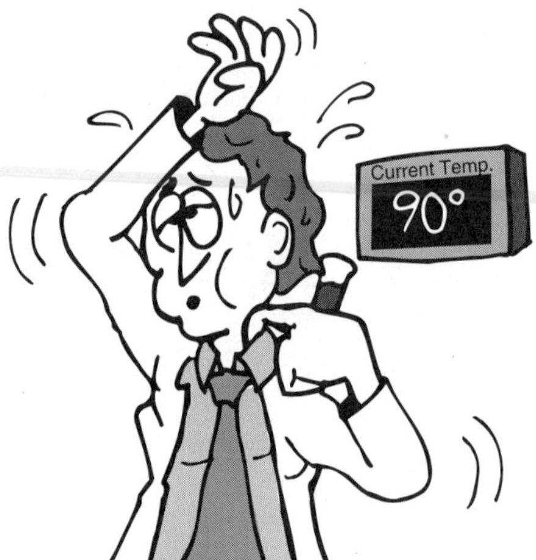

Activity 6: Getting Ergonomically Fit

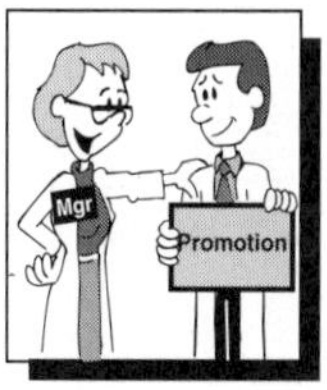

After reviewing the section on ergonomics, consider what practices a manager and other employees could develop to counteract situations potentially capable of causing injury.

Situation	*Action to avoid injury*
Sitting down for long periods of time	______________
Slumping	______________
Bending over a keyboard	______________
Data entry	______________
Telephone user	______________
Reaching for supplies when seated	______________
Reaching for supplies when standing	______________
Repetitive motion	______________

See Activity Discussion 2 at the end of this chapter.

Other considerations that require managers' and employees' attention include needs of physically disabled individuals, accidents not a result of simple clumsiness, awareness of hazards, and lack of safety devices and environmental safety procedures. Education and training, surveillance and reporting, responses and improvements will result in reduced injuries and employee comfort.

Resources Necessary for Work Performance

Depending on services offered by the laboratory, materials (including reagents, supplies, equipment, and instruments) will be identified. Once space is designated, managers must decide on instrument acquisition and inventory maintenance. Trends focus on leasing or renting equipment and instruments. Managers now consider the total cost to generate bigger cost savings and better use of products rather than individual product price.

MATERIALS MANAGEMENT

Practices that contribute to *good material management* consist of the following:

1. Ordering and paying for materials may be beyond an employee's or manager's authority. These processes are carried out most often by purchasing departments handling orders and accounts receivable departments handling all payments. The laboratory manager's responsibilities include communica-

tion with both departments and a follow-up or trigger system to track "lost" orders and approval.

2. Based on annual assessment of need and usage, procedures should be established for ordering and delivering every two weeks, once a month, or quarterly. Inventory management methods maintain adequate supplies and control costs. Establishing the *reorder point* can be based on quantity, when the volume of the item reaches a certain level, or when a designated time is reached (usually at the end of a month, after 30 days, or a combination). Exceptions might be allowed for purchasing more than one product from the same vendor when the price is reduced for both (quantity purchasing) or when a group purchases a larger quantity to reduce the price, or if the vendor is promoting a product and will discount it for a certain volume or period of time.

3. Deviating from procedures based on quantity or time needed to order materials is always expensive. Manufacturing and delivery costs can be exorbitant. Good planning and an inventory monitoring system promote ongoing success.

4. Establish a good working relationship with vendors assigned to your laboratory or area. Manufacturers want to produce and ship materials to receive payment and reduce their own storage time and inventory. Vendors want to serve their customers well.

5. Keep exact records of tests performed by quantity and frequency, supplies consumed, and costs incurred for specific periods. Adjust ordering accordingly if prices can be reduced not only for the item but for the delivery. Order more than one item from the same supplier and share the product with other laboratory sections.

6. Ensure accurate ordering of supplies by maintaining complete detailed records for each item: name (brand and generic), description including amount or number of the item in a single container, manufacturer, catalog number, packaging information (quantity in a box, package, or unit), list price and paid-for price last time purchased, and special ordering instructions. Additional information includes amount used during last period (2 weeks or 30 days) and average use during same period, expiration date if applicable, storage requirements and location, and lead time (longest time lapse between order and receipt). A record-keeping form is shown in Chart 13–1.

7. Investing in computer programs that use bar codes expedites inventory monitoring and managing.

Supplies, Equipment, and Instrumentation

General guidelines used for classifying materials identify *supplies* as those items that are consumable; whose storage lives are a year or less, and/or costs are less than $500. *Equipment and instruments* are those items with an extended use-life, no expiration date (storage life), and/or a cost of more than $500. A diluter costing $475 with a use-life of 5 years is classified as a supply item. It can be ordered directly from a manufacturer and is not depreciated over time. Rather, it is "expensed off" at the end of one year.

Selecting products based on reputation and manufacturer's name often is sufficient. Advertisements promote an item's striking features, but it is

CHART 13–1 RECORD KEEPING FORM FOR MATERIALS MANAGEMENT

Item Inventory Records

Section: Hematology

Materials Manager: *M. Smith*

Item	Unit Count	Usage per Month	Delivery in Weeks	Storage: Location and Requirements	Comments
Acetic acid AR	pint	1	1	acid cabinet	Also used in chemistry
Filter paper	box	1	1	store room	Also used in immunology
Sickle Cell kit	kit	3	1	refrigerator	Also used in PST laboratory
Pipettes	box	250	2	store room	Also used in immunology

Adapted with permission from GPG-A. Inventory control systems for laboratory supplies; Approved guideline. NCCLS, 940 W. Valley Rd., Suite 1400, Wayne, PA 19087. 1994; 14(3): 19–20.

managers' and employees' responsibilities to determine needs and assess whether or not a particular product fulfills that need. Favorable experience with an item provides reasons for buying it again.

"Buy to own" is being replaced by a "lease to upgrade" philosophy, as there are rapid advancements in technology and computerization of equipment and instruments. Standard instrumentation often becomes obsolete within a year. Equally rapid changes come from the transition of research as analyte studies and methodology-analyte studies become clinically significant.

Criteria for acquiring equipment and instruments involve cost and whether or not it has a depreciable life. For example, if an analyzer costs $1,200 with a use-life of 3 years, it will be classified as capital equipment. Capital equipment budgets are usually approved by the organization's board of directors and purchase requires (hospital or financial) administration authorization. The value, beginning at $1,200, is depreciated at the end of each of the first 2 years, ending at zero value the third year.

Five steps provide the rationale for equipment or instrument selection. The first step targets the facility and its strategic plans and needs, projected test offerings, and desired objectives such as improved quality, efficiency, and cost savings. The second step incorporates the specified need requirements gathered previously in developing a request for proposal. Information related to instrument characteristics and features is also sought (Chart 13–2). The third step involves trial of the actual instrument. Comparing currently used instrumentation and prospective replacements assists in determining certain criteria, including accuracy and precision of test results, reliability of opera-

CHART 13–2 REQUEST FOR PROPOSAL QUESTIONS

General
Manufacturer name and location, contact person
Instrument name and model number
Features: standard and optional
Specifications: Dimensions, power, environment

Costs
Price: Purchase/lease/rental agreement
Reagent and supplies price per test
Estimate life length (trade-in/upgrade program)
Other costs: service contract, training fees and expenses

Reagent
Type/s
Volume supplied
Storage: specifications (stability), life/use life within instrument
Consumption per test
Monitoring: supply (low), cross-over (contamination)
Dispensing process—pipettor with vacuum, pressure, etc.
Discard system

Optics and electrical
Light source
Optical system
Electrical requirements
Power surge control

Installation and training
Delivery time (How long before we get it?)
Pre-install environment requirements
On-site or off-site training
Knowledge and skill of trainer
Time required for training
Special requirements (easy or difficult)
Training manuals
Additional personnel: cost and location

Other
Users (Can visits be arranged?)
Use record (query downtime reasons and support) access to comparisons

Characteristics
Tests available: current/future, options (profiles or panels)
User choice of methods: principles of analysis
Throughput: theoretical and actual STAT capability
Processing: discrete or batch
Maintenance: daily start-up, preventive, shutdown
Accuracy and precision of test results

Sample
Type/s
Volume per test (minimum required)
Accessibility
Contamination and evaporation prevention
Dispensing process: auto or manual
Monitoring: amount (short sample)
On-line tray capacity
Auto dilute accessibility

Service
Warranty
Service:
- availability and limitations
- contract and exceptions
- telephone support
- accessibility of service representative
- availability of (repair) supplies and parts

Maintenance system
Reliability record

Supplies
Sample cup
Pipette and tip
Cuvette
Reagent supply system (lines or tubing)
Other

Computer/data management
Type
Storage capacity
Memory (patient files and results)
Delta checks options
Display unit type
Output printer or reader type
Interface mode/requirements
Self-diagnostic capability
Calibration capability
Quality control capability

Trial opportunity

tion, stability of sample and reagents, validity of information that the manufacturer provides, ease of operation, and operator acceptance: what the employees want/trust. The fourth step involves calculating the cost-of-operations and cost justification based on return of investment for each instrument. Comparison of the current instrument to the prospective one follows.

Now make the decision. (The decision-making process is discussed in Chapter 15). Objectivity from using a point system facilitates the process. Points can be allocated for each criterion desired and ranked by importance. Assess the strengths and weaknesses of each instrument, and determine a point value for each strength and weakness offered for each instrument. Consider the acquisition options. Include any other aspects associated with strengths and weaknesses. Tabulate the points. Prioritize the selection.

Organizing Activities and Events

New graduates rarely expect to be given these responsibilities. In the Introduction, the new technologist was told to start a molecular laboratory. Methodical preparation helped this employee to select the equipment, reagents, and instruments needed and to write procedure and SOP manuals.

Organization of a laboratory section or work cell might be improved on the basis of work experience from other situations. Again, new graduates wonder whether their ideas and suggestions are of value. It is not what you tell someone but how you tell them that makes something work. A generalist technologist working the afternoon shift and taking graduate classes in microbiology transferred to the virology laboratory. As he was trained, he quickly saw the inefficiency in the room layout and work flow in this slow-paced, individualized testing laboratory. He learned that all of his coworkers were specialists in microbiology and had worked exclusively in virology for many years. He examined potential changes and cautiously suggested improvements with explanations in work cells when his training was completed in each. As acceptance and trust were gained from his coworkers and the supervisor, he occasionally made the improvement, did his work, and then showed the others how much better the work could be done. Two approaches were used side-by-side by two different technologists with a new combined approach emerging.

Activity 7: Organizing Activities and Events

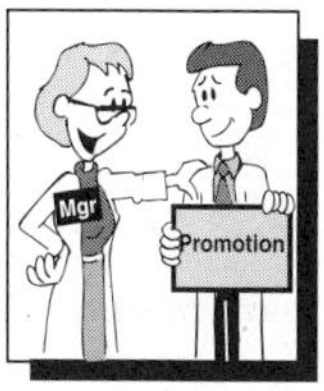

Working in small groups, select a laboratory procedure. Review literature about the test. Identify all resources needed: space, equipment and supplies, reagents, instruments, manuals and other instructions, safety supplies, and equipment. Diagram a possible laboratory section layout, and show items in their designated places.

None of these activities (see Activity 7) were actual changes in steps of the testing procedures or represented noncompliance with safety protocol: the changes were only in manipulations (altering habitual motions), supplies, equipment replacement and location, reagent storage, and record keeping.

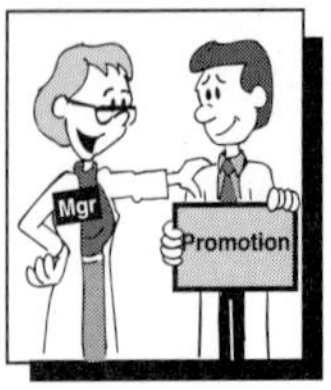

Activity 8: Work-flow Operation

For this activity, work in small groups. Identify an existing laboratory with which you are familiar or have access to: small to mid-size is recommended. Sketch the floor plan and existing fixtures, counters, and cabinets. Use graph paper and estimate sizes. Observe activities occurring in the room, and diagram using arrows for traffic patterns of workers (students) for 1 hour. Compare similarities and differences among types of testing, specimens, methods of testing, equipment, and instruments required. Discuss repetitive and excess movements of the workers. Note times between collecting of specimens, arrival of specimens in the laboratory, and reporting of results on the patient's chart (or to the physician). If using a student laboratory, modify the collection of times according to the activities that are real for this laboratory.

Summary

The organizing function of management constantly changes owing to new and better materials and resources. While striving for efficiency and cost effectiveness, managers face such problems as assessing the needs of customers to be served, selecting and acquiring materials and state-of-the-art instrumentation, and maintaining a smooth flowing and successful operation that achieves the organization's goals.

Selecting tests, job functions, and tasks, establishing a time frame and location when tests need to be done, and identifying personnel to do them are forces to be reckoned with as the laboratory business changes. Opportunities such as outreach programs that laboratories are engaging in dramatically influence change in laboratory operations. Organizing knowledge and skill enables managers to maneuver through unusual and critical circumstances to provide essential services for patient care.

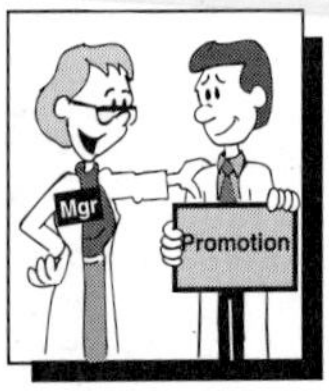

Activity Discussion I: Turnaround Time Improvement

Objective desired	Actions taken	Data collected; statistics evaluated
Fasting AM blood sugar (FBS) results on patient's chart 15 minutes before breakfast tray delivery	1. Begin phlebotomy 0500 2. Tube FBS specimens to lab 3. Run FBS samples on XYZ analyzer in Main Chemistry Lab 4. Verify results in LIS	*Collect data:* 1. Time FBS collected 2. Time FBS specimen received in lab and computer (accessioned) 3. Time FBS results entered in LIS; on patient's chart

5. LIS interfaced with HIS; patient's results available at nursing unit (i.e., on patient's chart)	4. Time breakfast tray delivered to patient *Evaluate statistics:* 1. Number of times FBS results were not on patient's chart 15 minutes before breakfast tray delivery

Activity Discussion 2: Getting Ergonomically Fit

Situation	Action to avoid injury
Sitting for long periods	Do not cross legs (could cause swelling or edema in lower extremities; heart works harder and blood pressure rises). Keep shoulders down and back; avoid hunching over. Adjust chair to fit you. Tilt work surface toward you; right angle is optimal.
Slumping	Gently pull shoulders up to earlobes, hold for 30 seconds, relax shoulders completely; spine will also be pulled up and straightened.
Bending over a keyboard	Sit straight and bend from the hips (prevents pressure on tendons of the shoulder, which could lead to a torn rotator cuff in later years).
Data entry	Position keyboard and wrist rest to appropriate height for you; position monitor and worksheets at appropriate tilt and distance from eyes; after 15 to 20 minutes of concentrated typing, look up to the ceiling or at something 10 to 15 feet away. Take short breaks (3 to 5 minutes) no less than every hour; go to the restroom, drinking fountain, or copier.
Telephone use	Cradle the receiver/mouthpiece on a telephone rest or use a headset. Wipe off the earpiece and mouthpiece after use (by one person) with disinfectant.
Reaching for supplies	Limit reaching to 16 inches beyond work area while seated. Do not lift heavy objects while seated or with one hand. Limit reaching beyond work area to 20 inches while standing. Stand on antifatigue floor mat (maximize foot pressure).
Repetitive motion	Take a break. Vary position of hand or wrist. Stretch extremity slowly.

Review Questions

1. Authority versus responsibility or power means that the person in charge has the
   a. right to direct, invoke compliance, allocate resources.
   b. ability to influence behavior.
   c. obligation to execute tasks and work.
   d. control of finances for income and expenditures.
   e. title, which means employees must do as told.
2. Redesigning a laboratory in order to achieve dramatic improvements in cost, quality, service, and speed is known as
   a. cost containment.
   b. quality assurance.
   c. reengineering.
   d. ergonomics.
3. Using an inventory of supplies method for ordering, stocking, and control, the reorder point is best determined based on
   a. manufacturer's production.
   b. standing orders shipped per month.
   c. quantity needed.
   d. price per item.
4. Of the five steps addressed in the selection of instruments, which of the following should be considered first?
   a. Trial of several instruments in your own laboratory.
   b. Request for proposal submitted to hospital administration.
   c. Visiting other laboratories to see what they are using.
   d. Review of (your) facility's strategic plans.

See p. 410 for answers.

References

1. Snyder JR, Senhauser DA. The nature of management in the clinical laboratory. *In* Snyder JR, Senhauser DA, eds. Administration and Supervision in Laboratory Medicine. 2nd ed. Philadelphia, JB Lippincott, 1989, pp 9 and 34.
2. Hemphill B. Taming the Office Tiger. Richmond, Kiplinger Books & Tapes, 1996.
3. Szilagyi AD, Wallace MJ. Organizational Behavior and Performance. 3rd ed. Glenview, IL, Scott, Foresman, & Co., 1989, p 451–453.
4. Larsen AL, Larsen AL. Authority and delegation. *In* Snyder JR, Senhauser DA, eds. Administration and Supervision in Laboratory Medicine. 2nd ed. Philadelphia, JB Lippincott, 1989, p 137.
5. Lott JA. Quality control and method evaluation. *In* Snyder JR, Senhauser DA, eds. Administration and supervision in laboratory medicine. 2nd ed. Philadelphia, JB Lippincott, 1989, pp 279–284.
6. Hammer M, Champy J: Reengineering the Corporation: A Manifesto for Business Revolution. New York, Harper Collins, 1993.
7. Johnson E, Lang JA, Wilson C. As we see it: reengineering our laboratories. Clinical Laboratory Management Review 1995; 1:60–64.
8. Hall G, Rosenthal J, Wade J. How to make reengineering really work. Harvard Business Review 1993; 6:119–131.
9. Hunter C. BioFit Engineered Seating Company, Waterville, Ohio.
10. Gile TJ. Ergonomics for the laboratory. Clinical Laboratory Management Review 1994; 1:5–7, 10, 12–15, 18.
11. Inventory control systems for laboratory supplies; Approved guidelines. GP6-A. Villanova, PA, National Committee on Clinical Laboratory Standards, 1994, p 14.

Suggested Reading

1. Brzezicki LA. Conquering the causes of cumulative trauma. Advance/Laboratory 1994; 3:20–23.
2. Castañeda-Méndez K. Reengineering: Is it right for your lab? Advance/Laboratory 1994; 6(9):16–21.
3. Cortizas ME, Shea M. Specimen processing: Centralized or decentralized? Clinical Laboratory Management Review 1996; 10(3):221–230.
4. Drucker PF. The new society of organizations. Harvard Business Review 1992; 70(5):95–104.
5. Editors. Technology. Answering the call of ergonomics. Advance/Laboratory 1994; 6(3):24–25, 58.
6. Hammer M. Reengineering work: don't automate, obliterate. Harvard Business Review 1993; 71(4):104–112.
7. Hemphill B. Taming the Paper Tiger. Richmond, Kiplinger Books & Tapes, 1995.
8. Johnson E. Reengineering the laboratory: strategic process and systems innovation to improve performance. Clinical Laboratory Management Review 1995; 9(5):370–380.
9. Lamm RD. Health care heresies: tomorrow's health care reality. Clinical Laboratory Management Review 1995; 9(9):88–89.
10. Lang JA. Laboratory restructuring at United Health Laboratories: a move to self-directed teams. Clinical Laboratory Management Review 1995; 9(5):423–429.
11. Lathrop JP. Restructuring Health Care: The Patient-Focused Paradigm. San Francisco, Josey-Bass Publishing, 1994.
12. Manganelli RL, Klein MM. The Reengineering Handbook: A Step-By-Step Guide to Business Transformation. New York, AMA-COM, 1995.
13. O'Brien CO. This month, fifteen years, and after. Ergonomics 1984; 28(8):831–832.
14. Polancic J. CLIA '88 compliance: Verification of methods. Clinical Laboratory Science 1994; 7(2):79–82.
15. Stewart TA. Reengineering: the hot new management tool. Fortune 1993; 8:40–48.
16. Winston S. The Organized Executive: New Ways to Manage Time, Paper, People and the Electronic Office. New York, W.W. Norton & Co. Inc., 1994.

Additional Reference

U.S. Department of Labor. Occupational Safety and Health Administration. Federal Register 29 CFR 1910. Ergonomic Safety and Health Program Management Guidelines. Jan. 26, 1989; 54(16):3904–3916.

14

Directing: The Third Management Function

OBJECTIVES

Upon completion of this chapter, the reader should be able to:

- Define directing and explain the value of effective directing on personnel and productivity.
- Describe three supervisor skills that enhance understanding of employees and colleagues.
- Explain the process of effective communication.
- Select communication techniques appropriate for particular situations based on their advantages and disadvantages.
- Define motivation and describe how an employee becomes motivated by both external and internal influences.
- Given selected "dissatisfiers," describe how each can be controlled or altered in order to prevent declining employee morale.
- Describe the process of delegating.
- Given a list of tasks, select those appropriate for the supervisor only and those appropriate for delegates. Briefly explain reasons for your choices.
- Compare and contrast benefits and drawbacks of delegating.
- Compare and contrast managing behaviors versus coaching behaviors; explain the effectiveness of each approach based on their similarities and differences.

KEY WORDS

directing

communicating

motivating

delegating

coaching

Introduction

Keep in mind that the primary goal of management (supervision) is effective work production. Regardless of the type of work involved, the process of producing work must be *directed*. Managers and supervisors guide employees on what the work is, how it should be done, and how the results will be measured as the essential foundation for the directing function.

Tools, techniques, and other resources for doing the work must be available for employees, and employees must be trained to perform assigned functions and tasks in order to accomplish the work. They must also demonstrate appropriate attitudes (Affective Domain, see Chapter 4). Guidelines, consisting of clear directives, provide employees with knowledge and essential skills necessary to perform their work. Directives, which often come from top-level administration and owners but emanate from external sources as well as from within the organization, assist managers in establishing the directing process.

In this chapter, four elements of the *directing* function are explained: communicating, motivating, delegating, and coaching. Because human interaction exists throughout each day for most people, heightening this experience by removing barriers and overcoming misunderstandings will generate more effective communication. Getting people to do their best or what will achieve the organization's goals, that is, what's "good for them" or what will satisfy customers, offers more challenges. Principles and methods of motivation are described. Delegation supplies efficiency and effectiveness to work operations while promoting skill development and professional growth for many laboratorians. Accomplishing desired outcomes at the optimal level, in a timely manner and efficiently, mandates skillful coaching by the boss/manager or co-worker/leader.

The Directing Function: Essential Skills

Directing implies concern for the operation and the process of running it smoothly. Successful directing arises from a human relations approach to management. Attitudes of managers and supervisors support the concept that people like to work and want to work when their goals are compatible with those of the organization.

Directing consists of issuing orders, conveying expectations, sharing organizational goals and objectives, and emphasizing the need for employees to work. When communicating with the employee, the supervisor should give directions that are clear and readily understood, explicit reasons why work must be done, logical applications in completing the work, and encouragement to employees to use their own creativity and imagination. At one time, many employees were commanded to do their work. Now, employees are directed to be involved when managers and supervisors incorporate empowerment strategies into their approach. Empowerment—giving of responsibility and authority as a "direction"—enables employees to develop their own work, monitor their own productivity, and assess outcomes themselves.

The human element in the directing process must involve sincere understanding among managers, supervisors, and employees. This includes recognition of their differences, styles of work, needs, sources of motivation, and responses to each other's style. Awareness of the knowledge, skills, abilities, interests, and special talents of employees produces significant advantages for supervisors and managers in the workplace. As the most complex interpersonal aspect of management, this does not happen overnight, nor is it easy. When effort is exerted to achieve this basic relationship, employees enjoy their work and feel that their contributions are important and valued. The results of effectively directing work are measurable:

- The operation will begin and end on time.
- Absenteeism and avoidance of work will decrease.
- Potential problems can be prevented.
- Solutions to problems will be offered.
- Results will reflect an increase in quantity and quality of services or products.

Directing becomes the catalyst, the enzyme, and the link between the beginning functions (planning and organizing) and ending functions (coordinating and evaluating) of management. It is like someone hitting the "Go" button to start the roller coaster up the ramp.

COMMUNICATION, THE KEY ELEMENT OF *DIRECTING*

Communication exists as a process for people to relate to each other in the workplace, at home, at school, and throughout the community. The number of books in libraries and bookstores, articles in journals and popular magazines, and expensive seminars demonstrates the growing concern regarding effective communication.

Nature of Communicating

We communicate to disseminate facts, share ideas, gain approval, refute disapproval, and dispense assignments. The manner by which one person communicates to another helps establish rapport with that person. Business consultants vouch that communication is the number one problem in most workplaces; counselors reiterate that communication is the number one problem for interpersonal relationships. Communication processes can be viewed as several channels: multidirectional, going from the top down, side-to-side, down up to the top, and diagonally across levels (Fig. 14–1). Multiple efforts throughout an organization are organized to maintain communication for all affected, including the "customers"—patients and their families, physicians and vendors, and the community at large.

Becoming adept at the art of communication takes practice. Efforts to develop and maintain open communication lines prevent communication breakdown and the possible downturn effect on productivity. Managers spend 85% in a single day in some form of communication: primarily speaking and listening and, to a lesser extent, writing and reading. All phases of the management process depend on some mode of communication. Equally important in the communicating process is *listening* and seeking feedback to validate that the message was understood.

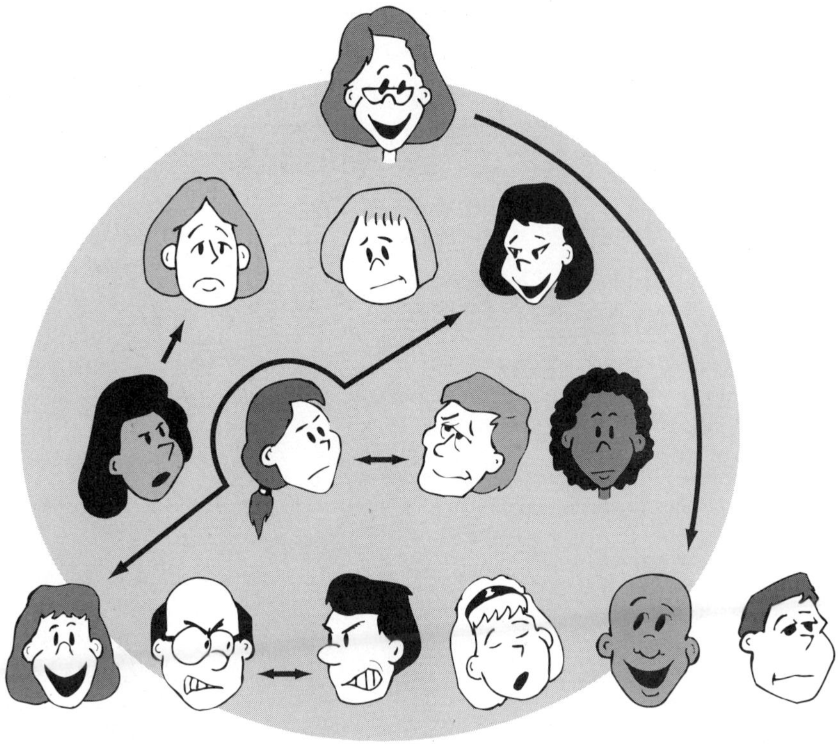

Figure 14–1 Formal communication channels.

Methods of Communicating

Communication flows from the "sender" as a transfer of information to a "receiver." Most often, senders speak or write their messages. Receivers listen or read in response. Methods, called *channels* or *media*, may vary according to style of the sender, the situation, and the content of the message itself.

Use of *verbal* communication fulfills a sender's objectives immediately. *Written* communication provides documentation: that is, a paper trail. The sender has proof of the message. In Table 14–1, advantages and disadvantages

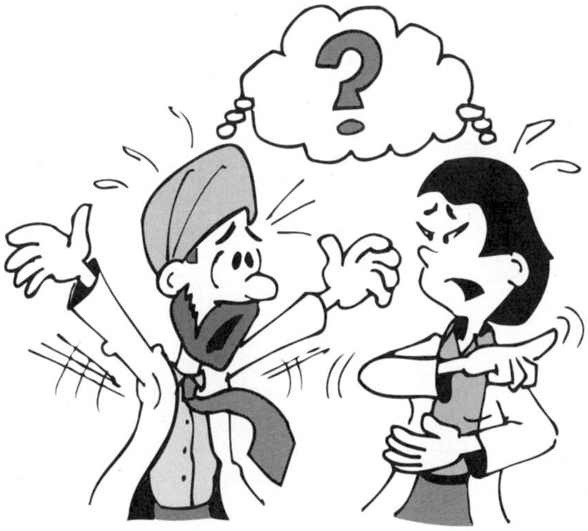

Table 14–1
COMPARING SPOKEN VS WRITTEN COMMUNICATION TECHNIQUES

Spoken
Pluses
Immediate feedback
Quick; saves time
Can engage other(s) for exchange of information
Can be warm, motivating, inspiring, friendly
Can capture attention of receiver
Reinforced by other techniques: body language, tone of voice, eye contact, phrases
Minuses
Jargon or idioms can confuse
Cannot save perceptions
Intended message may not be interpreted the same by all receivers
Other techniques (body language, written) may confuse receiver if different from words
Cannot retract words once said
Receiver may not be able to control sender's style without being equally rude, rambling, condescending, or chauvinistic
Written
Pluses
Paper trail: documentation of communication
Same message to many receivers
Convey multiple facts at one time
Allows reader to review, reconsider, rethink before responding
Messages can be consolidated, succinct, and direct
Can support with drawings, diagrams, and the like
Minuses
Feedback delayed
May be perceived as impersonal
May not capture attention, interest, or response of reader
Takes time
Need for clarification is unknown
Final

Table 14–2
OTHER COMMUNICATION METHODS

Body language	Stance or sitting; posture; moving or holding arms, hands, legs and (even) feet
Facial expressions	Movements made with eyes and mouth, chin, and forehead tell a lot. A stern look can mean disapproval while a smile is the opposite: approval.
Nonword oral expressions	Grunts, chuckles, smacking lips, grinding teeth
Pictures or graphics	Photographs, paintings, diagrams, designs, squiggles, doodles, cartoons, caricatures
Silence	Absence of not saying or doing anything often conveys significant positive and negative information.
Sounds	Music, air, noise (made by people) such as tapping (or drumming) fingers on a table, clapping hands (as in applause), whistle

Table 14–3
TEN TIPS ON TALKING

1. State *one* idea at a time
2. *Develop* the idea by explaining, illustrating, inviting questions
3. *Restate* it—check for understanding; listen
4. Say it *simply* and *clearly*
5. Make it *brief* and to the point
6. Relate it *specifically* to the person and the workplace
7. Get *acceptance* of this idea; listen
8. Pay attention to *emotions*
9. Call for *action*: agreement, commitment
10. *Encourage, reassure, praise*

of using these two predominant methods are listed. Other methods of communicating are highlighted in Table 14–2.

More than words convey a message. Several techniques work well for both outgoing, friendly people and shy, quiet people in relating to others. These skills encourage feedback and response.

Spoken Communications. Several logical steps that make up a spoken message are listed in Table 14–3. What is not said can be as important as what is said. Use *silence* to indicate: "I want you to tell me more," or "I'm thinking about what I will say to you," or "You have my attention, but not necessarily affirmation (agreement)." This is especially effective during an interview.

Include a *pause* when delivering a message to allow it to "sink in." A slow, deep, quiet breath helps vocal and delivery problems. It also allows a shift in theme or momentum of message delivery, or a break in tension if emotional levels escalate.

- *Think* before speaking (even when writing); then *rethink*: "Is this what I really want my audience to know?"
- *Define* your meaning. *Denote* or be explicit: *mother* is the term/noun for female parent. *Connote* or suggest/imply: the term *mother*, noun or verb, conveys love, tenderness, care.
- Use *courtesy*. This is one of the best ways to convey appreciation and respect of others.

Telephone talking leaves a different impression between the sender and receiver. Courtesy ranks highest on the telephone etiquette list. Identify yourself and verify the identity of person on the line. Be personable to create rapport and develop trust. Voice tone, rate of speech, and volume tell much about the interest and sincerity of the speakers. When leaving a voice-mail message, follow memo/e-mail suggestions, steps 1 through 5 under Tips for Writing your Memo and E-Mail; see boxed area. Keep in mind that the person (receiver) can only *hear* your message. It's important that you plan what you are going to say before dialing rather than rambling on and on and on when you're on the line. A succinct but detailed message prepares the receiver to respond. Caution: your message may be heard by persons other than the intended receiver.

Genuine *listening* includes using ears, eyes, and heart—an activity that requires particular skills to understand the real meaning of what we hear and observe—and what we *don't* hear but sense: silence, omissions, trust between individuals, body language, and appearance of eyes. Active listening tech-

TIPS FOR WRITING YOUR MEMO AND E-MAIL

1. Address *one* idea per message. Indicate the topic in the "Re:" line; this alerts the receiver to what the message concerns.
2. Describe the issue in the first paragraph.
3. Get to the heart of the message. Are you asking for a response? Do you want the recipient to take action? If the message is "for your information (FYI)" only, reconsider sending it.
4. Add any support information or detail in subsequent paragraphs. Don't include minor or irrelevant information.
5. Keep it readable; that is, use a font appropriate for business messages (Courier, CG Times or Universal versus script, italics, shadowed) and lower case. All upper case letters wear out one's eyes. Keep paragraphs short and use bullets to identify key points.
6. Read your message.
   - Is it clear? Will the receiver understand it?
   - Check spelling, grammar, and punctuation (although this is less important).
7. Save a copy of your message (if important) for yourself. (Although it is commonly thought that business electronic messages are saved somewhere, somehow within the institution as required by "communications" licensing, this may not be true.)

Table 14–4
FIVE FACTORS FOR FAVORABLE LISTENING

1. Eliminate physical barriers
   - Move out of busy area
   - Remove furniture between you and others (desk, chair)
   - Circle chairs for a group
   - Adjust physical distance (not too close, nor too far)
   - Ensure privacy
2. Listen to words and behaviors
   - Separate fact from gossip and opinion from hearsay
   - Identify emotional content
   - Confirm that observed behavior matches verbal message
   - Identify what real message is if delivery is covert (concealed)
   - Hear at 400 words per minute, and speak at 170 words per minute, so you've got lots of time to think
3. Restate what you heard
   - Validate intent and content
   - Confirm accuracy of facts
   - Be active in the communication process
   - Identify perceptions
4. React to message
   - Verify understanding: nod, smile, frown, say "go on"
   - Remain objective, neutral
   - Identify what the sender wants from you
   - Avoid evaluation and defensive responses
5. Summarize
   - Brief review
   - Who will do what
   - When will action be complete

niques use concentration on the sender; reduction of "distractors" from one's self, the setting, or others; and the giving of feedback for understanding. Burley-Allen advises a communicator to start listening to the inner self and to remove negative influencers, then to focus on others.[1] Listening also takes practice (Table 14–4).

Nonverbal Communications. Use *body language* to duplicate or reinforce a spoken message. Avoid sending a conflicting message that confuses the receiver. A person displays confidence and calm when standing or sitting erect: back straight, chin level with the floor, shoulders back, tummy pulled in, arms and hands relaxed at one's side, feet flat on the floor. Good posture indicates interest and enthusiasm and projects self-esteem.

Eyes making contact, especially during lectures and talks, express the point, "I'm interested and I think what you have to say is important." Avoiding eye contact signals uncertainty of the receiver's position relative to the sender. Employees sense unconcern or lack self-confidence with them when managers don't look them in the eye.

Activity 1: Interpreting Body Language Messages

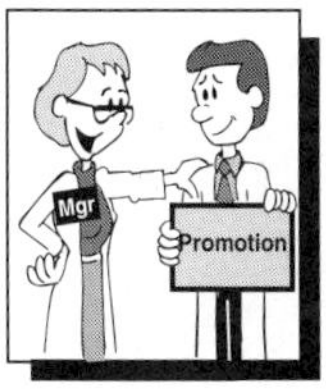

Discuss the message you think each of the following illustrations sends:

1. Posture
   - hand on hip
   - droopy eyelids → asleep
   - arms crossed
2. Gesture
   - finger on chin, against cheek
   - hand on head, leaning sideways, elbow on chair arm
   - pointing finger
   - hands clenched
   - drumming fingers on chair arm
3. Facial expression
   - smile
   - big eyes, mouth in an "O"
   - eyebrows tightened, corners of mouth down
   - stoic
   - blank, staring
4. Eye-to-eye contact
   - looking away
   - looking at watch or clock

5. Body image
   - far apart/almost touching
   - leaning toward other person
   - both seated at same level
   - sender standing (receiver sitting)

Written Communications. Memo and e-mail communications, even though intended for only *one* person, should *not* be considered confidential! The writing style one uses for either of these quick and direct contacts with another person differs from that used with other written modes (Table 14–5).

Informal Communications: The Grapevine. Often called the nervous system of an organization, the grapevine exists as a fact of life. The grapevine is an informal channel of communication among employees: managers recognize that they cannot control it. However, with certain skills they can influence it. Not much different from formal channels of communication in the workplace, the grapevine transmits information and carries attitudes. A grapevine is fast and nonselective: any message at any time to anyone might be carried. Information passed informally instead of through timely formal communication can lead to repercussions: employees can be misinformed, become disgruntled, and tolerate obstruction of their work production. Attuned managers understand their organization's grapevine and simply ask of trusted, conscientious employees, "What do you hear that I should know?"

Patterns. Formal and informal communication diagrams, called *patterns* (Fig. 14–2), represent structured as opposed to loose configurations. The effectiveness of each depends on the work environment and the specific situation.

Table 14–5
SEVEN CLUES FOR WRITING

1. Use the following techniques to secure attention:
   - **Bold typeface**
   - Underlining
   - S p a c i n g
   - *Italics*
   - Page set-up (use a box)
   - Colored paper (create a trademark—mine's purple)
   - Symbols, icons, caricatures
2. Adapt for the reader.
3. Be tactful, courteous, use good taste.
4. Material should be clear, precise, no jargon, readable: geared to reader's ability.
5. Use the appropriate style
   - Conversational
   - Forceful
   - Persuasive
   - Active or passive
   - Humorous
6. Be helpful.
7. Leave the reader with a favorable impression.

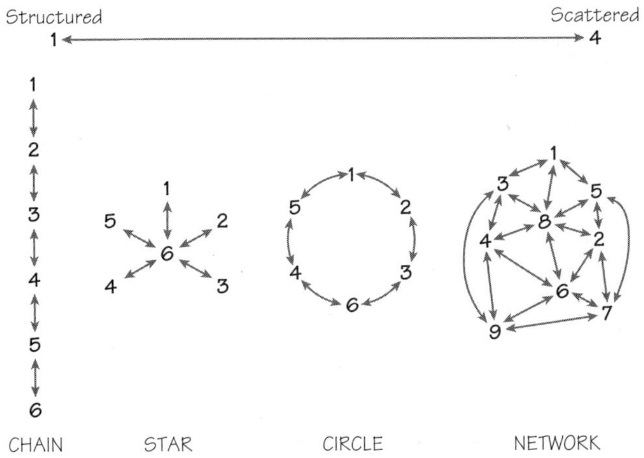

Figure 14–2 Patterns of communication.

Activity 2: Methods of Communication

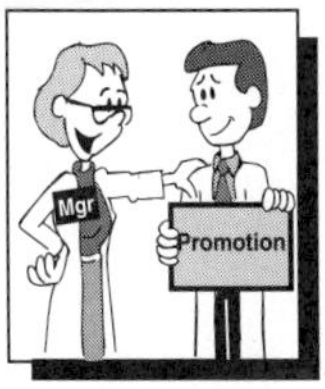

Describe methods of communication that you use derived from your own experiences. Explain the methods and descriptors that give pleasure or happiness, are positive, and encourage or uplift feelings. Just the opposite, which ones make you unhappy or feel negative or sad? What other emotions and reactions might be triggered by communication? Discuss with your group methods that are better for work and professional situations than for family and personal situations. Describe those important for use by health care professionals and ones that might be more closely associated with religion, politics, or news (TV or paper media). Discuss situations in which managers need (or should have) or lack (or should squelch) a grapevine.

Barriers to Effective Communication

Difficulties found within the communication process come about through barriers. What are these and why do they happen? Once a manager is aware of a barrier, his/her task becomes focused on dissolving or controlling it. Barriers detected and removed easily have been identified as *physical*: noise on the telephone line, static across the TV screen, too small type or print, electrical interference on a computer screen, colors in a room (walls, ceiling, and flooring), improperly using or not using a hearing aid, poor furniture or work equipment arrangements, uncomfortable temperature of a room, and even a seat that's too hard.

Other less detectable or correctable impediments consist of *verbal* modes of delivery that encompass speech patterns such as ending a statement on a high note (translates the statement into a question); using a condescending or patronizing tone of voice, soft or loud/gentle or harsh pitch of voice or slurred words; facing and talking to the chalkboard by an instructor; and using incomplete sentences or inadequate vocabulary.

Semantic barriers specifically regard language. The listener (receiver) who is unfamiliar with the English language cannot discern shades of meanings. Jargon (slang), obscure symbols, idioms, colloquialisms (words or phrases peculiar to a region or locale), or graphics might be difficult for someone to interpret. *Psychological* barriers encompass those based on the nature of individuals: preconceived expectations, self-awareness, assumptions by either the sender or the receiver or both, or attitude regarding the sender's opinion ("I'm not wrong!"). Others include lack of attention, selective screening of information before passing it on, power and status perceptions, lack of empathy, threat of change, a defensive mind set, misinterpretation, negativism, and jealousy. Even humor added with best intentions, if offensive to the receiver, can destroy the intended message.

Personality characteristics influence communication: the person who jumps to conclusions, who is closed or narrow minded, has tunnel vision, listens only to words, or reads only what is written. If these characteristics are to be altered, managers must use perseverance and exceptional skill: convince, cajole, and motivate.

Other barriers that can affect the context of messages include ethnicity, leadership and managerial styles, age, and education. Reports indicate that men and women communicate differently. Both sexes use humor and small talk in different ways to generate a comfortable atmosphere. Men tend to be direct and more to the point, whereas women tend to be subtle and provide detailed explanations to arrive at their points.

Phrasing questions and choice of verbs can deter a response. Certain words block persuasion; examples are "should," "have to," "must," and "ought to." By culture and socialization, senders use these words but receivers turn off the rest of the message.

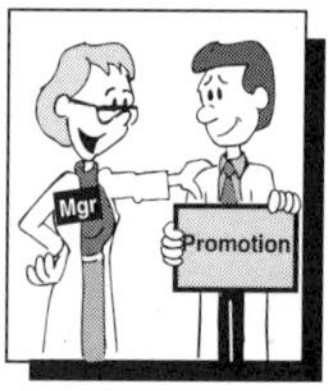

Activity 3: Barriers to Effective Communication

Describe barriers you've observed or encountered. How did you become aware of them? Describe techniques to effectively overcome barriers.

Advice For Better Communication

Supervisors should plan and organize the environment and time for exchange of communication. They can control the receptiveness of employees to the communication by acting in a supportive and positive manner. All three conditions (place, time, and attitude) should be mutually acceptable before the exchange.

Determining the most effective method requires thinking about the situation. The following questions help determine the controlling process. Who will be involved? Where should the communication take place? Is an immediate response or action needed? Is the message private—that is, intended for one person or designated individuals only? What resources are available for sending the message if not face-to-face communication? Finally, what assurance should be obtained that the message was both received and understood?

When messages are not understood, managers and supervisors must try to communicate again, either by clarifying the original message or by using a different method. Sometimes, acknowledging differences without trying to change the other person or adapting to the other person's situation are sufficient to prepare to send the message again. As effective communicators, managers acquire a variety of communication skills and learn when to use the appropriate one. They figure out how to deal with people whose personalities aren't likable. They make it a point to become known for their courtesy, professionalism, interest in employees, and ability to make correct interpretations.

Occasionally, a receiver thinks the sender wants a response that is an opinion, a judgment, or approval or disapproval. It requires skill to identify when feedback—especially evaluation—isn't really wanted at all: for example, when the sender really only wants someone to listen.

Why Communicate?

All of these tips, tricks, and techniques involve the use of common sense about courtesy toward others. Communication between managers and employees supports performance and work. With practice in these techniques, skills expand and comfort increases; interactions improve and mistakes can be avoided. Others will be convinced of your sincerity and will respond favorably. The goal of getting the work done will be achieved.

MOTIVATING: THE INSPIRATION ELEMENT OF *DIRECTING*

Motivation is defined as a condition of influencing oneself to move or act in a given direction.[2] Motivation stems from what a person wants or needs. Figure 14–3 shows a model of the motivating process. A person becomes motivated through initial awareness of a need, identifying it, selecting strategies to satisfy it, acting out the chosen strategy, and evaluating whether or not it worked.

Managers, through supervisors, provide tangible motivators: environment, conditions, resources, and rewards. They can also provide intangible motivators: encouragement, praise, and recognition. Motivators can precipitate good behavior and acceptable performance **or** noncompliance, bad behavior, and poor performance by a person. The laboratory, although devoted to relatively strict policies and methodologies for doing the work, can become an environment favorable to high morale. The difference is made by people. Psycholo-

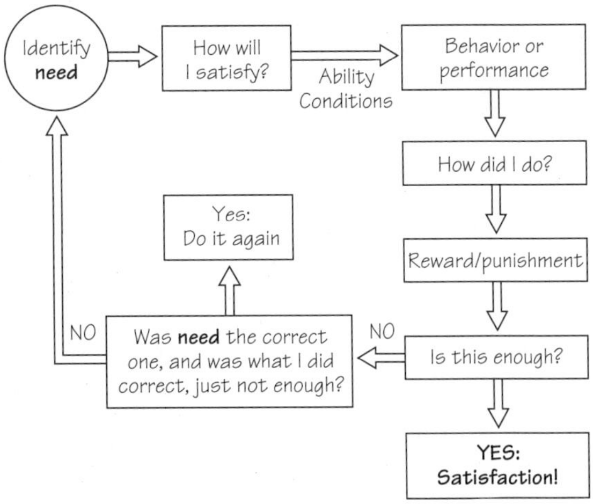

Figure 14–3 Basic motivational model. (Modified from Szilagyi AD, Wallace MJ, Jr: Organizational Behavior and Performance, 3rd ed. Glenview, IL: Scott, Foresman and Co; 1983.)

gists advise: What gets rewarded, gets repeated. What gets ignored, doesn't get done.

Motivation Theories

Several theories promote various motivational factors. One of the first researchers, Frederick Taylor, studied work as the factor that controlled worker efficiency primarily through pay. This approach was termed *scientific management.* Douglas McGregor subsequently espoused the human element in this approach through two theories. Theory X characterized traditional beliefs that people disliked work, needed to be forced to work, and wanted close supervision. Theory Y characterized opposing beliefs that physical and mental effort for work was as natural as it was for play; people would work if they were committed to organizational goals and rewarded for achieving objectives. They desired responsibility and opportunity to be creative because they weren't taxed intellectually doing modern industrial work. This theory remains valid today, although goals are often personal rather than those of the organization.

Theories were reported regarding factors that start, arouse, or energize human behavior. Abraham Maslow based his studies on three hypotheses: (1) needs influence the behavior of people, (2) needs rank in order of importance, and (3) people progress from basic to complex needs when the needs at each level are minimally satisfied. From these assumptions, Maslow derived five levels of needs: physiological, safety and security, social, ego and status and esteem, and self-actualization (Fig. 14–4).[3]

Frederick Herzberg proposed two distinct motivational factors. One, hygiene factors, refers to extrinsic conditions that, even if present, do not motivate; this leads to job dissatisfaction. Job-related conditions consist of salary, job security, working conditions, fringe benefits, status, company policies, and quality of worker relationships. The second, intrinsic conditions, called *motivators*, similar to Maslow's higher-ranked factors, helps build motivation and increase work performance, hence job satisfaction. These are less easy to define: achievement, recognition, the work itself, responsibility, advancement, and personal growth and development.[4]

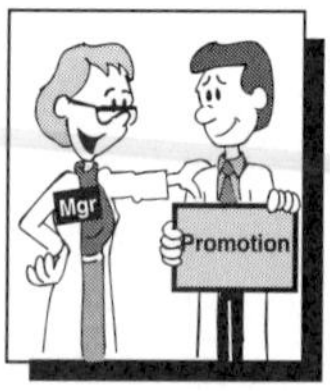

Activity 4: Fulfillment of Needs

Write a brief outline of your needs at this stage in your life. Describe what fulfills each of those needs for you. Discuss for laboratory professionals—phlebotomists, technicians, technologists, supervisors, educators, managers, and pathologists—how their needs at each level might be fulfilled.

Among other theories, the reinforcement theory related to learning concepts will be briefly described. Reinforcement emphasizes objective and measurable behaviors such as quantity of work accomplished, faithfulness to budget, and time and plans versus intrinsic ones such as motives and desires.[5] Four types of reinforcement can modify an employee's motivation: (1) *positive*: praise or pay raise for exceptional performance to increase repetition of the good behavior; (2) *punishment*: denying requests or privileges (pay deductions, loss of continuing education opportunities) informs employees that

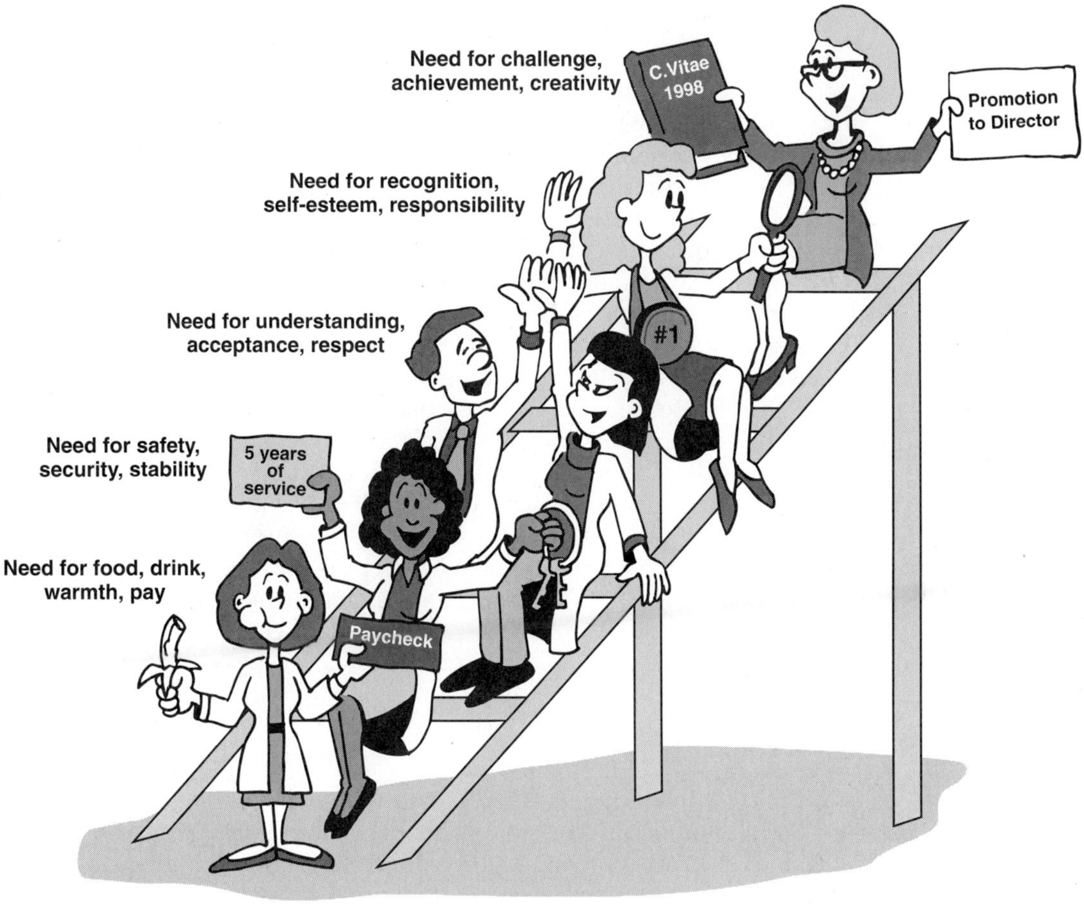
Need for challenge, achievement, creativity
C.Vitae 1998
Promotion to Director
Need for recognition, self-esteem, responsibility
Need for understanding, acceptance, respect
#1
Need for safety, security, stability
5 years of service
Need for food, drink, warmth, pay
Paycheck

Figure 14–4 A hierarchy of human needs. (Data from Maslow A: Motivation and Personality. New York: Harper and Row; 1970.)

their behavior is unacceptable and should be decreased or not be repeated; (3) *negative*: strengthens desired behavior similar to positive reinforcement but the employee works harder to avoid the consequences such as reprimands or criticisms; and (4) *extinct*: withhold or deny the reinforcer. In one situation, to cut costs, administrators stopped awarding gift certificates for yearly perfect attendance. Employees then perceived that absenteeism was acceptable, and sick-time increased significantly among the employees. The cost-savings strategy backfired because a desirable behavior was stopped. Preferred *extinct* reinforcers eliminate undesired behaviors such as loss of telephone privileges for making (excessive) personal phone calls during work time.

Note that of the four reinforcers, three suggest actions by managers, without careful thought and planning, that produce undesired behaviors by employees. This helps explain why it is so difficult to maintain high efficiency and high levels of productivity.

Principles of Motivation

Four categories describe fundamental principles of motivation (see Four Principles of Motivating). These principles take into account the people chosen for a specific task, expectation of how it will be done, and effectiveness of their work and the product, service, or result. Empowerment and delegation differ in the authority extended to employees. *Empowering* employees gives them the privilege to choose assignments among themselves and make decisions for which they have (almost) complete authority. *Delegation* refers to handing over designated assignments to selected employees, who perform various duties ranging from basic to complex with minimal supervision.

Recognition of some kind should exist for all activity and work performance. It should not be based on an "all or none" philosophy. Partially completed or tried and failed attempts should be appropriately recognized. Positive aspects of work and strengths gained by employees should be emphasized. Rewards or other recognition should correspond to the activity or work.

The *self-fulfilling prophecy* purports that whatever the expectations, opinions, thoughts, or beliefs are of another or of oneself will come true or be verified as true. Telling someone, "Of course, I know you can do it!" gives him/her confidence to do the task. Asking someone, "I value your opinion; what do you think of this situation?" encourages that person to think and contribute. Made by a manager known for his high standards and employee recognition, the statement "Our goal is to increase productivity by 20% for the next quarter," will generate a frenzy among the employees to reach 120%! A supervisor who is in school can encourage an employee to enroll in graduate classes. The employee will think, "If the supervisor can do it with his other commitments, so can I!"

Motivators and Reinforcers

Convinced that motivation comes from within a person and is intrinsic, most managers leave their employees alone. Others corral colleagues and employees and set about to create an atmosphere that stimulates achievement. They advocate this as their primary responsibility, and it takes 70% of their time. This activity "sends" positive messages that the manager cares, is paying attention, will help resolve problems, communicates expectations and the role employees play in achieving them, and praises for work done well. It remains with the employees to fulfill the expectations.

For certain tasks—particularly sales, marketing, and scores on exams—rewards should be identified at the onset of performance and distribution of rewards clearly described. Tangible rewards, usually gifts, if appropriate for the task, are valued by employees. Some administrators prorate rewards among workers so that everyone receives something; they give higher-valued rewards for significant productivity and lesser-valued but useful items for completion of any of the quarterly goals. Tangible rewards might be lunch or dinner or tickets to a hockey game, congratulatory letters, or thank you notes. Intangible rewards include praise, compliments, and applause.

Regardless of the theory or the methods of implementing motivating

FOUR PRINCIPLES OF MOTIVATING

1. Empower employees.
2. Delegate work.
3. Recognize employees' accomplishments.
4. Positive feedback becomes a self-fulfilling prophecy.

factors selected, rewards should be contingent upon employees' performance rather than nonperformance-related behaviors (what a person does outside of the workplace). Recognition programs for employee productivity and satisfaction should be implemented.[6]

Activity 5: Motivating Workplace and Professional Factors

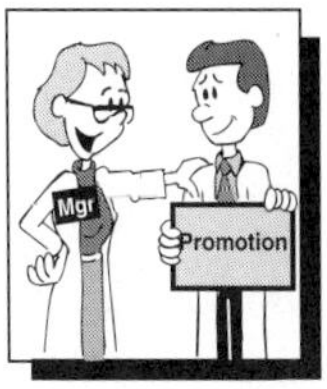

Identify tasks and activities that laboratorians perform in the clinical laboratory and as leaders in professional societies. Describe at least one tangible and one intangible motivating factor for each and an appropriate reward or recognition. Discuss what "motivates" laboratorians to do quality work and be involved and professionally active.

"Dissatisfiers"

Various factors in the workplace can cause dissatisfaction among employees, which leads to reduced incentive to perform or excel. Awareness of new behavior patterns, not typical of employees, should trigger concern. Employee complaints, absenteeism, resignations, or mistakes are symptoms of dissatisfaction. Attentive supervisors will attempt to uncover aspects of the work environment as potential causes (unless the cause is the supervisor). Review Maslow's need hierarchy (see Fig. 14–4). Psychological work factors can become dissatisfiers. Employees tolerate working short-staffed for only a limited period. Some will work for less money initially, then expect compensation for their experience, and if compensation is not forthcoming, will leave. When general working conditions become poor, or what was promised does not materialize, employees will react negatively.

Additional factors include threatened job security, reduced benefits (decreased or eliminated pay raises or earned time off), increased cost of health care coverage, harassment, unfair policies, favoritism demonstrated by supervisors, or inadequate training (with resultant incompetence). Dissatisfiers result from higher level needs not being met: lack of professional recognition, especially if not noted on performance appraisals; minimal or no growth potential; poor relationships with coworkers or superiors; inept supervisor/management; or difference between one's own philosophy and the management's values or work ethics.

One major obstacle to satisfaction for laboratorians and other health caregivers stems from minimal creative contribution available to them. Because the laboratory work requires structure and attention to detail, tolerance for creativity can be low. Economic constraints and productivity demands drive laboratory professionals to rethink how they work. These changes can develop into dissatisfiers without management planning and intervention.

Activity 6: Motivational Intervention

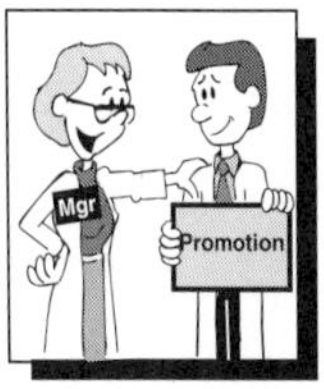

From the descriptions of motivators and dissatisfiers presented, select five and describe methods that managers, supervisors, and team leaders might use to stimulate the motivators and reduce or eliminate the dissatisfiers.

The job of motivation by managers and supervisors is never-ending. Ascertain for every employee which factors motivate them, encourage them, and make them feel valued. These strategies, implemented with sincerity, produce exceptional results.

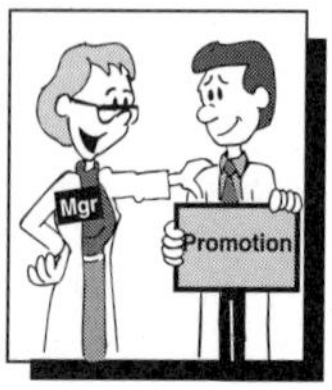

Activity 7: Nonwork Motivators

Form a group to do a nonwork-related activity. Write out the purpose and obtain approval from the necessary officials. Using some of the ideas listed above, identify a contribution each member of the group could make. Discuss whether or not enthusiasm was generated and why.

DELEGATING: THE CONVINCING ELEMENT OF THE *DIRECTING* FUNCTION

Delegating is getting things done by getting other people to do them. This means supervisors entrust some of their responsibility and authority to someone else, not just give away work. Delegating becomes necessary when the workplace demands that overlapping projects be handled by supervisors. Rather than frustration, supervisors can use the art of delegation. Delegation allows them to divide and share responsibilities. It becomes a method of achieving greater productivity and morale among employees. Supervisors also gain rewards from promoting their employees through a sense of accomplishment as more jobs are completed. The results? An energized work atmosphere where everyone is less grouchy and less tired when they start their work day. Job satisfaction and fun can prevail.[7]

Effective Delegation

Effective delegation begins with decisions about which projects, tasks, and jobs can be handed over to someone else. Certain activities come under the purview of supervisors owing to the sensitivity of the issue, confidentiality, organization or department policies, or objectivity required. Preparing an outline or a description of (1) the assignment with deadlines and timeframe; (2) possible resources; (3) relevance to organization, department, or staff; (4) responsibility and authority to be delegated; and (5) the essential skills required to complete the assignment provides a much clearer idea of what to do next (see Steps for Effective Delegating).

The nature of the work to be done sometimes calls for more than one individual if various specific skills, knowledge, and abilities are needed. For example, the delegate with analytical skills but no experience at writing may collect data regarding purchase of a new instrument. Then the supervisor and delegate will write the proposal.[8] Asking if the employee wants to undertake the responsibility is the next step. Honesty in detailing criteria and outcome along with promise of support as needed for unplanned incidents or unexpected barriers also helps obtain acceptance from the best employee. Communication of a realistic deadline must be established. Records should be kept of meetings, discussions, progress, and stages of completion of the job between supervisor and delegate. The delegate must realize that the supervisor will be

STEPS FOR EFFECTIVE DELEGATING

1. Decide what can be delegated
2. Prepare an overview
   - Deadlines
   - Timeframe
   - Essential skills required
   - Possible resources
   - Relevance to organization/department/staff
   - Responsibility and authority
   - Handling barriers/incidents
3. Select employee—someone who already has the skills/potential to acquire
   Did he/she accept or reject?
4. Allow time for assignment to be done
   - Support as requested by delegate
   - Monitor progress as preplanned
5. Give recognition
   - Others should know who is doing what
   - Documentation of meeting organization objectives
   - Reward

held responsible and ultimately accountable for the job. A list of supervisory tasks with selected examples is shown in Table 14–6.

Even new supervisors learning their jobs can assimilate delegating into their agendas. One key to successful delegating requires knowing the skills needed to do your job.

Activity 8: A Supervisor's or Delegate's Task?

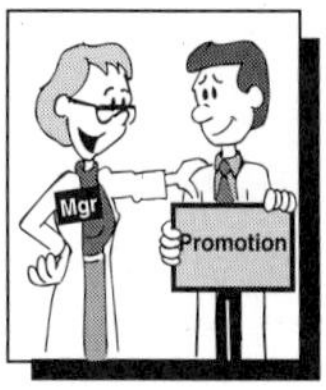

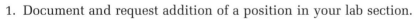

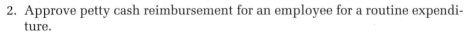

For each of the following tasks, should you, as the supervisor of a lab section, do it yourself or should you delegate it? Briefly explain why.

1. Document and request addition of a position in your lab section.
2. Approve petty cash reimbursement for an employee for a routine expenditure.
3. Review end-of-month reports and ascertain progress toward your lab section objectives.
4. Reduce expenses in your lab section by 5% for the remaining 4 months of the fiscal year.
5. Interview a prospective employee referred to you by a neighbor.

6. Attend a seminar on new instrumentation sponsored by a manufacturer.
7. Explain to one of your employees why he/she is receiving a raise.
8. Ask an employee his/her thoughts regarding your idea for his/her work area.
9. Lunch with a manufacturer's sales manager to negotiate service contacts on three automated chemistry analyzers.
10. Give a presentation on lab careers to community chamber of commerce.

See Activity Discussion 1 at the end of this chapter.

The Art of Delegating. Recognition of the value of employees can be demonstrated through delegation. Delegating is an art. The nuances of successful delegation change depending on the job, the people involved, and the situation. It supports professional career development in others. Using good decision-making skills may result in the elimination of jobs deemed inappropriate, worthless, or expensive. The good jobs are retained to be shared by good employees.[9]

Supervisors who disregard this vital tool of delegation and then later find themselves needing help have to convince their employees of the benefits of helping out.[10] When employees are persuaded to accept that benefits will follow from their involvement for the organization, its customers, and themselves, they will alter their behavior from not cooperating to even suggesting new projects. Supervisors must use their communicating and motivating skills to secure respect and collaboration from their employees.[10]

COACHING: GETTING TO NUMBER ONE

Coaching correlates to teaching and developing. More often, we associate coaching with sports and competition rather than work and productivity. Similar results are desired in both situations. Like teachers or coaches, exceptional managers and supervisors effectively and continually catapult their workers to perform beyond what they expect even of themselves. How can employees be influenced to do something considered distasteful, difficult, dangerous, or menial?

Coaching Analysis

Reports about peak performers relate their honest interest in their team(mates), employees, or players; the importance of the work to be done; and the value of the individuals performing the work. Keys to coaching for this peak performance are outlined in Table 14–7. Coaches inform the team (employees) (1) what is expected of them and the desired results, (2) how the job could be done and the available resources, and (3) power they have to do the job (responsibility and authority). An analysis of the whys of coaching is diagrammed in Figure 14–5, modified from several sources.[11] Initially, performance of the individual, employee, or student, is assessed, specifically in comparison to competency standards. Then each step requires consideration for action and consequences. Note that the significant activity throughout the whole process demands skillful communication generated by the "coach" with the individual. Listening becomes important for the recipient.

Action conducive to behavior change or improvement of (work) perfor-

Table 14–6
SUPERVISOR TASKS WITH SELECTED EXAMPLES

Supervisor only	Delegate	
*‡	‡	Mission, goals, and objectives for department or section
*‡	‡	Budget for department or section
*	†	Chair meetings of department or section
*	†	Attend executive meetings as representative of department
*‡	‡	Job description
*‡	‡	Performance standards and responsibilities
	*	Schedule employees time and dates to work
*		Approval
	*	Schedule employees to work station or assignments
*		Approval
*§		Hire: Interview, check references, pre-employment assessments
*‡	‡	Orientation
*		Performance appraisals
*		Counseling
*		Discipline
*		Commendation
*§		Terminate
*§		Transfer
*	*§	Employee competence assessment
*	*	Department proficiency testing
	*	Develop and write reports
*		Approval
	*	Inventory
	*	Select supplies, reagents, equipment, instruments
*		Approval
	*	Purchase supplies, reagents, equipment, instruments
*		Approval
*	*	Committees, chair and/or member
*	*	Safety
*	*	National Medical Laboratory Week
*	*	Continuing education
*	*	Employee orientation, training, education
*	‡	Quality assurance
*	*	Task forces, chair and/or member
*	*	Cost containment
*	*	Training
*	*§	Public relations
	*§	Special projects: Work flow analysis, employee and customer satisfaction surveys, computer needs assessment
*		Approval of report

* Perform task alone
† Perform task under direct supervision
‡ Perform task as a team member
§ With restrictions, special training, or assistance (Human Resource Dept.)

mance by the individual involves goal setting between both parties: establishment, assignment, and agreement. Discussion focuses on what is needed and expected (good for the company)—with clarity, level of difficulty, challenge, standards of performance (peer competition). Outcomes desired include task performance and satisfaction.

Mentoring

Mentoring returned to vogue when cooperation, team work, and investing in each other for profit and collegiality (financial and otherwise) became a way

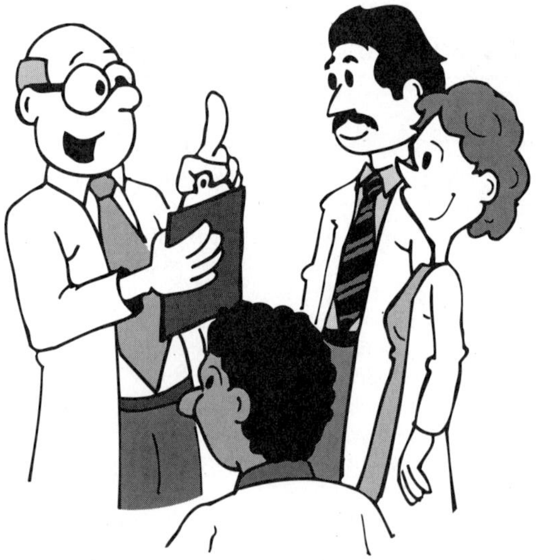

of succeeding in the workplace. Defined as trusted counselor or guide, a mentor supports, nurtures, and assists a protégé. Within the work or professional environment, a senior employee (manager or technologist) may observe the potential in another person. Taking an interest, the mentor offers support and the person responds. Thus, a special relationship begins that is based on trust. Sharing not only information but also work ethics, professional behavior, and work experiences, each person will learn from the other. On the other hand, an employee may seek a mentor and find someone through observing and listening. What does that person do that impresses and appeals? Sustenance for the relationship comes from both parties.[12]

Nurturing a working relationship often results in friendship and camaraderie that transcends the workplace in situation and time. Value from the mentoring process most often is not money, reward, or promotion. Intrinsic compensation comes as the employee develops and tries new endeavors. The greatest compliment comes when an employee tells you, "I want your job." As a mentor, a person not only provides ideas and suggestions but also points out both opportunities and essential attributes needed to secure those opportunities. Open to new and different ideas and offering their own, em-

Table 14–7
KEYS TO COACHING SUCCESS

Create conditions: communicate and be sensitive to attitudes that affect decisions. Answer the "Why bother?" question.

- Generate trust: Relationships are based mainly on trust. Intervene when trust issues impede work; be responsible for preserving the dignity of others.
- Support acceptance: Help to accept shortcomings and fear of change so that employees move on and learn.
- Promote autonomy: Encourage honest communications and exchange of ideas.
- Ask rather than tell: Question in order to help find more effective ways to work.
- Accept emotional aspects of work: Work-related emotions as part of human communication may reveal larger issues and information that can affect productivity.

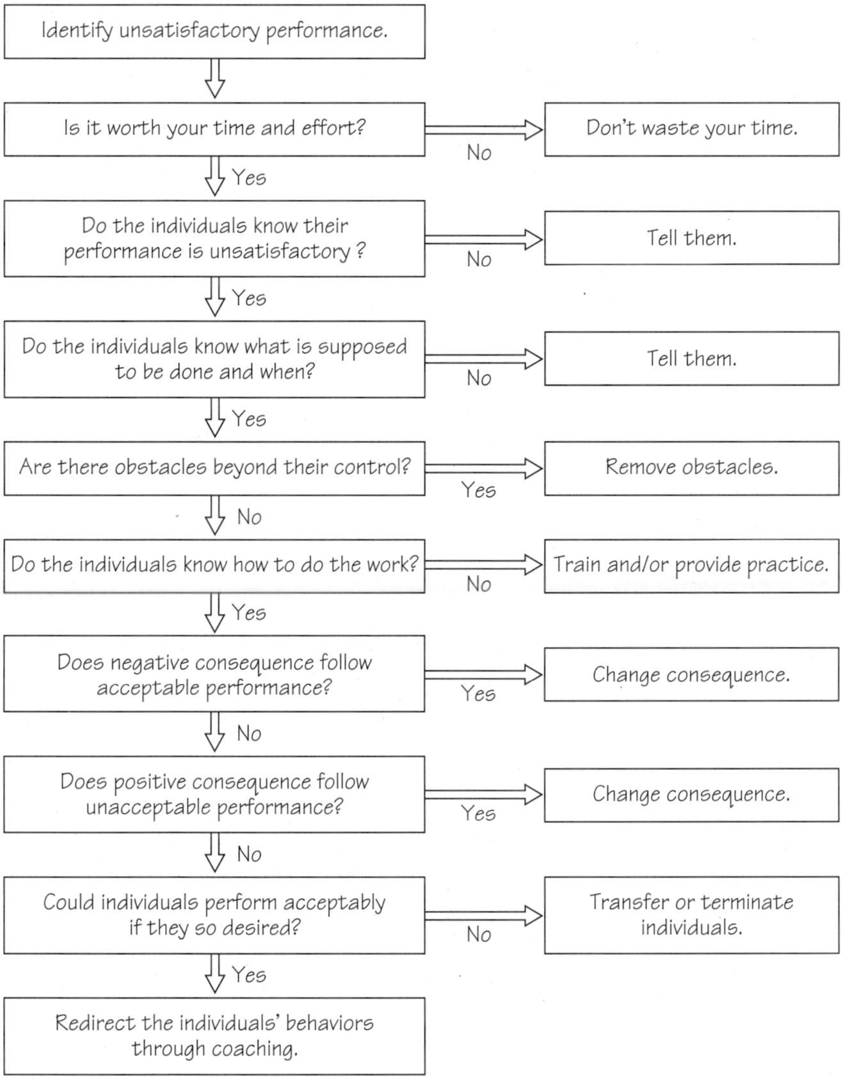

Figure 14–5 Coaching analysis.

ployees enhance the mentoring process. They take responsibility for what they undertake. When they achieve success, they let their mentors know the outcome of their influence.

From Greek mythology we learn that Mentor, a friend of Odysseus, was entrusted with the education of his son Telemachus. Can you imagine anything more important than the lifetime education of people? Mentoring is a wonderful gift regardless of where it is given: workplace, home, community, or professional arena.

Summary

Directing should appear to you now as a comprehensive activity related to people; an exchange of ideas and information between manager and employee, mentor and protégé, senior and junior; and a sense of expectation and fulfillment through accomplishments. An awareness of factors, both positive and negative, and the force with which change can be wrought in the workplace creates challenges for managers and employees. Effective direction requires constant observation—close or distant, overt or covert (in-view or unobtrusive)—and unremitting support of the work process and how work is performed. For new supervisors, learning basic and common sense approaches of communication, motivation, delegation, and coaching helps tremendously in understanding their employees and themselves as well. *Efficiency is doing things right; effectiveness is doing the right things.*

Managers hold a twofold responsibility: the first is to manage the work and workplace, work processes and work systems; and second, by investing time and effort in employees, to encourage and allow them to further develop their skills and abilities. Both guarantee that the goals of the organization will be fulfilled.

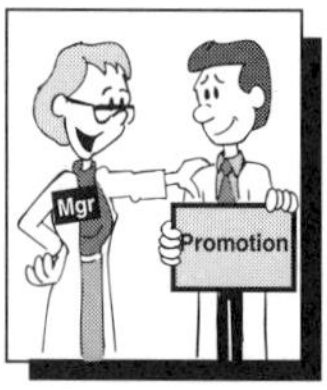

Activity Discussion 1: A Supervisor's or Delegate's Task?

For each of the following tasks, should you, as the supervisor of a lab section, do it yourself or delegate it? Briefly explain why. (W = work task, E = explanation.)

1. W = Document and request addition of a position in your lab section.
   E = Supervisor should do it as it relates to organization structure, workload and potential additional increase, and personnel costs.

2. W = Approve petty cash reimbursement for an employee for a routine expenditure.
   E = Delegate: Secretary or clerk could handle this, as the expenditure is routine and accounted for in the budget, and the supervisor reviews monthly financial statements.

3. W = Review end-of-month reports and ascertain progress toward lab section objectives.
   E = Supervisor should do, as this is an evaluation of work and the supervisor would write a report on progress or variance from expected performance.

4. W = Reduce expenses in your lab section by 5% for the remaining 4 months of the fiscal year.
   E = Supervisor is responsible for outcome and report but could lead a small group of employees in a brainstorming discussion on how to do this.

5. W = Interview a prospective employee referred to you by a neighbor.
   E = Supervisor should handle regardless of referral; this is a personnel issue.

6. W = Attend a seminar on new instrumentation sponsored by a manufacturer.

E = Delegate would be more motivated and enthusiastic; criteria should exist that all delegates report verbally to others, and in writing to the supervisor, what is technically new.

7. W = Explain to one of your employees why he/she is receiving a raise.
   E = Supervisor should do this, as it is a personnel issue related to motivation and salary.

8. W = Ask an employee his/her thoughts regarding your idea for his/her work area.
   E = Supervisor should include employees involved with work they are responsible for by initiating communication. Motivation plays a factor if intent is to seek participation now in order to obtain acceptance later.

9. W = Lunch with a manufacturer's sales manager to negotiate service contracts on their automated chemistry analyzers.
   E = Supervisor should handle negotiation, as this falls under the budget category, unless instruments are assigned responsibility to a technical employee, in which case it should be a team effort.

10. W = Give a presentation on lab careers to community chamber of commerce.
    E = Delegate with enthusiasm and positive presentation skills could do this and gain recognition outside the organization. Supervisor should assist in acquisition of resources and request a report afterward.

Review Questions

1. Explain why *directing* is acknowledged as the most important step in the management process.
2. What forms the basis of successful directing?
   a. Strong ties with upper management.
   b. Advanced management education and training.
   c. A process-oriented approach.
   d. A people-oriented approach.
   e. Desire of both managers and employees for high profits.
3. Bias as a barrier to good communication is considered to be
   a. Physical.
   b. Cultural.
   c. Psychological.
   d. Semantic.
4. Describe at least three examples in which "silence" is incorporated in a conversation.
5. Briefly describe, in your own words, the four theories of motivation presented in this chapter. Explain the merits of each regarding application in the clinical laboratory today.

See p. 410 for answers.

References

1. Burley-Allen M. Listening. New York, Wiley & Sons, 1995.
2. Tootle B. Leadership for leaders, seminar. New Orleans, LA: Delta Gamma Fraternity National Convention, 1994.
3. Szilagyi AD, Wallace MJ, Jr. Organizational Behavior and Performance, 3rd ed. Glenview, IL, Scott, Foresman and Co., 1983, pp 82–87.
4. Szilagyi AD, Wallace MJ, Jr. Organizational Behavior and Performance, 3rd ed. Glenview, IL, Scott, Foresman and Co., 1983, pp 88–91.
5. Szilagyi AD, Wallace MJ, Jr. Organizational Behavior and Performance, 3rd ed. Glenview, IL, Scott, Foresman and Co., 1983, pp 103–108.
6. Pacetta F, Gittines R. Don't Fire Them, Fire Them Up. New York, Simon & Schuster, 1994.
7. Wilkinson I. Delegation 101. Clinical Laboratory News 1994; 20(9): 26–27.
8. Umiker W. Delegation: how to make yourself dispensable—and promotable. Medical Laboratory Observer 1982; 14(6): 63–68.
9. Weiss WH. Supervisor's Standard Reference Handbook, 2nd ed. Englewood Cliffs, NJ, Prentice Hall, 1988, pp 38–51, 65–68, 87–109, 244–251.
10. Ladman AJ. The art of delegating. Clinical Laboratory Management Review 1988; 10(1): 193–195.
11. Fournies C. Coaching for Improved Work Performance. Blue Ridge Summit, PA, Liberty House, 1978.
12. Mostrous SJ. PRO Files: Mentoring. The Anchora of Delta Gamma. Columbus, OH, Summer 1992.

Suggested Reading

1. Bradford L, Raines C, Martin J. Twentysomething: Managing and Motivating Today's New Workforce. New York, Master Media, 1992.
2. Cheevers AH, ed. Creating and motivating a superior, loyal staff. National Institute of Business Management, 1101 King Street, Alexandria, VA 22314, 1994.
3. Davis K. Management communication and the grapevine. Harvard Business Review 1988; 66(1): 84–90.
4. Frey R. Empowerment or else. Harvard Business Review 1993; 71(5): 250–258.
5. Frings CS. President, Chris Frings & Associates, 633 Winwood Drive, Birmingham, AL 35226–2837. 205/823–5044.
6. Ginott H. Between Parent and Child. New York, Macmillan, 1965.
7. Gordon T. Leader Effectiveness Training. New York, Wyden Books, 1977.
8. Gray J. Men Are from Mars, Women Are from Venus. New York, HarperCollins, 1992.
9. Ricard VB. Developing Intercultural Communication Skills. Malabar, FL, Krieger Publishing Co, 1993.
10. Tanner D. Talking from 9 to 5. New York, Avon Books, 1994.
11. Tear J. Gender Dynamics. New York, William Morrow & Co., 1995.
12. Scott C, Jaffe D. Empowerment: Building High-Commitment Workplaces. Los Altos, CA, Crisp Publications, 1991.

Resources

CareerTrack. 3085 Center Green Drive, Boulder, CO 80301–5408 1–800–334–6780, http://www.careertrack.com

Seminars International. 8780 Mastin, Overland Park, KS 66212 1–800–843–8084

15

Controlling: The Fourth Management Function

OBJECTIVES

Upon completion of this chapter, the reader should be able to:

- Differentiate work standards from work compliance.
- Describe 10 requirements of work performance measures.
- Present an appropriate PDCA cycle for specified clinical laboratory preanalytical, analytical, and postanalytical problems.
- Given a laboratory situation, describe the problem, develop possible solutions, and explain what results might be obtained for each solution.

KEY WORDS

work standards
performance standards
work measures
productivity
quality assurance
PDCA cycle
decision making
problem solving

Introduction

The controlling function of management consists of ensuring that the work to be done gets done correctly, in a timely and cost-effective manner. Employees must realize what constitutes their work and associated responsibilities; likewise, they must understand that they are accountable for their own performance and completion of their duties. In the controlling function, managers and supervisors prepare employees for their assignments and monitor the process of work.

In addition to specific assignments or tasks, work standards (performance standards) and work measures (productivity) must be developed and employees informed of these expectations. Employees can participate in continuous quality improvement (CQI) methods: *P*lan, *D*o, *C*heck and *A*ct (PDCA) activities. Quality management systems determine what needs to be improved, when to do it, and how this will be accomplished. The work process and results (outcomes) can be monitored and evaluated through quality assurance (QA) programs.

Health care services and costs, under close scrutiny for appropriateness and control, are destined for rapid and significant changes. Astute managers prepare plans and implement changes to address situations that fail to achieve the objectives of the organization. Identifying an inefficient work process or system, then determining feasible solutions, requires knowledge and skill in decision-making and problem-solving processes. A few basic guidelines along with practice will develop confidence in taking the initiative to improve the work process and organization's services. Action, reaction, and anticipation improve results and outcomes for customers and employees.

Work Standards

Usually, administrators and customers project their desires and needs that impact on establishing standards and the criteria and level or degree of each. Increasingly, employees are encouraged to provide input into their work standards and criteria for the quality of work they do. Table 15–1 presents

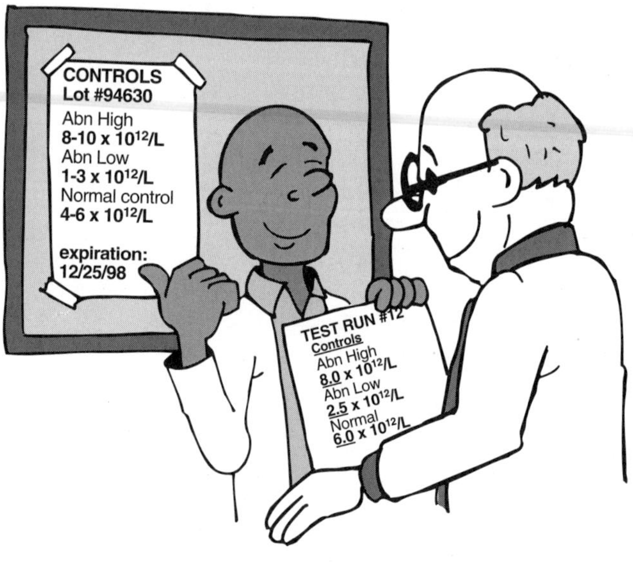
CONTROLS
Lot #94630
Abn High
8-10 x 10^12/L
Abn Low
1-3 x 10^12/L
Normal control
4-6 x 10^12/L
expiration:
12/25/98
TEST RUN #12
Controls
Abn High
8.0 x 10^12/L
Abn Low
2.5 x 10^12/L
Normal
6.0 x 10^12/L

Table 15–1
WORK STANDARDS

Components of Work Systems	Setting Standards
Employees' abilities	Develop orientation, training, education, and competence assessment programs. Document participation and completion. Establish number of tasks that should be completed in a given amount of time.*
Supplies, materials, equipment, instruments: readiness and functionality*	Utilize inventory records, maintenance records, quality control records and charts—in a given amount of time.
Work to be done*	Monitor TAT (increase speed), volumes (for growth), errors (for reduction); accuracy and precision of work measurements.
Finances	Personnel costs associated with regular and overtime pay and benefits; resource costs for maintenance and operation; cost per test and cost per batch/run; cost variability of same analyte tested on different instruments (methods); improved cost effectiveness/savings; correct billing for tests; appropriate payment for tests.

*Documentation for each shift, day, week, month, quarter, semiannual, and, for certain criteria, annual.

examples of work standards derived from components necessary for work systems. Longest reported methods for developing work standards: (1) analysis of past production records, (2) time analysis, (3) work sampling, (4) time study, and (5) motion study.[1] Various combinations of these methods better serve to establish standards and specific performance criteria.

Activity 1: Performance Expectations

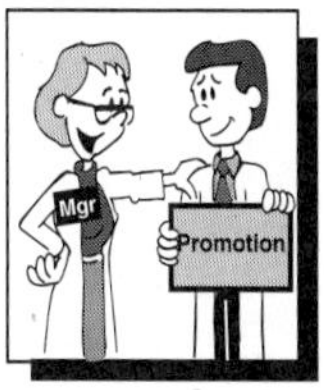

Write three to five statements describing your expectations in doing a job (at school, at work, or at home). Compare yours with others: your teacher, boss, or parents. What basis formulated your standards? Think of situations when you didn't achieve your expectations and others when you exceeded them. Describe your feelings. What standards do you project on others for similar work? Describe your reactions when they meet your expectations and when they do not.

Three points related to work standards require clarification. First, standards must relate to the work itself and be realistic. No matter how much hospital or laboratory administrators desire 100% or absolute precision, all the components in performing work by *people* rarely support attaining this level. To achieve *no* errors, *true* values, *faster* than time allowed, *below budget*, at *all times*, by *all personnel*, and in *all patient cases* (normal/healthy and abnormal/diseased) remains impossible. Standards must not only meet regulations and rules and fulfill customer satisfaction but also must be feasible.

Second, standards differ from compliance. Many laboratory situations require strict safety protocols; for example, work with infectious agents or

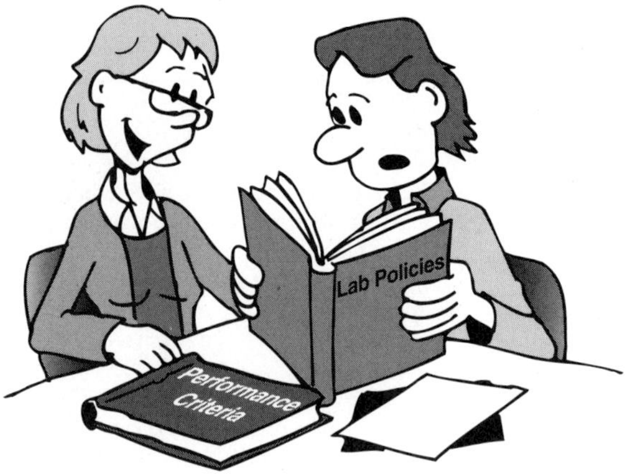

radioisotopes. An employee with excellent technical skills may identify the correct organism but fail to obey specific safety rules regarding working with specimens and media containing suspected organisms in a ventilated hood. He therefore exposes himself to potential contract of disease. A standard might state, "All employees will follow all safety rules at all times when working with . . . ." Compliance requires each safety rule to be executed even when supervisors are not watching.

Third, *work standards* differ from *technical standards* (also called *essential functions*) that describe those abilities and functions which the employee must be able to perform physically, mentally, and emotionally. The National Accreditation Agency for Clinical Laboratory Sciences (NAACLS) requires clinical training programs to publicize specifications for prospective students.[2] Table 15–2[3] lists the essential functions and technical standards that form the basis of the curriculum for all programs designed for the training of students in the field of laboratory science.

Managers' responsibilities include communicating standards, developing performance criteria, and formulating policies. To be effective, managers may have to communicate in more than one mode, at more than one time, and in more than one learning domain (refer to Chapter 14 for communication ideas).

Table 15–2
ESSENTIAL FUNCTIONS FOR MEDICAL TECHNOLOGY STUDENTS

- Comply with policies and procedures.
- Display manual dexterity.
- Show visual acuity for microscopic entities, computer screens, small-sized charts, tables and devices.
- Distinguish and discriminate colors and shadings used in stains and chemical reactions.
- Use reasonable judgment under stressful conditions.
- Demonstrate basic to more complex thought processes including assimilation and interpretation of data through appropriate problem-solving skills.
- Have physical, mental, and emotional health to perform productively, with accuracy, and in feasible time allowance.
- Communicate with patients; medical, scientific, nursing and allied health caregivers; and administrators and supervisors via authority protocols.

From Klosinski DD, et al. Essential functions. *In* School of Medical Technology Student Brochure. Royal Oak, Mich: William Beaumont Hospital, 1996.

Table 15–3
TEN REQUIREMENTS OF APPROPRIATE WORK MEASURES

- Correlates with work
- Provides prompt reports (data)
- Forecasts with anticipated margins of error rather than solely previous information
- Is objective
- Is adaptable
- Differentiates exceptions at critical points
- Is cost-sensitive
- Is understandable
- Indicates possible corrective action
- Forms a link to organizational framework

WORK MEASURES

Managers frequently face serious concerns regarding work productivity and the effect of laboratory work on patient care. Measurement of work that is either performed by employees or produced by machines generates information to compare against predetermined standards. Because objectivity is highly desired, quantifiable criteria should be assessed as much as possible. In Table 15–3, requirements of appropriate measures are identified.

One example of primary data helpful to "measure" work productivity is *turnaround time* (TAT). Factors which affect TAT include staffing, test ordering as routine versus STAT, instrument availability, and the various shifts (day, afternoon, night, or weekdays versus weekend). Looking at a test TAT provides a starting point to further investigate to find the real problem.

Activity 2: Turnaround Time (TAT) as a Work Measure

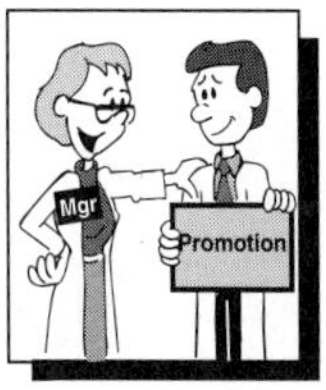

A hospital laboratory manager received complaints from the Chief of Medicine that certain test results were consistently reported much slower on the afternoon and midnight shifts than the day shift. Obtaining TATs for each test per shift was fairly easy from the laboratory informative system (LIS). Compare TAT averages reported in minutes for glucoses and CBCs for three shifts for one month. Are the data and your analysis of TATs sufficient? What else should be considered for any of the shifts?

	Glucose TAT	CBC TAT
Days	38	42
Afternoons	38	42
Midnights	42	52

See Activity Discussion 1 at the end of this chapter.

Productivity data influences decisions in several areas: staffing (when and where employees are needed and the number of persons to perform the work), personnel skill mix (such as technologists, technicians, and assistants),

Table 15–4a
LABORATORY MANAGEMENT INDEX REPORT RATIOS

Productivity Comparison Ratios
Measure how effectively the laboratory is using its most valuable asset—labor.
Utilization Comparison Ratios
Examine how medical staff physicians order laboratory tests.
Cost-effectiveness Ratios
Explore effective use of personnel, supplies, and equipment.

Data from College of American Pathologists. Laboratory Management Index Program. Northfield, IL, 1993.

problem areas, test menu adjustment, testing dates and times, and equipment and instrument selection changes or intervention. Studies conducted intradepartmentally (hospital) and interinstitutionally generate comparisons for productivity assessments; all should be based on anonymity for optimal objectivity. Work has been described as "a closed-loop process . . . that connects a customer and a performer" with performance linked to customer satisfaction.[4] The College of American Pathologists (CAP) provided a program, the Workload Recording Method for collecting data, designed to measure personnel productivity from subscribing laboratories and publishing comparisons.[5] In 1992, the CAP introduced a comprehensive program, Laboratory Management Index Program (LMIP), comparing various factors to further measure work productivity between laboratories; see Tables 15–4a and 4b.[6]

Conversely, other factors beyond the assignment itself and related to the employees themselves influence productivity. How employees feel and think about their work and their employers, managers, and supervisors all affect their productivity.[7]

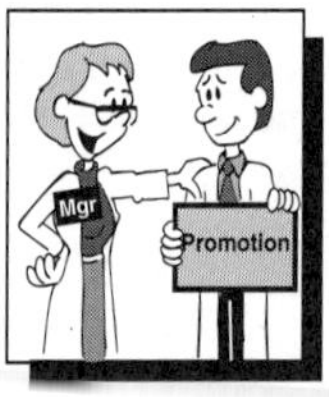

Activity 3: Factors Influencing Productivity

Rank the following factors in order of importance to you: 10 = most important to 1 = least important. Ask 10 or more co-workers, friends, or classmates to also rank the factors. Average the rankings for each factor. Discuss what you learned about the factors that affect productivity the most and the least.

_______ Company policies and rules

_______ Peer and group relationships

_______ Pay and monetary reward (bonuses)

_______ Opportunity for professional growth and promotion

_______ Sense of achievement

_______ Recognition of work done well

_______ Job security

_______ Working conditions and environment

_______ Interest in the work itself

_______ Importance and responsibility

Are there any factors not listed here that would be important to you? If so, describe them. Refer to the Activity Discussion 2 for additional rankings.

Table 15–4b
LMIP PRODUCTIVITY RATIOS: ONE EXAMPLE

Productivity Comparison Ratios
1. On-site billable (ordered) tests per FTE
2. On-site billable (ordered) test per technical FTE
3. Percent technical FTEs/total FTEs
4. On-site billable (ordered) tests per worked hour
5. On-site billable (ordered) tests per paid hour
6. Total labor expense per on-site billable (ordered) tests
7. Consumable expense per on-site billable (ordered) tests
8. On-site billable (ordered) tests per 100 workload units
9. Depreciation expense per on-site billable (ordered) tests
10. On-site billable tests per total on-site tests

Quality Assurance

In addition to reviewing work processes, targeting the workload of employees, clarifying expectations regarding work performance, and designing tools to measure productivity, managers become involved in developing plans to enhance the quality aspect of work. *Quality assurance* (QA) encompasses more than review of work processes, workload, performance, and productivity to incorporate revisions for work improvement. A division of the quality process, *quality control* (QC) demonstrates the quality of work results reported at the end of the analytical (testing) phase. Quality control measures indicate when problems exist by allowing the review of values from normal and abnormal controls for accuracy and precision of the testing procedure including instrumentation—and really little else. The Centers for Disease Control and Prevention (CDC) has proposed new systems controls to resolve regulatory issues for QC requirements (Table 15–5).[8, 9] These systems extend beyond traditional QC. A complete QA program incorporates QC of test results along with additional steps for preanalytical and postanalytical phases: specimen acceptability and outcome measures. Quality assurance programs allow more thorough investigations of problems and resolution opportunities and implementation of actions to reduce and remove problems. Objectives of QA programs focus on three areas: (1) early detection and reduction of *errors*; (2) utilization of *resources* that contribute to cost effectiveness (materials, procedures and manuals, and personnel); and (3) accreditation and licensure *approval.*

Laboratorians and other health caregivers identify monitors to assess significant concerns periodically. Table 15–6 shows examples from a large

Table 15–5
EXAMPLES OF QUALITY CONTROLS

Test system controls	Electronic checks Battery checks Sample or reagent level checks Optic checks Self-diagnostic systems Flags for improper sample flow Flags for incorrect use of components
Environmental controls	Temperature change flags Internal checks on adverse humidity conditions Built-in controls that check the integrity of reagents
Operator* controls	Simple test system operation training† Periodic assessment of performance

*Individuals who use equipment, operate instruments, perform analyses.
†Many managers and supervisors plan regular and as-needed in-service sessions for employees.

Table 15–6
EXAMPLES OF QA MONITORS

Tabulated Number of Incidents Per Month:

GENERAL

1. No wristbands on patients for whom orders to collect blood specimens were issued.*

COAGULATION

1. Specimens clotted; zero acceptance, redraw always required.*

TRANSFUSION MEDICINE/BLOOD BANK

1. Specimens received in error should be less than 1% with zero critical errors (wrong name and/or hospital identification number). Noncritical, but very important, errors consist of wrong or missing wristband number, phlebotomist's signature illegible or ID omitted, time drawn missing, misspelled patient names, wrong tube, hemolyzed, QNS.*
2. Disposition of O negative red cell units should be less than 10% of total transfusions and greater than 65% O negative units should be transfused to O negative patients.†

MICROBIOLOGY

1. Strep gram-positive A rapid antigen test TAT within 20 minutes with no more than 2% exceeding standard.
2. Expectorated sputum specimens of which at least 65% are acceptable by stain screening for culture and 60% yield a pathogen.†

CHEMISTRY

1. Blood gas TAT should be less than 20 minutes with no more than 10% exceeding time.*
2. Insulin intensive therapy glucose results of 100% reported 30 minutes prior to dietary tray.*‡

HEMATOLOGY

1. Bone marrow pack completeness: correct number of equipment, correct wrapping, technologist's initials.
2. Clerical errors in typing hematopathology special reports from transcription: accuracy of identification number; absence of typographical, omission, and spelling errors; other errors.

*Enumerated according to nursing unit. QNS = Quantity not sufficient.
†Physician orders.
‡Other information such as tray delivery time.
NOTE: These few QA monitors were selected to represent the cross-section of personnel performing work in a health care setting.

hospital laboratory.[10] QA, considered less effective as a reactive method by some (Miller and Clark[11]), still generates solutions to problematic tasks.

Plan, *Do*, *Check*, *Act* (PDCA)

Continuous quality improvement principles address an anticipated problem in a multistep process. Usually a team or committee of managers and employees selects a situation that they determine needs attention. They envision that the work process could be more efficient or that it is too costly; it may be that customers have complained about the work results or outcomes. The team considers ways to improve the situation. Plans are proposed and prioritized together with an order of implementation of each revision. Then the team observes results from each revision to assess any improvements in the situation. They formulate the reasons for maintaining the status quo or continuing to implement revisions.

Dr. W. Edwards Deming advocated the *P*lan-*D*o-*C*heck-*A*ct cycle (PDCA), known also as the *Shewhart Cycle*. The *p*lan phase of PDCA "establishes an analytical design that includes basic definitions, monitors (quality improvement criteria), and restrictions."[11, 12] In the *d*o phase, the team collects data according to established procedural policies (criteria, standards, and time period). The *c*heck phase requires the team to analyze the data. In the *a*ct phase, the team devises and implements new procedures and/or policies. Repeating this cycle (see Fig. 15–1) continues the process of seeking and instituting improvements in the workplace.

Activity 4: PDCA Applied to a QA Monitor

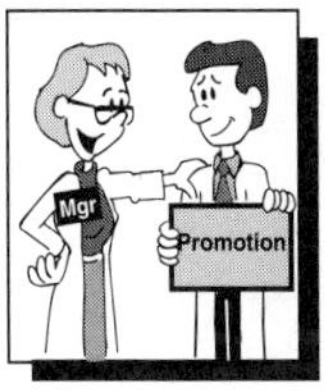

Select one QA monitor from Table 15–6. Discuss the PDCA cycle for it. Note any assumptions you would have to make in this example. Describe possible outcomes that a successful as well as an unsuccessful new procedure or policy might cause.

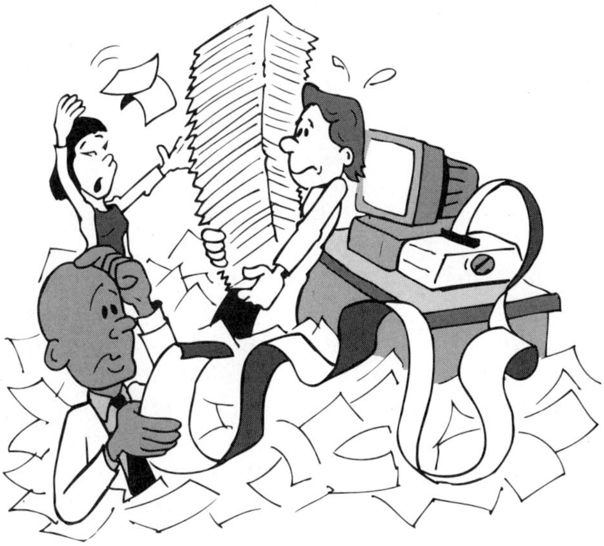

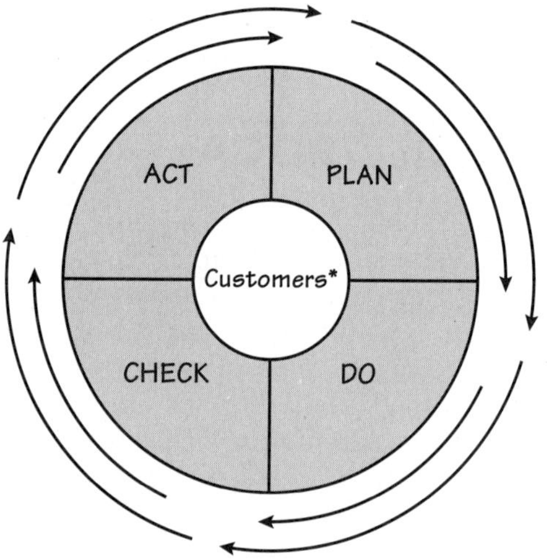

*Customer Service ⇒ Customer Satisfaction

Plan	Identify area for improvement. Why is this area (customer or employee complaints) costly? What is current procedure? Collect data to establish a target. Analyze causes of the problem—root causes with greatest probable impact.
Do	Implement improvements (changes, interventions), identify the who, what, why, when, where, and how to correct the problem.
Check	Analyze the results. Did changes produce expected results? Have root causes been decreased or eliminated? What is the difference between "before" and "after" values with the goal? Are any additional solutions needed?
Act	Standardize the process to hold the gain. What other changes would increase margin of improvement?

Figure 15–1 PDCA cycle.

Statistical thinking will one day be as necessary for efficient citizenship as the ability to read and write.—H. G. Wells

Statistics confirm the need to act: to revise; to demonstrate validity, accuracy, and precision; to account for costs (expenses and savings); to measure productivity; and to evaluate the impact of problems and potential solutions. Several tools are commonly used to visualize mathematical comparisons. Some of these are cause-and-effect chart, flow diagram, Pareto diagram, trend (run) chart, histogram, scatter diagram, control chart, and check sheets. See Appendix 15–A for chart and diagram examples.

In some situations, quantitative studies provide sufficient data for change: inventory control, estimates of costs (purchase, lease, or maintenance of equipment), number of patients seen in the OP lab, and accounts receivables. Basic bar diagrams, histograms, or Pareto charts display this information adequately. Other situations depend on the identification of the "cause," which often can be investigated and confirmed with statistical information.

Quality programs should be set up for more reasons than to "pass a test" (meet accreditation and licensure standards). Successful organizations hold a very real quality philosophy. Crosby states, "I know of about 10 companies that deliver defect-free products and services to their customers."[13] He advocates that management's job should be to:

- Develop clear requirements that employees, suppliers, and customers can understand.
- Train people and provide resources (for these people) to meet requirements.
- Educate themselves to become examples of those who prevent mistakes and avoid production of defective work.
- Set performance standards at "defect-free."
- Review finance department reports as indicators of quality.

Decision Making and Problem Solving

Decision making refers to the process of choosing among several alternatives. *Problem solving*, which consists of multiple steps, refers to the process of recognizing that a problem exists, defining it, determining what happened to cause it, and what steps will be necessary to solve it (possible solutions). Additionally, consideration must be given to the question: *if* a solution is implemented, *then* what will happen? Study potential solutions through an "if—then" analysis process. Scientists who think analytically ponder these steps thoroughly before taking action. The antithesis to effective problem solving occurs when the characteristic of perfectionism hinders someone from making the final decision—choosing which solution to implement. Determining choices based on their importance by using weighted values and predetermined rankings makes action selection and implementation easier.

> With some reflection and effort, we can solve the wrong problem.
>
> —Anonymous

Sirkin[14] characterized four cycles of "problem-fixing" similar to the steps described above. During the first cycle, correct identification of the problem must occur. Situations that result in failure, in productivity at substandard levels, or in products and results of poor quality warrant immediate attention.

In the second cycle, attempts are made to prevent problems. Attention given to control of situations, productivity, products, and results through monitoring processes usually prevents problems from occurring. The objective is to prevent old problems from recurring as well as new ones from beginning.

The third cycle involves the investigation of possible underlying causes of previous problems. Essential input often comes from employees who perform the technical work, because they understand the work methods and instruments. They are quick to find root causes and develop means of eliminating them in order to make their work-lives better. A by-product of this strategy can be seen in positive attitudes and rising morale as success is marked in retaining customers, and obtaining new ones.

The fourth cycle engages these experienced problem-solvers, the technical employees, to anticipate improvements. Throughout the process, cooperating toward setting common goals of survival and growth necessitates that managers and employees listen to one another. Exploring multiple interventions as possible strategies or solutions and discussing possible pitfalls and advantages that point to the implementation of changes must be a continual team effort. When a particular solution is selected, the action must be communicated to all involved; their commitment and enthusiasm must be secured. Once interventions are in place and activated, the noticeable improvements of higher profit margins and faster turnaround times provide positive feedback that the change was indeed the right one. The more employees become involved, the less managerial involvement is needed to make decisions. Decisions considered major, in the third and fourth cycles of problem solving, which most often involve changing protocols and policies (making exceptions to rules) or spending money, rest almost exclusively with management.

Employees included in decision-making and problem-solving processes may require preliminary instructions in order to function effectively. During team-building meetings, managers must provide to them the parameters of their role and activities in the process. Beginning with the situation (problem) to be addressed, resources that they might need are offered, and then responsibility is allocated to select and implement solutions. The group leader, if not the manager, determines the rules for the group and the members, chooses the decision-making method, and establishes communication between group members and the manager.[15]

Perceptive teams develop an alarm system that sets control actions in place when deviations start to occur. With experience they learn when to initiate triggers to enact solution(s) just when a problem begins. (Refer to group and team development and skill building in Chapter 16.) Much of this appears to be common sense. However, education is necessary, even in home situations. A teenager explained her inability to solve a personal problem by saying to her parents, "You want me to come up with *solutions* to my problems? I only know about solutions from my chemistry class."

Imagination and creativity help during all decision-making and problem-solving steps. Preston emphasizes the importance of creativity to meet the demands—especially the unforeseen demands—of today's chaotic health care environment.[16] Practical advice is to dialogue, diagram, dream, and then decide.

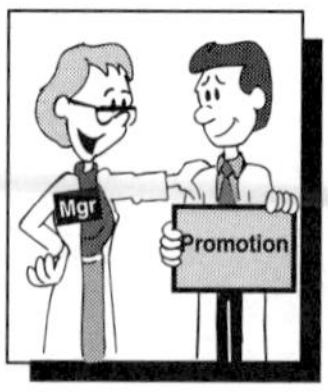

Activity 5: PDCA Strategies

Students in management classes during their junior year identified problems they had encountered in their work experience. Very few had ever worked or were working in clinical laboratories. From the abbreviated list, which is in random order, select five problems to discuss, using the PDCA cycles and problem-solving strategies.

Declining productivity

Spotty attendance

Poor morale

Inaccuracy

Poor management

Lack of defined procedures

Bad interdepartmental relationships

Training: lack of, inappropriate, inconsistent, not validated

Variable reliability

Lack of motivation

Poor communication

Lack of cooperation between workers

Too much managing

Bad intralaboratory relationships

Managers taking advantage of their authority

Tardiness

Lack of following procedures

Undeveloped interpersonal skills

Too many managers/supervisors

Approaches to Implementing and/or Controlling Programs

Whether managers are implementing methods for work standards and measures, quality assurance and processes, or safety, decision making and problem solving require them to focus on two approaches. The first approach deals with human relations: dialogue, convince (the "tell and sell" approach), educate and train, and encourage employees, colleagues, employers, and customers. These tasks consume 90% of a manager's time. The second approach concentrates on facts: collecting data, displaying information, and performing statistical analysis. These tasks consume the remaining 10% of a manager's time. Spending most of the time on the wrong approach will result in chaos. Experts state the maxim, "You cannot manage what you cannot measure."

Managers and supervisors should keep in mind that if they think people are the problem and get rid of them, they will probably be left with a situation that they did not expect—the problem remains. Experts contend that problems stem from process failure and not from people.

Summary

The controlling function of management creates processes to ensure that work gets done correctly and in a timely and cost-effective manner. Employees, working with managers, are accountable for their own performance and completion of their duties. Managers and supervisors in the controlling function prepare employees for their assignments and monitor the process of their performance by work standards and work measures. Work processes and results can be monitored through quality assurance systems. Continuous quality improvement methods such as the *P*lan, *D*o, *C*heck and *A*ct (PDCA) cycle help determine when and how to improve work and results.

Laboratorians—managerial and technical personnel alike—have to learn decision-making and problem-solving strategies. They must become aware of when it is necessary to change and then to implement the necessary changes! Confidence and intuitiveness develop with experience.

The basic guidelines studied and practiced in this chapter will help the reader take the initiative to identify and then solve problems related to improving work. Likewise, developing attitudes and knowledge that promote problem prevention enhances a successful process.

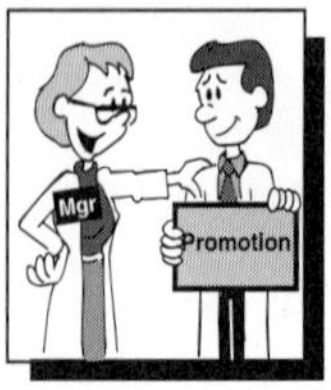

Activity Discussion 1: TAT as a Work Measure

Since the average TAT for the midnight shift is higher than for days and afternoons, it would appear that the complaint is legitimate. However, additional information per shift should be considered:

1. Total number of tests performed.
2. Total number of test results within reference range (normal) and the TAT for this group.*
3. Total number of test results outside reference range (abnormal) and the TAT for this group.
4. Total number of tests ordered STAT and the TAT for this group.
5. Review TAT averages for the past six months. If similar, accept TATs for the month under consideration as valid. If any values appear significantly different, continue data collection.
6. Review instrument logs for problems or downtime.
7. Review staffing schedules for problems caused by lack of employees or deficient training.
8. Review (critical) incident reports indicating personnel performance problems during the month.
9. Review report documents for any/number of result corrections, repeat testing, specimen problems requiring recollection.
10. Review LIS logs for problems or downtime.

Activity Discussion 2: Factors Influencing Productivity

Average of rankings gleaned from previous classes, 10 = most important to 1 = least important. Compare your information with information from your classmates.

1. Interest in the work itself
2. Working conditions and environment
3. Opportunity for professional growth and promotion
4. Sense of achievement
5. Company policies and rules
6. Peer and group relationships

---

*Looking at only TAT numbers without considering other factors and accepting complaints as valid may result in making changes that do not really solve the problem. If no other factors influence the data, then you would accept the complaint as valid and must address it as a serious problem warranting resolution. Depending on the laboratory, the afternoon shift may process more normal specimens from outpatients collected in doctors' offices (an outreach program). Usually the midnight shift consists of minimal numbers of technical personnel who perform STATs in higher volumes.

7. Pay and monetary reward (bonuses)

8. Importance and responsibility

9. Recognition of work done well

10. Job security

Review Questions

1. Work standards fulfill organizational objectives when they are
   a. Measurable.
   b. Objective.
   c. Relate to specific tasks.
   d. Economical.
   e. All of the above.
2. Consider this work measure for safety: "Wear gloves, protective cover and face shield when handling specimens in open containers." What mode(s) of communication of management's expectation of compliance by employees could be used?
   a. Urgent message on the LIS.
   b. Copies inserted in the front of all Policy and Procedures manuals.
   c. Memo posted on bulletin boards requiring employees to initial after reading it.
   d. Told to all employees at Safety meetings.
   e. Copies filed in all supervisors' manuals.
3. Describe the value of monitoring turnaround times of glucose testing on insulin intensive therapy (IIT) patients.
4. In using a PDCA cycle, which of the following statements best describes problem solving for improvement?
   a. Collect data for review to determine the responsible person.
   b. Develop a plan to change a step in a (selected) process and make sure it works.
   c. Plan to make a change(s) based on analysis of data and selection of appropriate policies.
   d. Use problem-solving strategies to select criteria to measure the improvement.

See p. 410 for answers.

References

1. Longest BB Jr. The controlling function of management. Cadence 1974; 5(1):37–51.
2. National Accrediting Agency for Clinical Laboratory Sciences. Essentials and guidelines of accredited educational program for Medical Technology. IV. Students 13. Program description K. Chicago, 1995.
3. Klosinski DD et al. Essential functions. In School of Medical Technology Student Brochure. Royal Oak, Mich, William Beaumont Hospital, 1996.
4. Denning PJ. Work is a closed-loop process. American Scientist 1992; 80:314.
5. College of American Pathologists. Manual for Laboratory Workload Recording Method. Northfield, Ill, 1991, pp 4, 157–160.
6. College of American Pathologists. Labora-

tory Management Index Program. Northfield, Ill, 1993.
7. Gvazdinskas LC, Maffetone MA. Employee satisfaction: an integral component of total quality. Clinical Laboratory Management Review 1995; 9(2):107–116.
8. Centers for Disease Control and Prevention. Atlanta, 1996.
9. Auxter S. CDC, CLIAC rethink quality control under CLIA '88. Clinical Laboratory News 1996; 22(8):1,16.
10. Monthly Quality Assurance Monitors. Department of Clinical Pathology, William Beaumont Hospital, Royal Oak, Mich, 1996.
11. Miller LJ, Clark GB. Quality improvement in cutaneous micrographic surgery laboratory. Quality management series. Clinical Laboratory Management Review 1994; 8(6): 578.
12. Maxwell KR, Stevenson TD. Quality assurance and peer review in the clinical laboratory. *In* Snyder JR, Senhauser DA (eds). Administration and Supervision in Laboratory Medicine. Philadelphia, JB Lippincott, 2nd ed. 1989, p 375.
13. Crosby PB. Completeness: Quality for the 21st Century. New York, Dutton, 1992, p 119.
14. Sirkin H, Stalk G Jr. Fix the process, not the problem. Harvard Business Review 1990; 68(4):26–33.
15. Gill SL. Groups and decision making: skills and strategies for group leaders. Clinical Laboratory Management Review 1995; 9(6):464–476.
16. Preston P. Breaking down barriers to creativity: encourage innovative problem solving. Clinical Laboratory Management Review 1995; 9(6):449–455.

Suggested Reading

Work Standards and Measures

Berte LM. Developing Performance Standards for Hospital Based Personnel. Chicago, ASCP Press, 1989.

Comer DR. Improving group productivity by reducing individual loafing. Clinical Laboratory Management Review 1994; 8(4): 252–253.

Schaffer RH. Demand better results—and get them. Harvard Business Review 1992; 70(2): 142–149.

Schwabbauer MH. Learn to do more with less. Advance for Medical Laboratory Professionals 1996; 8(2): 10–12.

Quality Assurance/TQM/CQI

Clark GB. Quality assurance, an administrative means to a managerial end. Part IV: Choosing quality improvement indicators in a TQM and CQI environment. Clinical Laboratory Management Review 1992; 6(4): 426–440.

Dobyns L, Crawford-Mason C: Quality or Else: The Revolution in World Business. Boston, Houghton-Mifflin, 1991.

Eckhart J, Gilbert P. Improved Coumadin therapy using a continuous quality improvement process. Clinical Laboratory Management Review 1996; 11(2): 153–156.

Nardella A. Seven steps to quality improvement. Laboratory Medicine 1995; 26(3): 172–174.

Scherkenbach WW. The Deming Route to Quality and Productivity: Road Maps and Roadblocks. Washington, CEEPress Books, 1992.

The Transition from QA to CQI. An introduction to quality improvement in health care. Oakbrook Terrace, Ill: Joint Commission on Accreditation of Health Care Organizations, 1991.

Welborn AL, Collins JB. Creating the environment for process improvement. Clinical Laboratory Management Review 1995; 6: 477–489.

Williamson JW, Hudson JI, Nevins MM. Principles of Quality Assurance and Cost Containment in Health Care. San Francisco, Jossey-Bass Publishers, 1982.

Decision Making and Problem Solving

Baer DM, Galey WT, Morehead L. How to solve problems using the labor-management partnership. Medical Laboratory Observer 1996; 26(6): 80–83.

Castañeda-Méndez K: Reducing costs by improving quality. Advance for Administrators of the Laboratory 1994; 2(3): 30–32, 59.

Lemery LD. Logical Thought Processes: A Guide to Effective Problem Resolution. Management and Education Tech Sample No. MGM-1. Chicago, American Society of Clinical Pathologists, 1993.

Peters T. Judging judgment: ouch! *In* Peters on Excellence. CAP Today 1991; 5(6): 62.

Roseman E. The individual versus group approach to decision making. Medical Laboratory Observer 1995; 27(3): 50–53.

Roseman E. Using analytical tools to make big decisions. Medical Laboratory Observer 1993; 25(8): 42–46.

Sirota D, Wolfson AD. Pragmatic approach to people problems. *In* People: Managing Your Most Important Asset. Boston, Harvard Business Review, 1988, pp 10–18.

Statland BE. Assessing the quality of management decisions. Medical Laboratory Observer 1994; 26(10): 24–28.

Weiss RL, Ahlin PA, Hawker CD, Schumm CL. Transition in quality: from quality assurance to strategic quality management. Clinical Laboratory Management Review 1995; 9(1): 27–45.

APPENDIX **15–A**

Seven Basic Statistical Visual Aids

1. Cause-and-effect diagrams show causes of a specific problem grouped into categories, most often "methods," "management," "material," and "machinery." Also called *fishbone diagrams* from the shape, or Ishikawa diagrams for Kaoru Ishikawa, the man who created them.

2. Flow charts delineate steps of a process; these are very helpful in service industries where work processes involve unseen steps. Key symbols are:

⬭	Start or stop
→	Direction of flow
▭	Process step
◇	Decision point
○	Evaluation point

3. Pareto charts (simple bar charts) show causes in rank order, based on data collected for each cause, which equals 100%.

4. Run or trend charts show results or data of work plotted per unit of time; for example, number of drugs tests performed for 24-hour period per month.

5. Histograms, another form of bar charts, demonstrate frequency of events; for example, number of specimens collected which have errors from specific nursing units.

6. Scatter diagrams illustrate the relationship between two variables; for example, t-test or comparison of results obtained from two methods.

7. Control charts, complex versions of run charts, show data plotted within statistically calculated upper and lower limits, referred to as "range." Daily, per shift, or per batch of tests use of controls demonstrates where normal and abnormal control results fall. If within the range, the method (and instrument) system is considered "in control" and results can be reported. Any point falling outside of the range, called an outlier, requires investigation for causes of unusual or serious nature.

16

Coordinating: The Fifth Management Function

OBJECTIVES

Upon completion of this chapter, the reader should be able to:

- Describe the various personnel who would be needed to perform laboratory procedures for a variety of work (laboratory) environments.
- Identify job characteristics based on duties and responsibilities.
- Write acceptable and lawful questions to ask an applicant in an interview.
- Discuss reasonable accommodations for disabled employees who would work in a laboratory setting.
- Compare rationale for traditional and contemporary schedules for laboratory personnel.
- Develop a technical personnel work schedule when given information regarding staff requirements.
- Describe the aspects and subsequent benefits of working together in teams, work groups, committees, or task forces in health care.

KEY WORDS

coordinating
interviewing
preplacement assessment
hiring practices
personnel staff
scheduling staff
teamwork

Introduction

Laboratory services now extend beyond the traditional hospital setting. This is because changes in the focus of health care dramatically impact how patients receive care. The emphasis on cost effectiveness (see Chapter 18), staffing, and efficiency of services provided continues to increase. Reengineering strategies dictate establishing new laboratory locations, changing personnel requirements, and redesigning work systems (see Chapter 13).

The laboratory services that begin with patient identification, including specimen collection and processing, test analysis, and result reporting, must be studied. Goals and objectives, written during the planning process, have impact on how the coordinating function will be carried out. Responsibility for the total laboratory operation (all processes and test results) rests solely with the laboratory director (or owners). This implies significant oversight of personnel by managers and supervisors, senior technical personnel, and others as designated. (Various regulations are discussed in Chapter 17.)

This chapter focuses on the coordinating process for all laboratory personnel. The manager's responsibilities in coordinating people who help and support as well as actually perform laboratory work include determining the number and type of staff needed and their schedules. Providing adequate staff consists of developing and utilizing multiskilled workers, leading teams, and hiring personnel (including health care givers who may not even work in the lab or for the manager). Managers also are responsible for establishing a productive workplace environment.

The Coordinating Function

Coordinating consists of implementing the planning, organizing, directing, and controlling functions of management. Balancing people and work, resources and procedures, (customer) demands, and productivity requires the constant attention of managers. Managers are challenged to skillfully coordinate laboratory services performed in various places by a range of personnel: for example, which tests (work) will be done, how it will be done, where it will be done, when it will be done, and who will do it. They must integrate general and specialized laboratory activities in systematic and efficient ways.

Patients needing laboratory services and other diagnostic tests no longer stay in hospitals during these procedures. Laboratories for most routine testing, or at least specimen collection stations along with other facilities, are located anywhere the customers are: hospice and nursing facilities, short-stay and extended care facilities for people who don't necessarily require regular medical attention, doctors' offices, exercise clubs, workplaces, school (preschool through university) health centers, pharmacies, walk-in medical centers, patients' homes, and even shopping malls. Special, unique, complicated, and esoteric laboratory procedures are performed on delivered specimens in large commercial and reference laboratories, often quite a distance from patients or their doctors.

Community businesses want their employees to maintain their health. Businesses promote wellness and preventive medicine programs either on the premises or nearby.[1–3] Successful programs produce greater worker attendance and productivity, safer working conditions, and lower medical expenses paid out by employers. Periodic physicals, including laboratory testing, increase the incidence of early detection of disease. This allows employees to be monitored if they show evidence of preclinical disease states or are in high-risk categories for certain diseases. These employees can receive more effective therapy at the appropriate time.

Coordinating involves establishing policies to promote the standards and objectives of the organization and department. Managers also coordinate systems including workflow, data management, relationship of work and sites and personnel, and separation or integration of dissimilar or similar functions and tasks.

Managing Staff: Getting the Job Done

The manager sees to it that the right work is done, and the supervisor sees to it that the work is done right.[4] Managers assess the education, training, and experience of personnel and determine further training and in-service or continuing education needs. Personnel in combination with other resources are utilized in coordinating the work process. This knowledge allows managers and supervisors to switch from being *firefighters* dealing with crises and constantly "putting out fires" to becoming *lifeguards* providing resource and backup assistance. The Joint Commission on Accreditation of Healthcare Organizations (JCAHO) so strongly advocates this principle that individual chapters in their accreditation manuals are devoted to the education, orientation, and training of employees.[5]

Laboratory managers also must prepare their employees for new tasks and opportunities that the employees will be offered. Some of these roles will provide much more patient and other health care giver contact. Knowledge in advanced topics of laboratory science and medicine, pathophysiology, and therapy monitoring will be expected. These employees will use skills requiring adroit manual deftness, especially in performing molecular diagnostic testing and capabilities of performing multiple tasks simultaneously. Their attitudes must expand to accept change, to be flexible and adaptable, and to seek higher standards (in their own performance and the work they produce).

LABORATORY PERSONNEL

Laboratory science academic and clinical practicum program curricula require study in all major and most minor subjects of clinical laboratory science (Table 16–1). Until recently, most laboratory science graduates secured positions limited to one (possibly two or three) discipline(s) and concentrated on acquiring advanced knowledge and skills related to that position.* Now laboratorians find themselves in new roles.[6–8] Opportunities have emerged for technologists and laboratory scientists in areas of patient-focused care teams, training and managing new laboratorians and other health care givers to perform laboratory tests and provide laboratory-related services, marketing and consulting, health care/insurance finance, and information services (computers). Technicians perform many of the high-volume routine and automated

*Certain exceptions exist for personnel with associate and baccalaureate degrees in histotechnology and cytotechnology. Also, masters and doctoral degrees offer specialized studies in clinical chemistry, microbiology, hematology, hemostasis, virology, mycology, parasitology, and molecular biology (plus management and education).

Table 16–1
CURRICULA FOR MT/CLS AND MLT/CLT CLINICAL PRACTICUM PROGRAMS*

	MT/CLS	MLT/CLT
Blood bank†	Yes	Yes
Chemistry	Yes	Yes
Hematology	Yes	Yes
Microbiology	Yes	Yes
Immunology	Yes	Yes
Body fluids/urinalysis	Yes	Yes
Coagulation	Yes	Yes
Phlebotomy	Yes	Yes
Parasitology	Yes	Introductory
Mycology	Yes	Introductory
Virology	Introductory	No
Flow cytometry	Introductory	No
Toxicology	Introductory	No
Endocrine tests	Introductory	No
RIA	Introductory	No
Molecular pathology	Introductory	No
Management	Yes	No
Education	Yes	No
Computers (LIS)	Yes	Introductory
Quality assurance, safety, ethics	Yes	Yes

*This model represents general information rather than a specific program. Knowledge and skill levels to be taught for any subject would correspond to appropriate professional standards.
†Immunohematology or Transfusion Medicine.

laboratory procedures. Other trained laboratory personnel have preanalytical (before testing) and basic (waived) testing responsibilities. Nonlaboratory health care workers performing ancillary and support laboratory tasks are among the personnel reporting to laboratory managers. Clerical, data processing, phlebotomy, specimen processing, and courier duties require personnel to be trained in areas of safety, universal standards/precautions, patient confidentiality, and laboratory information systems (LIS). Figure 16–1 depicts laboratory personnel stratification and career development that has existed, for the most part, for more than 25 years. Laboratory facilities undergoing physical (structural) or work redesign have instituted cross-training or retraining of personnel for more generalist positions or for assignments including another (laboratory) discipline. Objectives of this kind of personnel development include mobility to staff workstations as needed and flexibility to rotate to various shifts as workloads demand.

Government regulations have defined criteria for personnel who perform laboratory procedures. Laboratory tests are now grouped into waived, provider performed microscopy procedures (PPMP), moderate- and high-complexity classifications under Clinical Laboratory Improvement Amendments (CLIA '88).* Waived and PPMP tests can be performed and results reported by nonlaboratory personnel who have been trained and have their competence assessed (annual requirement). Nurses, nurse practitioners, physician assistants (PAs), allied health practitioners such as respiratory therapists and car-

*Additional classifications such as the accurate and precise technology (APT) are being considered by the federal government and associated agencies.

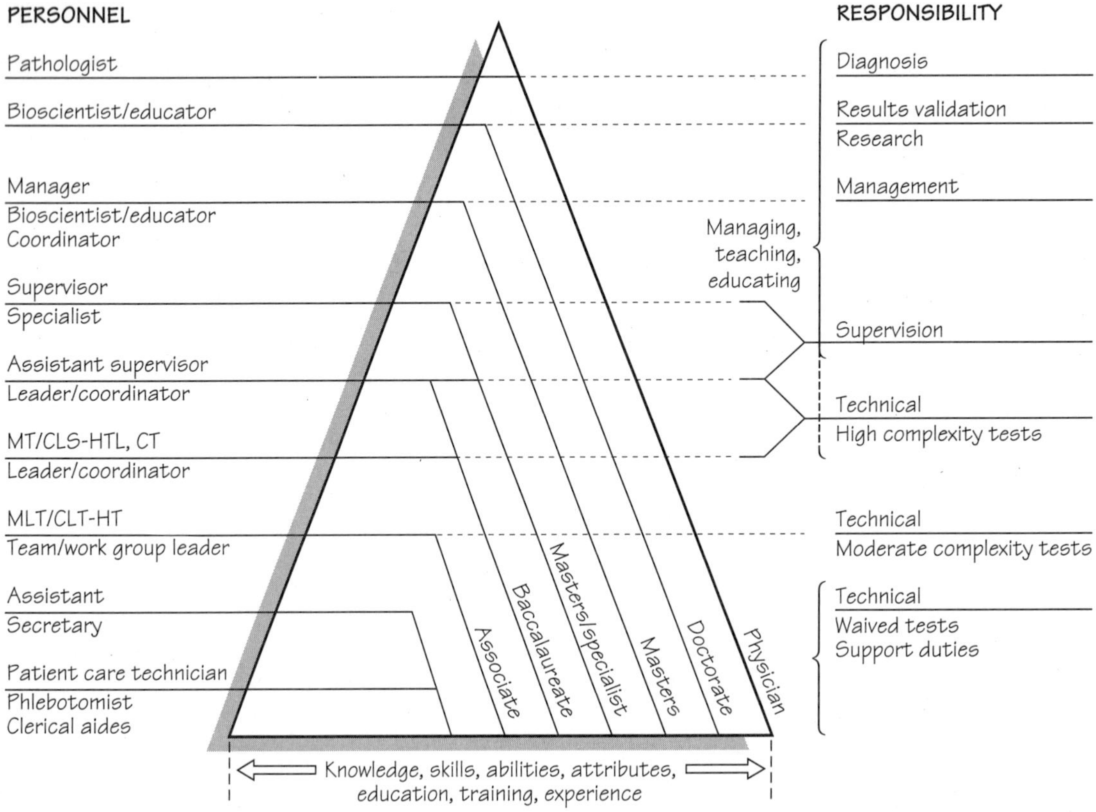

Figure 16–1 Stratification of laboratory personnel. (Modified from Tomlinson R: Conceptual model for considering utilization and education of medical laboratory personnel. American Journal of Medical Technology 1970; 36(2): 67–74.)

diac catheterization technologists, and patient-focused care technicians are performing these tests. Home-care services use nonlaboratory personnel also: for example, physicians, nurse-midwives, and dentists. Laboratory regulatory and accrediting agencies, such as Health Care Finance Administration (HCFA), JCAHO, and the College of American Pathologists (CAP), require verification of training and competence of any persons performing laboratory tests.

In optimal circumstances, oversight and management of laboratory testing procedures and "testing" personnel regardless of location is handled by laboratorians. Such departments or sections, called ancillary site testing (AST) or point-of-care testing (POCT), must adhere to stringent JCAHO, CAP, and, in some cases, state regulations. Laboratorians knowledgeable about policies, procedures, training, and quality control/assurance find themselves very busy fulfilling assignments of monitoring, documenting, evaluating, and training nonlaboratory "laboratorians" in these nonlaboratory "labs."

MULTISKILLED WORKERS

Acquiring additional skills became popular when rural and large medical facilities experienced shortages of health care workers. Health care educators worked with administrators to identify needs and develop training modules. Employees studied new skills, and when they could demonstrate competence in performing tasks, they were given additional and different assignments.

These modules were designed so that one individual (or *teams* or *work groups*) would deliver many patient "bedside" services, such as performing electrocardiographs (EKGs), taking x-ray films, collecting blood specimens and performing (waived) laboratory tests, reading blood pressures and temperatures, bathing and taking care of personal hygiene needs, administering certain medications, and performing other basic tasks. (All tasks must meet nonlicensure criteria.)

Cross-training activities for laboratorians are being implemented in various health care settings. One type of cross-training, called intrasection, appears obvious for laboratorians and consists of acquiring and maintaining competence at all workstations within a laboratory discipline (transfusion services). A second type, intersection, dominates non–day-shift laboratories and other health care settings with personnel rotating across disciplines: perhaps working in hematology one month, STAT chemistry the next, and transfusion medicine the third. The third type, interdepartment, refers to competence in providing a broader scope of medical care, spanning two or more disciplines. Rarely does a health care worker with a baccalaureate degree obtain the education and training to perform multiple tasks in other medical-related disciplines. The extensive and divergent training required in health professions rarely supports performing combined tasks such as moderate- to high-complexity laboratory tests and radiation therapy, histotechnology and mammography, nuclear medicine imaging procedures and physical therapy exercises, or respiratory therapy and cardiac catheterization. Most often individuals will *add* knowledge and skills if they desire more patient contact or want to apply their knowledge in a different medical venue, such as a medical technologist who becomes an orthopedic nurse, a radiation therapist who becomes a family practice physician, or a cardiac catheterization technologist who becomes a nurse anesthetist.

Another viewpoint of multiskilled attributes addresses the education, skill, and experience that medical technologists/clinical laboratory scientists possess. With competencies in organization, troubleshooting and problem solving, quality control, and analytical thinking, they can perform additional tasks outside the laboratory. They can readily assume responsibilities per-

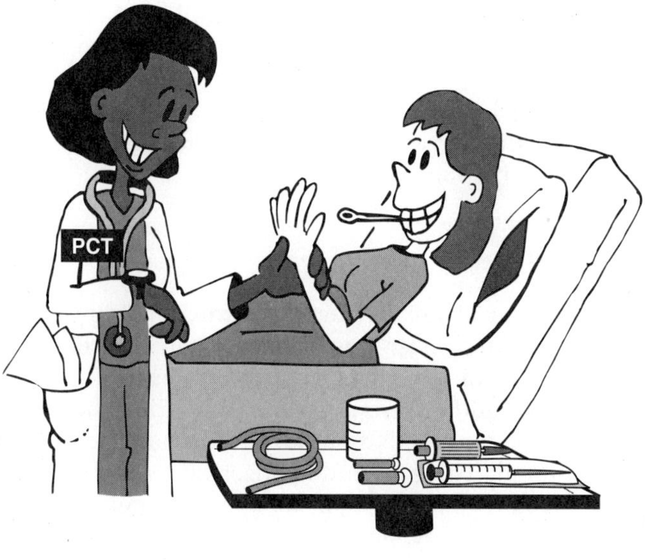

forming tasks in new and different areas. Examples of careers that use laboratory science knowledge and skills include specialized medical areas such as epidemiology and in-vitro fertilization; specialized science areas such as forensic and archeology molecular pathology, and toxicology in sports competitions and centers; community health such as public health, regulatory agency inspectors, and occupational and environmental health and safety; research; education; and management.[9]

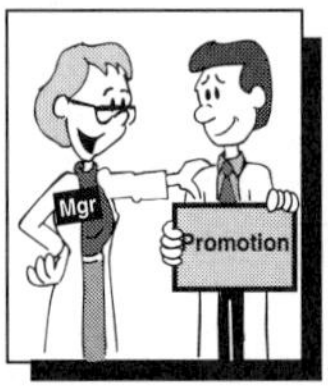

Activity 1: Value of Multiskilled Health Care Givers

Consider the situation in which a patient bedridden at home needs blood pressure and temperature readings, physical therapy exercise and massage, medications given orally and by injection, oxygen treatments, an EKG, and regularly timed blood tests to monitor therapy. Given the range of care required for this patient (and licensure of medical personnel), discuss the feasibility of reducing the number of health care givers to two or three who would perform all necessary procedures in a limited number of visits. Describe potential benefits and disadvantages regarding costs, time, exposure (control of nosocomial infections), and attention to the patient.

Hiring Practices

Multiple steps engage managers in the hiring process: recruiting, interviewing ("tell and sell" the job and the organization), assessing abilities of the applicants, checking credentials and references, selecting the candidate(s), offering the position, negotiating wages and work if necessary, assessing medical status to work, and setting the start date. Selected topics are addressed in this section, including the interview, preplacement assessment, and requirements to accommodate disabled employees. Because jurisdiction over hiring practices extends to federal as well as state laws, managers should discuss any additional information and policies with the organization's human resource department (HRD) and attorneys to ensure compliance in all areas. If they lack HRD or legal assistance, managers should contact appropriate government agencies.

It is advisable to seek additional specific information on the many aspects and details of hiring the "best" employee available in other resources (see Suggested Readings and Appendix 16–A).

THE INTERVIEW

Skillful interviewers can glean pertinent information from applicants. They can plan the interview from several aspects by creating a setting conducive to interaction; writing a list of questions to be asked regarding knowledge, skill, and affective behaviors; and developing the information they want to provide to the interviewee as a prospective employee. Certain techniques encourage the applicant to respond. These include pauses and silence; asking questions that require an explanation rather than a "yes" or "no" response; watching body language for contradictory signals; and actively listening both to what is

Table 16–2
SAMPLE WEIGHTS FOR WORK BASED ON IMPORTANCE AND TIME

Medical Technologist/Clinical Laboratory Scientist (MT/CLS): Duties and Responsibilities	Job Description Weights, Total = 100%	Performance Appraisal Weights, Total = 100 Points	Candidate's Profile Weights (Interview)
1. Performs complex clinical laboratory tests safely, with accuracy and precision, following accepted standard of practice; demonstrates ability to relate theory to test procedures and make appropriate clinical interpretations.	40%	20	
2. Reviews test results for accuracy and reasonableness; verifies accuracy of results as reported either manually or by computer.	20%	15	
3. Performs quality control testing/evaluation on equipment and reagents, according to standards of practice.	10%	10	
4. Operates, maintains, and troubleshoots highly sophisticated laboratory equipment and instrumentation.	10%	10	
5. Demonstrates effective interpersonal skills to work with others within the section between sections and throughout the facility.	5%	15	
6. Manages time effectively, completes assigned daily tasks within a reasonable time frame; overtime, when used, is well justified and assigned work that cannot be completed is reported to supervision; upon early completion of assigned tasks, helps co-workers.	5%	15	
7. Instructs students, residents, and new employees according to established policies and programs.	5%	5	
8. Readily assumes additional duties and professional responsibilities.	5%	10	
TOTALS	100%	100 points	

being said and what isn't said directly but rather implied. Initially, interviewers should concentrate on conducting a fair interview until they gain confidence in their roles and a higher level of comfort.

In addition to the job description of the duties and responsibilities, developing a job profile of the personal characteristics required to do the job (work) provides another guide. Objectivity in selecting prospective employees can be increased by assigning "weights" to each job duty/responsibility based on the importance and/or time of each (Table 16–2).

Activity 2: Technical Job Characteristics

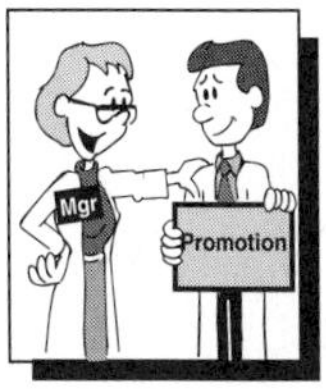

For a technical position in a clinical laboratory, describe 10 characteristics that you think are important to be demonstrated by the employee. Discuss your list with others in your class. Select the five characteristics that most of you have listed. Compare the compiled list and your own list with the duties and responsibilities identified in Table 16–2.

Creating a written interview guide of appropriate questions and key points related to the applicant's abilities becomes easier with these resources. Certain questions are considered discriminatory and illegal to ask (Table 16–3). Information gathered should enable the manager to assess whether or not the applicant can perform the duties and responsibilities based on performance in other positions (or training if the person has not yet worked in a laboratory). Use the written interview guide to maintain fairness with all applicants and to ensure that each has the same interview opportunity.

These questions will help avoid inadvertently asking improper questions or putting the applicants on the defensive. Interviewers should maintain control of the interview. If the applicant becomes nervous or aggressive, it is important to remain calm and bring the interview to an end in as neutral an atmosphere as possible.

Inexperienced interviewers may prefer to openly use the interview guide and write brief notes on it as the applicant talks or during pauses. Usually the job profile is not shared, as it serves as the tool for final selection. Handing out the job description is appropriate, especially if the work requires special activities or involves demands under unique circumstances (for example, the

Table 16–3
SAMPLE INTERVIEW QUESTIONS

Acceptable	Unacceptable (Unlawful)
Describe your knowledge and skills relevant to the job.	Do you work any extra jobs?
Demonstrate your ability to perform essential functions.	Do you have any disabilities? What is your ethnic background?
The days and times you would be scheduled to work are ______________. Can you meet these expectations?	Are you married, divorced, or widowed? Do you have children or plan to have any? What religion do you practice? What is your credit (financial) status?
Can you meet the job requirements legally?	Are you healthy?
Can you prove your age, as you must be 18 years to perform ________.	How old are you? With whom do you live?
Show proof of certification or license.	What does your spouse do?
Have you ever been convicted?	Have you been arrested for an alleged crime?
Show proof of legal status to work in the U.S.	What country are you from? Give me a photograph of yourself. Are you male or female?
Have you been or are you a member of ASCLS, ASCP, AACC, CLMA, or other laboratory professional organization?	Tell me about clubs and community organizations of which you are a member.
What instruments (equipment) can you use? Minimal experience or proficient?	
Can you perform this job with or without reasonable accommodation?	Do you need reasonable accommodations to perform this job?
Can you meet the attendance requirements of this job?	How many days were you sick last year?

The policy is a simple one: If a question is not directly applicable to the hiring decision and relevant to the job, it cannot be asked.

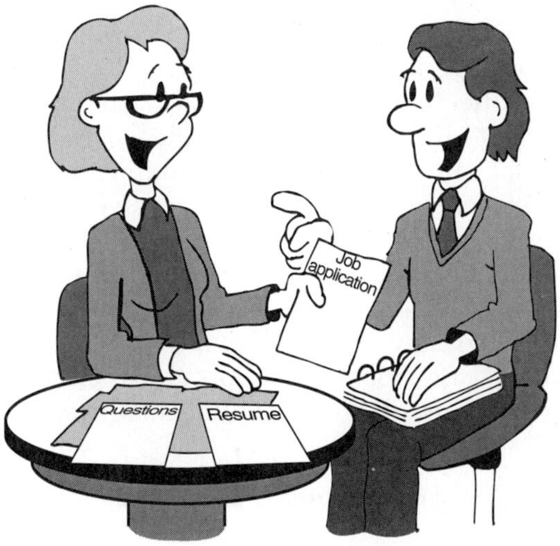

laboratory work is from an unusual customer source such as pediatric oncology). Most HRD directors prefer managers to discuss the organization's performance appraisal forms and process with employees during orientation.

In planning the interview, first look over the applicant's resume, curriculum vitae, and/or application. Prepare explanations to questions the applicant might ask. Start the interview on time. Conduct it in a quiet, comfortable, and private room. If in an office, turn the phone off (send calls to someone else), shut the door, and use a "do not disturb" sign. It is important to pay attention to the interviewee. This can be done by pronouncing the person's name correctly or asking how to pronounce it. Another important feature is for busy managers to control their own body language and to avoid wiggling in the chair, crossing and uncrossing arms and legs, tapping fingers together, and glancing at the clock. Stick to the time frame, especially if others will be interviewing the applicant also. Show enthusiasm and caring about the work and employees. Acting natural is acceptable; just be professional about it!

During the interview exchange, think about your language. Avoid idioms; slang terms; nicknames of tests, instruments, or activities peculiar to your laboratory; and local or regional geographic expressions. Speak clearly. If the applicant speaks English as a second language, make sure he/she understands your questions.

Activity 3: Writing Interview Questions

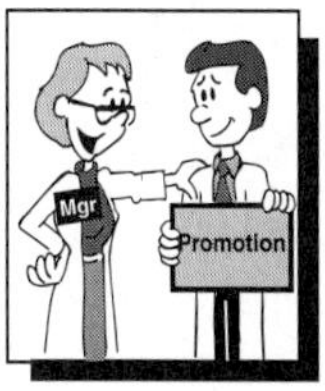

As a group, write a question for each of the five predominant characteristics selected in Activity 2. Review them for impropriety. Review them again as queries that lead applicants to tell you "the right answer" or "what they think you want them to say." Rewrite those that are unacceptable. Compare your questions with those in Table 16–3.

PREPLACEMENT AND HIRING ASSESSMENTS

Preplacement assessment of knowledge and skills *relevant* to the job can be accomplished in various ways, including a written quiz, unknowns for actual analysis, or results for interpretation. All assessment tools must be validated by ensuring that employees already performing the work can answer the questions or perform the "unknowns" correctly. All applicants for the same position level must be allowed to take identical tests related to the tasks they will perform. Consult your department administration and HRD before implementing a preplacement assessment policy. In laboratories with clinical training programs, supervisors often develop variations of the quizzes and practicals used with students for employee preplacement assessment tools.

Necessary information may be asked *after* the individual is hired (Table 16–4). Some information may be used for federal reports such as those required for affirmative action or equal opportunity employers, medical and other insurance applications, and documenting qualifications for employment.

Diversity and the Americans with Disabilities Act (ADA)

Traditionally, diversity in the United States represented people from different racial and ethnic backgrounds who conformed to images and rules in the workplace. They retained their language, their values and beliefs, and individuality at home and in their communities. No longer does conformity or uniformity achieve corporate goals or produce dedicated employees. People no longer want to just do a job but want to contribute and make a difference!

Attempts are clearly under way in corporations for inviting, supporting, and managing diversity in the workplace. Certain traditional management styles of successful managers enable them to maintain their effectiveness with a diverse workforce: communication skills showing clear speaking and active listening; equal and consistent expectations of performance, honesty, and respect for others; acting in accordance with what they say; and, above all, valuing the person as a human being who has the right to perform work regardless of his/her religion or ethnicity.

Another federal legislative development in hiring practices stemmed from many employers' lack of compliance with older laws such as allowing disabled persons the right to work. Today, increasing numbers of disabled workers are being hired for positions in businesses where they are succeeding and contributing to the organization.

Disabilities are categorized (then considered "qualified") based on (1) a physical, mental, or psychological impairment that substantially limits one or

Table 16–4
QUESTIONS APPROPRIATE TO ASK *AFTER* HIRE

What is your date of birth? (Ask for FICA and Social Security purposes.)
Will you provide me with a photograph of yourself?
Who should be contacted in case of emergency?
What is your marital status?
What is your ethnicity? (Ask if required by human resources or an external agency.)
Are you unable to work certain days of the week or holidays based on your religious practices?
What are specifics of your medical history that warrant any special accommodations?
Will you agree to the following tests?
  A. Drug testing (System must follow confidentiality protocols with testing performed by an external, unaffiliated laboratory.)
  B. Color-blindness test (May be required in order to adjust test analysis procedures.)
What special accommodations might you need in order to perform work? (ADA requirements)

Table 16–5
ADA ACCOMMODATIONS

In	Out
Levers	Doorknobs
Automatic opening/closing of doors	Revolving doors
ADA compliance officers	Human resource generalists
Confidential medical files maintained separately from departmental personnel files	Medical files in personnel records
Paper cups at drinking fountains	
Reasonable accommodations	Proclaim, "It's not in the budget."
Workability programs	If cannot do job, stay home.
Return-to-work programs	Extended workers' compensation leaves
ADA Seminars	
Terms:	Terms:
"Individual with a disability"	"Handicapped"
"Able-bodied person"	"Normal person"
Assessment of essential functions	Prejob offer for physical exam
	Asking applicant about his/her workers compensation or medical history

Modified from Halliday J: Worksite: ADA. Crain's Detroit Business 1992; 8(26): 13–18.

more major life activities; (2) a record of substantially limiting impairment (medical history); and (3) consideration of having a disability (by an employer). For individuals with disabilities, accommodations that are considered reasonable must be made according to the ADA. Reasonable accommodation indicates modification or adjustments to the workplace or the work process to enable a qualified person with a disability to do the work. It also refers to changes that must be made for employees with slight-to-severe hearing impairments. Table 16–5 presents a short list of ADA-enforced and acceptable accommodations.

Activity 4: Identification of Reasonable Accommodations

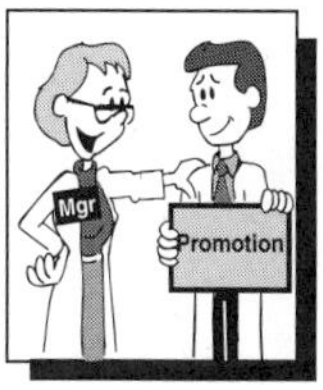

Describe disabilities* and suggest reasonable accommodations that might be made in a laboratory in order for someone to do the work. Consider individuals in wheelchairs, with only one arm, and with shortened arms due to polio or other disfiguring medical conditions. Consider prospective employees with arthritic hands, limited vision, hearing aids, speech impediments, dyslexia, or those who are color blind.

*Exclude those disabilities that truly would prohibit someone from fulfilling the essential functions.

Accommodations that might be necessary include those for a technologist in a wheelchair, a technician who uses crutches occasionally because of a leg prosthesis, someone who wears glasses with very thick lenses because of visual impairments, an administrator and a clerk who wear hearing aids, a blind telephone operator/clerk who schedules appointments, an employee who returned to work from a mental health medical leave, a woman who is in therapy owing to the murder of her daughter, and so forth.

Staffing and Scheduling

Laboratory managers previously scheduled employees according to predicted maximum hospital inpatient and outpatient census and workload. The peak of work most often occurred during the day shift, Monday through Friday, and was handled by technologists who worked as specialists in one or two laboratory sections. Most of the support staff of phlebotomists, clerks, and aides also worked days. Sufficient staff usually was available to cover all workstations on all shifts even during illnesses and vacations, and for special activities such as method evaluations and training of new personnel. With workload shifts, staff reductions, and automation increases among the many factors altering workloads, scheduling staff now frequently challenges the most experienced supervisor.

Planning for the necessary staff requires identification of *all* functions by task analysis (skill necessary to perform and time required to perform the task), establishment of priorities to produce results, and determination of critical pathways. *If* the test menu changes, especially by addition of complex manual procedures, *if* the workload does not lessen during a holiday season, or *if* productivity drops owing to inexperienced employees and increased training activities, *then* staffing patterns must be altered. Bennington and Westlake note that the proper scheduling of personnel has more impact than any other single parameter in determining optimal delivery of laboratory data and cost control.[10]

Unplanned or abrupt changes in service requests can throw managers and employees into a tailspin. Reasons for altering laboratory work and schedules include the following: (1) Phlebotomists no longer work primarily for the laboratory as they have acquired new skills, report to other managers, or have become members of patient-focused care teams; (2) test requests such as inpatient fasting blood glucoses are doubled or more and require blood collection before breakfast is served; (3) outpatient specimens arrive in the laboratory area after 1600 hours (4:00 PM) until midnight or later; (4) new facilities are installed in the hospital, such as for cardiac catheterizations and heart transplants; (5) the emergency center (EC) sets new goals to become a regional trauma center or a poison and drug testing center, handle an increase of

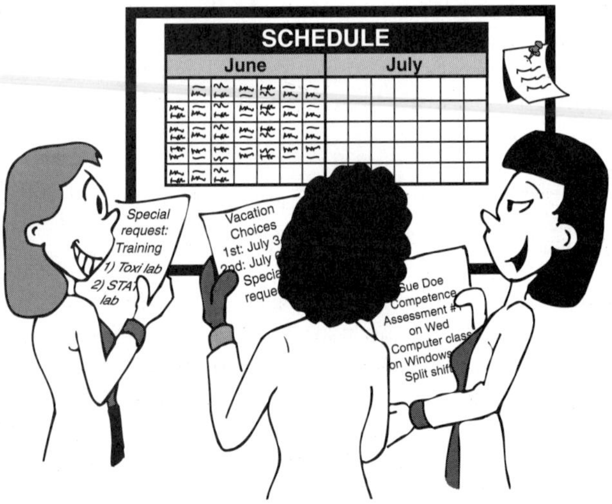

50% more patients, or reduce patient length-of-stay to 4 hours[11]; and (6) the laboratory sets a quality assurance objective to decrease laboratory STAT turnaround times for specific units (EC, ICU, nursery) or tests. Comfortable schedules and assignments may have to be reconfigured with minimal notice or preparation. Proactive laboratory directors and managers set objectives and change systems to improve laboratory services before mandates are thrust upon them. Careful planning, even developing alternate plans based on *if-then* assumptions, will prepare employees to adapt. Cognizant employees can facilitate a smooth work system, retain or possibly increase their productivity, and enhance their morale through job satisfaction.[12]

Activity 5: Laboratory Schedule Changes

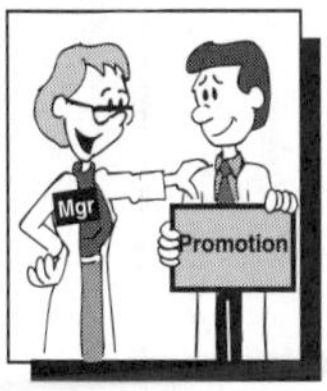

Discuss each of the reasons for redesigning laboratory work and schedules. Describe what laboratory managers might plan to do to meet each demand regarding personnel, instrumentation, site, and testing event time (of day and day of week).

See Activity Discussion 1 at the end of this chapter.

Altering staff patterns and schedules has become a major function of supervisors, especially in large laboratories with high volumes, varied customer bases, and specialized testing. STAT testing, when offered as a laboratory service, receives top priority and requires adequate personnel competent and trained to perform these tests. Table 16–6 shows average percentages of testing personnel needed based on the data in Figure 16–2. Supervisors use a grid format or computer program to assign personnel to workstations at the peak testing times (Tables 16–7 and 16–8).[13, 14] Monitoring testing volumes allows supervisors to project the *minimal* number of personnel needed per shift per weekday and for weekends and holidays. Flexible staffing implies 8-hour shifts, and full-time-equivalents (FTEs) have new meanings; a shift may span 3 to 12 hours, or two people may work sequential times to fill one full-time position. An axiom advises, "When work needs to be done, have people stay. When work is all done, send people away."

A well-planned, perfect schedule can be confounded by human-related factors: tardiness, absenteeism and illness, or emergency leave (employee's own medical or family). Other factors may be staff not yet adequately trained to handle unusual or abnormal tests, and personnel unwilling to work over-

Table 16–6
STAFFING NEED CHANGES

		Traditional	Contemporary
Day-shift specialists:	Technologists	70%	35%
	Technicians	5%	15%
	Lab assistants	5%	5%
Off-shift generalists:	Technologists	20%	20%
	Technicians	—	20%
	Lab assistants	—	5%

NOTE: Example represents possible changes in a large hospital laboratory.

Table 16–7

TECHNICAL STAFF SCHEDULE: LARGE HOSPITAL FULL-SERVICE CHEMISTRY LABORATORY

Workstation	Monday	Tuesday	Wednesday	Thursday	Friday	Weekend
STAT lab	3 MT 2 MLT	3 MT 1 MT train 2 MLT	3 MT 1 MT train 2 MLT	3 MT 1 MT train 1 MLT	3 MT 1 MT train 2 MLT	2 MT 1 MLT
Off-site labs: OR and PST	1 MT 1 MLT	1 MT 1 MLT	1 MT 1 MLT	1 MT 1 MLT	1 MT 1 MLT	1 MT
Automated instruments and cholesterols, irons	2 MT 1 MT train 2 MLT	2 MT 1 MT train 2 MLT (1 to PST lunch)	2 MT 1 MT train 2 MLT (1 to PST lunch)	2 MT 1 MT train 2 MLT	2 MT 2 MLT	1 MT and 1 MLT or 2 MT
Glucose, enzymes, CKMBs	2 MT 1 MLT	2 MT 1 MLT	2 MT 1 MLT	2 MT 1 MLT	1 MT 1 MLT-AM	1 MT
Electrophoresis, Sweat Cl^-, ALP Isoenzymes, L/S ratios, FSI tests	4 MT (1 to OR lunch)	4 MT 1 MT train	4 MT	4 MT	4 MT (1 to OR lunch)	2 MT
Specials, Toxi lab, Opiates/TCA	3 MT	2 MT	3 MT	3 MT	2 MT 1 MT-AM	2 MT
Front desk	1 MT (to PST lunch)	1 MT	1 MT	1 MT (to OR lunch)	1 MT	1 MT
Urines	1 MLT	1 MLT	1 MLT	1 MLT	1 MLT	1 MLT
Special assignments: lectures, competence assessments, computer/LIS/HIS and other training	1 MT AM lecture and Electrophoresis train in Afternoon	2 MT Competence assessments	2 MT Competence assessments	2 MT Competence assessments; 1 MT AM lecture	3 MLT train for Breath H_2	
TOTALS	25	27	28	26	26	13

NOTES: 1. Total technical personnel = 38; 26 MT/CLS and 12 MLT/CLT; plus 1 Supervisor and 4 Assistant Supervisors.

2. Day shift begins at 0530 hours with 2 MTs; others begin work 0600–0900 hours.

3. Saturday and Sunday staffing minimum is 13/day; holidays can be staffed with 10 to 12 depending on inpatient census and day of the week of the holiday.

4. Medical technology or medical laboratory technician students in their chemistry laboratory rotation can be assigned only to workstations where employees are not training or performing competence assessments.

5. Lunch coverage is indicated for special areas, Monday–Friday.

Table 16–8

TECHNICAL STAFF SCHEDULE FOR 2 WEEKS; SMALL TO MID-SIZED LABORATORY

Technologists—Lab Section	Su	M	T	W	Th	F	Sa	Su	M	T	W	Th	F	Sa
Chemistry	3	5	6	6	6	5	3	3	5	6	6	6	5	3
Hematology	1	3	3	3	4	3	1	1	3	3	3	4	3	1
Microbiology	1	3	3	3	3	3	1	1	3	3	3	3	3	1
Blood Bank	1	3	3	3	3	3	1	1	3	3	3	3	3	1
Immunology	*	1	2	2	2	2	*	*	1	2	2	2	2	*
Technicians—Lab Section														
Chemistry	1	2	2	3	2	2	1	1	2	3	3	2	2	1
Hematology	1	2	2	2	2	2	1	1	2	2	2	2	2	1
Microbiology	*	1	1	1	1	1	1	1	1	1	1	1	1	1
Immunology	*	*	1	1	1	*	*	*	*	1	1	1	1	*
Blood Bank	*	1	1	1	1	1	*	*	1	1	1	1	1	*
Urines	1	1	1	1	1	1	1	1	1	1	1	1	1	1
TOTALS: MT/CLS MLT/CLT	 6 3	 15 7	 17 8	 17 8	 18 8	 16 7	 6 4	 6 4	 15 7	 17 9	 17 9	 18 8	 16 8	 6 4

*Coverage by other staff working the same day.

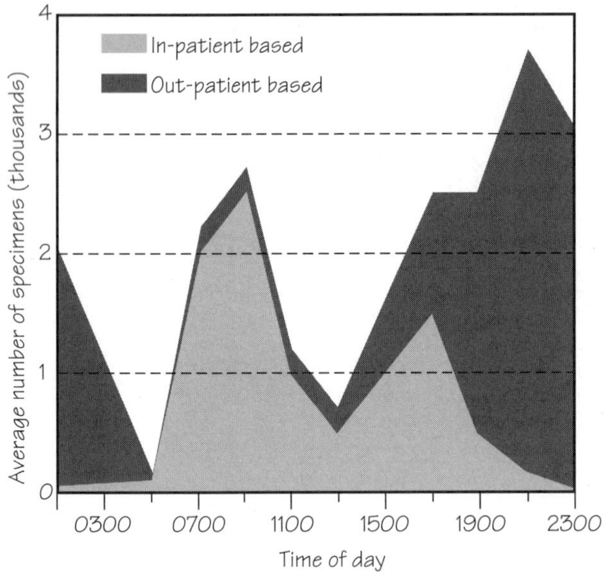

Figure 16–2 Testing volumes comparison.

time or extra time on a continual basis because of staff shortages or sporadically heavy workloads. Additional factors influencing schedules arise from training needs, especially when new procedures or testing services such as toxicology or molecular pathology, instruments, or an LIS are installed and implemented. Personnel may accumulate benefits such as vacation, unused sick time (saved as "banked" hours), and compensatory time if overtime is not paid, and may request this earned time to take all at one time.

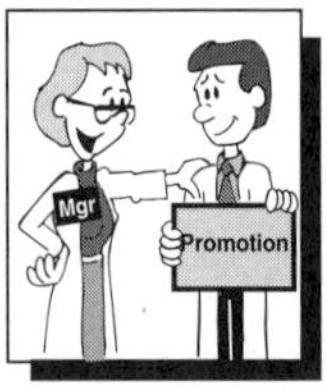

Activity 6: Adjusting Assignments

Review the staffing schedules in Tables 16–7 and 16–8 and discuss situations that would force supervisors to make adjustments in personnel assignments at the beginning of a work shift. Describe what changes might have to be made.

Inherently, personnel who contribute to scheduling decisions when factors warrant change will want to preserve quality, a professional workplace, and personal success and rewards, which will be evident by their attitudes. Levitt suggests these employees will "start with enthusiasm and then . . . approach each task with the passion of the scientist and the precision of the artist."[15]

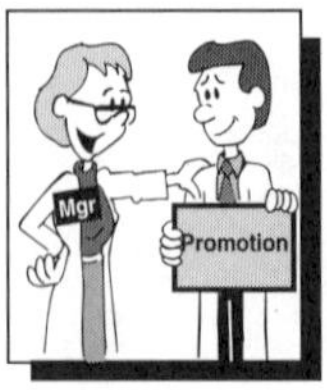

Activity 7: A Two-Week Schedule

In Table 16–8, the number of technical personnel are allocated for laboratory sections for a 2-week period. Develop a schedule identifying personnel to fill these assignments based on the following staff: 12 full-time technologists, eight part-time technologists, five full-time medical laboratory technicians, and four part-time medical laboratory technicians. No other time, such as personal time, vacation and training, needs to be considered.

Working Together

Although working relationships have existed casually among various hospital departments in providing patient care, with more patients (customers) receiving their health care outside of the hospital, formalized arrangements of health care givers working together have become essential. Providing patient care more efficiently *and* effectively can be accomplished by forming *teams* or *work groups.* In some cases, members trained and responsible for other duties, such as the few described for the multiskilled practitioners, facilitate the management of teams. One further benefit is the minimal number of personnel coming in contact with patients, with the exception of specific health care givers whose advanced skills may be needed.

Laboratorians must do more than just help their co-workers at various workstations on the afternoon shift or when a STAT chemistry lab is overburdened or when an instrument is malfunctioning. Truly delivering laboratory services in tandem with other patient care is now demanded of them. Receiving information regarding collection time of a drug level, performing the analysis, and reporting the results promptly and accurately becomes crucial, as these results determine the next dosage level of medication or admission to the hospital for other treatments. As Williams states: "The results of many far exceed the results of few."[16]

TEAMS, WORK GROUPS, COMMITTEES, AND TASK FORCES

A team prospers *first* of all because members desire to accomplish a common goal. Significant common goals might be to reduce patient days in the hospital or produce laboratory test results faster (turnaround time). The directive is clear and specific to all team members. *Second*, team members act according to certain rules and behave according to policies, most of which are official from the organization. Team members also adhere to a professional code of conduct that defines the affective behavior of a laboratorian: Come to work when scheduled; be on time; know how to do the work; understand methods, instruments, and checking and reporting results; and respect patient confidentiality. *Third*, teams follow protocols that are discussed in meetings: every morning to delegate assignments, weekly to share information and address problems and solutions, and monthly to discuss new tests and instruments to be evaluated. Protocols often include informal procedures such as a department newsletter, a National Medical Laboratory Week reception for laboratory employees, a summer picnic, or a winter holiday community service project. All get-togethers foster *esprit de corps* for team members. Real teams do not have to get along. They have to get things accomplished.[17] *Fourth*, team members play designated roles either officially by job title, job description, work activity or unofficially by election (by other members) to be leaders, inspirers, harmonizers, socializers, and ambassadors. Teams, not their members, compete. Team members cooperate, but, even more so, they must collaborate. They jointly share the desire to contribute of their talents to produce results.

In the workplace, many successful managers use tactics similar to sport teams coaches, posting popular slogans, such as "A **TEAM** succeeds because **T**ogether **E**veryone **A**ccomplishes **M**ore" and "Being there to pick up for a colleague is teamwork." Managers and supervisors use friendly gestures like a handshake or a gentle pat on the shoulder, a smile, a wave of a hand, giving a "thumbs up" sign, and sending verbal and written messages of support and understanding with a let's-go-for-it attitude. Managers let workers know of their importance, expected contributions, and value with notes of encouragement, letters of appreciation, and cards for their birthdays and anniversaries.

In the laboratory workplace, work groups are expected to function in ways similar to teams. Traditionally, work groups were assembled based on members' training and expertise according to laboratory discipline (hematology, microbiology, blood bank) with authority relegated to the most senior employees. As reengineering and downsizing takes place in health care organizations as well as in laboratories, work groups must change, with members able to use other talents in addition to their medical knowledge. In certain situations, work groups are "self-directed"; that is, leaders, rather than supervisors, act as facilitators and coaches. Progressive hospital administrators have reorganized medical departments, nursing units, and laboratory sections in both physical layout and personnel structure. Laboratorians are taking positions in new work groups, some of which solely serve a broad variety of laboratories, whereas others combine patient care responsibilities, working with nurses, physical therapists, pharmacists, and patient care technicians (PCTs). Laboratorians must now demonstrate interpersonal skills and abilities to communicate with patients and teammates, be capable of solving problems related to a patient's disease and clinical status, and use their laboratory science knowledge to collaborate with other health care givers and physicians regarding laboratory tests and other diagnostic and therapeutic protocols.

Successful work groups are composed of employees who want new or additional responsibility and seek empowerment. They understand group structure and roles, are willing to acquire collaborative and interrelationship skills, and will use trust and interdependency from all members.

Supervisors and managers play an important role by serving on committees. In hospitals and laboratories, several committees meet regularly according to their purpose and surrounding activities. A committee consists of a group of people charged to deliberate on, investigate, recommend and take action, or report on some matter. Examples of committees addressing subjects that necessitate constant surveillance and upgrading are listed in Table 16–9. Laboratorians, either by appointment or volunteering, represent their laboratory sections or work group. Involvement shows initiative and willingness to do more than just regular assignments.

The two characteristics differentiating task forces from committees are purpose and time span of existence. A task force often is identified to determine how an issue or concern might be resolved, and members are selected for their expertise, for balance, and to produce successful results. Assignments consist of producing recommendations and projections related to cost and efficacy benefits. Not all results produced by a task force are favorable: Recommendations might be positive for cost savings but negative in retaining jobs. The decision of what to do and how to go about doing it rests with management. This means that a task force submits findings and recommendations but rarely makes decisions about actions. This responsibility rests with the management. Subsequent implementation of the product usually continues by

Table 16–9
EXAMPLES OF COMMITTEES

Laboratory Committees	
Safety and chemical hygiene	Quality assurance
Competence assessment	Education and training
New employee orientation	Employee recognition
National Medical Laboratory Week	
Hospital Committees	
Safety	Quality assurance and utilization review
Patient confidentiality and ethics	Employee wellness (prevention of illness)
Accreditation	Holiday celebrations
Public relations	Volunteers
Bring your kids to work day	Recreation and wellness programs

NOTE: A committee may serve as the general or oversight committee with subcommittees existing in each laboratory section: for example, new employee education, training, orientation, and competence assessment.

a work group, team, or committee. Common laboratory task force assignments are needs assessment and feasibility studies for (education or training) programs, employee (student) recruitment and retention, computer software selection, robotics and automated systems feasibility, reengineering (total or specific laboratory section), LIS, or local area network (LAN).

Reaching decisions as a group may be achieved by consensus or majority vote. In the workplace, most decisions are made by consensus. For example, everyone agrees to some degree on the decision they rank first. Emphasis is placed on organizational needs rather than on individual needs. In professional organizations and other groups, parliamentary procedure determines that decisions will be selected by vote and majority rule.

Workgroup cohesiveness is characterized by trust, risk taking, mutual support, and (group) esteem. Groups effectively make decisions when members (1) use the resources of each other's abilities or expertise; (2) are focused on the assignment; (3) stick to the time frame; (4) are satisfied with their contributions; (5) identify a decision that is appropriate, reasonable, and feasible; and (6) believe that the decision is one that they can fully support.

Activity 8: Teamwork

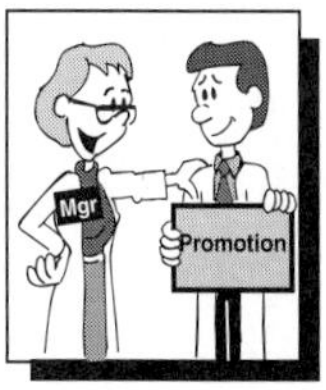

Within your class, create teams of five to seven members. Each team is to select an activity that is oriented to benefit your community, school, or organization and that can be accomplished in an hour or less. Decide how teams will function: as work groups, committees, or task forces. Write descriptions for your team following the four criteria presented above: results desired, rules to be followed, protocols for members, and roles of members—official and unofficial. What do you think is the last part of successful teamwork when the team has done its work?

See Activity Discussion 2 at the end of this chapter.

Note: With approval, this is an activity that students or employees could actually do.

Effective Coordinating Through Meetings

Meetings provide the most effective vehicle for communicating, planning, and coordinating. Identifying *purposes* for meetings becomes crucial to facilitate the occurrence of activities. Keidel advocates "three good reasons . . . to meet at work: create a forum . . . make decisions, and . . . build a team."[18] Therefore, when planning a work meeting, the purpose is selected first, and only those individuals who can contribute to achieving the purpose are invited. Even at work, meeting for a social purpose such as to celebrate achievements—for example, accreditation of the laboratory or employee recognition—is acceptable and, in certain cases, essential.

Regularly scheduled meetings between managers and supervisors, supervisors and employees, and among employees (forum meetings) serve the primary purpose of communicating: to tell and sell, disseminate information, and discuss issues and ideas. Participation should be encouraged if time can be provided—and *if* not at the immediate meeting, *then* time should be allotted for them at the next one.

Planning and preparing for a meeting should include the following four steps. First, *take care of premeeting details*: secure a site; distribute an agenda stating the purpose with information regarding place, date, time, and what participants should bring; assemble meeting materials; and order refreshments (if appropriate). Second, *begin the meeting* in an appropriate manner to set the tone. Offer friendly greetings to help establish rapport. Establish rules of conduct. Assign roles: (1) Leader–the person who actually runs the meeting; (2) Record keeper–notes significant information on chart, poster, or chalk/white board. If nothing new is said in the 5-minute period allotted, participants may be at a stalemate; the record keeper helps them stay focused; (3) Timekeeper–keeps meeting on track but moving forward; (4) Recorder–documents information including tasks to be done, who is responsible, when tasks are to be accomplished; and (5) Secretary–prepares minutes and distributes them with task information included. Third, *conduct the meeting.* A leader's function is to encourage participation, discourage contrary behavior by participants (in a nonthreatening way), influence attention to agenda, and support humor and creativity. Make sure everyone who wishes to contributes and believes that his/her attendance strengthened the purpose of the meeting. Fourth, *finish the meeting* with a review and summary: who is going to do what and when and how everyone will know what's going on. When decisions, assignments, and clarifications have been concluded, adjourn the meeting. "'Bye," and "Thank you for participating!" are simple but appreciated courtesies. Another courtesy to people using the facilities after the meeting is to rearrange the room to the original order and remove materials and supplies brought to the meeting.

More common courtesies enhance a good meeting. People should arrive on time and, if late, not ask questions about information already discussed. They should avoid interruptions such as phone calls and beepers or someone coming in to ask a question of an attendee. Meeting facilitators should be firm and direct, when common courtesy fails, to an attendee who monopolizes or tries to control the meeting (for his/her own hidden agenda), and whispers to others during the meeting. All attendees should finish on time and leave the room promptly after a meeting.

Decision-making meetings require members to prepare for the decision by studying alternatives beforehand and to come ready to participate. This means that the manager, leader, or president does *not* do the preparation, determine the decision, and tell members what to do. Talking freely about ideas as members discuss the issue to be decided, presenting concerns, considering alternatives studied, and reviewing options take some time and must be encouraged. Productive meetings require the meeting leader and members to do their homework *before* the meeting. Brainstorming before and during the meeting aids decision making.

Workplace Environment

Balancing the impact of change on laboratory personnel requires managers attend to the planning and coordinating functions consistently. Not all changes will be perceived as good or beneficial. If not anticipated, change can create a difficult work environment as employees struggle to learn and gain competence in new and different situations. Employees do not always behave as they usually do during stressful and uneasy or changing times. Managers are responsible for encouraging and supporting an atmosphere in which inappropriate and unacceptable behaviors are not tolerated.

Socialization of personnel becomes important in several respects: teamwork, handling of difficult co-workers and clients, empowerment with the authority to make decisions and act, coping with stress and change, and initiating actions that result in improvements in work and surroundings. Upsetting the balance can be detrimental to morale and productivity.

Through coordinating work groups, teams, meetings, and other activities, managers can establish a system for controlling balance in the workplace. Of similar importance, recognition of employees by honoring them privately and publicly demonstrates respect for them as people as well as their contributions.

POLICIES REGARDING BEHAVIORS IN THE WORKPLACE

Policies that are clear, strong, and well defined must be developed by human resource and organization administrators, including laboratory managers, who should explain inappropriate, unlawful, and unacceptable behaviors. Programs that protect and reduce risks must be developed to ensure compliance. These policies and programs are to be communicated to all employees at the time of hire and during their employment. If a manager or supervisor becomes aware of a situation and does not intervene, in certain situations, he/she may be held responsible and also liable for punitive damages even if not directly involved.

Policies must span the process before, during, and after hire (of employees). Legitimate practices address firing an employee also. Additional policies address violence in the workplace and sexual harassment. All policies must include a reporting and complaint procedure that is confidential and will be responded to immediately. Federal laws, presented in Appendix 16–A, provide the basis for policy making in the workplace.

The Occupational Safety and Health Administration (OSHA; see Chapter 17) introduced guidelines on March 14, 1996, for managers to use to help "reduce workplace violence to the greatest extent possible." Policies and programs should address (1) worksite analysis to identify high-risk situations; (2) prevention and control of hazards through appropriate physical designs and administrative practices; (3) employee training and education to recognize potential hazards and protect themselves and co-workers; and (4) management commitment and employee involvement through policies and practices. Usually, violent acts against health care workers consist of assault (being pushed, cursed at, bitten, hit, or kicked), most frequently by patients and public who are criminals, acutely disturbed (mentally ill), hostile, drug addicts, or very frightened, and happen in isolated or low-staffed locations.

Another concern is sexual harassment, which is defined in general but legal terms as "conduct which is unwelcome of a sexual nature which is severe and pervasive and interferes with a responsible person's ability to function at work." Often the individual is offended by a remark; the atmosphere in the workplace is threatening and hostile when co-workers tell raucous and obscene jokes, and a boss or superior makes explicit (direct) or implicit (suggested) comments that link a sexual favor to the employee's job.

Summary

The manager, in coordinating the functions of planning, organizing, directing, and controlling, becomes immersed in maintaining optimal laboratory operations. Knowledge and skill in hiring practices and balancing resources and work requests become paramount for the successful manager. External forces that are exerted on laboratory operations challenge all laboratorians regardless of their role: managerial, supervisory, technical, or support. Cooperative efforts through teams, work groups, committees, task forces, and effective meetings facilitate improvements when necessary and where most useful.

Working with individuals calls for managers who can see and be willing to fulfill the needs of employees within their span of control. Government laws and the organization's policies must remain foremost in every manager's mind. Courtesy and care in how employees are addressed and treated by the manager and co-workers alike must be kept constantly in mind.

Enhancing the workplace environment makes for a significant improvement for employees and therefore for production. Diversity of employees goes beyond numbers (of workers) but includes proactively soliciting and using their contributions. Managers have little choice but to value individuals for their contributions and efforts. Benefits desired—including financial—encompass personal and professional growth for *all* employees.

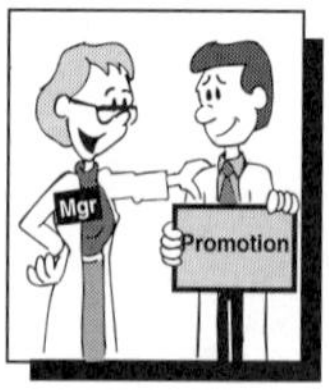

Activity Discussion 1: Laboratory Schedule Changes

1. Specify who will collect blood specimens and post assignments in the laboratory.
2. All personnel who collect blood specimens, deliver specimens to the laboratory, process specimens, or perform the test analysis and report results may be assigned to earlier work-start times (for example, 0530 hours).
3. Personnel may be assigned late evening or midnight shift start times.
4. Circumstances may require creation of a laboratory site within the cardiology department's suite.
5. Install a satellite laboratory in the EC and provide 24-hour testing staff; install a dedicated pneumatic tube system between EC and STAT labora-

tory; train laboratory personnel to increase their organizational and prioritization skills.

6. Develop a plan specifying alterations in the work system, communicate the plan to employees working on the specific units and in the laboratory, eliminate or control barriers, acquire more efficient instrumentation, train laboratory personnel.

Activity Discussion 2: Teamwork

The last element needed for successful teams is the recognition of their accomplishments. Although important for the team as a whole, recognition of individual effort, contribution, and credit for success outweighs the team. Congratulations should go to everyone by way of notices on bulletin boards and in newsletters, a party, and, when possible, bonuses and promotions. Of course, written recognition of outstanding or significant work should be filed in each employee's personnel record. Failure of the team's effort should be discussed with the whole team in attendance. Discussion regarding any particular individual's failing to contribute is done privately.

Review Questions

1. Coordinating as a laboratory management function requires careful consideration of all of the following *EXCEPT*
   a. Planning of meetings
   b. Building teams
   c. Organizing fund-raising activities
   d. Scheduling personnel according to workloads
2. Characteristics other than technical skills a laboratory supervisor might address with an applicant for a medical technologist position include
   a. religious activities.
   b. professional society involvement.
   c. registration for a particular political party.
   d. willingness to work overtime.
   e. disabilities that would require special accommodations.
3. When an applicant has been offered a position in a laboratory, describe questions that can be asked that would not be acceptable during an interview.
4. Identify 15 items for a checklist that should be covered before, during, and after a meeting.

See p. 411 for answers.

References

1. Perkins AG. Medical costs: saving money by reducing stress. Harvard Business Review 1994; 72(6): 12.
2. Ahern H. In vitro allergy testing is making its mark. Advance/Laboratory 1994; 3(3): 45–47.
3. Brzezicki LA. Drug abuse on the rise. Advance/Laboratory 1996; 5(7): 49–57.
4. Levitt R. Administration vs. management: convictions. Harvard Business Review 1989; 67(4): 8.
5. Accreditation Manual for Pathology and

Clinical Laboratory Services. Joint Commission on Accreditation of Healthcare Organizations. Oakbrook Terrace, Ill: 1993.

6. Davis JT. Staffing challenges for the POL. Advance/Laboratory 1994; 3(3): 12–13.
7. Kost GJ. Bedside know-how. Advance/Laboratory 1996; 5(7): 63–70.
8. Brzezicki LA. From microscopes to marketing. Advance/Laboratory 1996; 5(7): 77–78.
9. Klosinski DD. Cross-training: walking a new path. Clinical Laboratory News 1996; 22(11): 11, 13.
10. Bennington JM, Westlake GE. Responsibility scheduling. Laboratory Management 1978; February: 60–63.
11. Mohammad AA, Summers H, Burchfield JE, et al. STAT turnaround time: satellite and point-to-point testing. Laboratory Medicine 1996; 27(10): 684–688.
12. Gvazdinskas LG, Maffetone MA. Employee satisfaction: an integral component of total quality. Clinical Laboratory Management Review 1995; 9(3): 108–116.
13. Scheduling employees. Computer program: E-Squared Software. 1303 Orlando Drive, Fort Wayne, IN 46825.
14. Visual Staff Scheduler®. Pro (VSS). Atlas Business Solutions, Inc., Fargo, ND, 1996.
15. Levitt R. Attitudes, convictions. Harvard Business Review 1989; 67(4): 8.
16. William RL. Essentials of total quality management. New York, AMACOM, 1994.
17. Katzenbach JR. Seven experts discuss what teamwork takes. Harvard Business Review 1994; 72(6): 26.
18. Keidel RW. Meaningful meetings. Clinical Laboratory Management Review 1996; 10(4): 357–361.

Suggested Readings

1. Chervinski D. Drawing the line on workplace violence. Advance/Laboratory 1994; 3(9): 39–43.
2. Frings CS. Team building: setting a climate for motivating your team. Clinical Laboratory News 1996; 22(8): 21.
3. Garon JE. Resumes and cover letters: A guide. *In* Management in Action. Clinical Laboratory Management Review 1995; 9(4): 304–309.
4. Gore MJ. Self-directed teams: the new form for American work. Clinical Laboratory Science 1994; 7(12): 326–330.
5. Honen D, ed. Part-time employment as a full-time proposal. Managing laboratory personnel: The CLIA and OSHA manual. Thompson Publishing Group, Inc., 747 Third Avenue, New York, NY 10017: 1995; 2(3): 3, 7.
6. Jackman M, Waggoner S. Star Teams, Key Players. New York, Ballantine Books, 1991.
7. Katzenbach JR, Smith DK. The Wisdom of Teams: Creating the High-Performance Organization. New York, HarperCollins, 1994.
8. Kurec AS. Criteria-based job descriptions. Tech Sample®. Management and Education No. MGM-3. Chicago, ASCP, 1989.
9. Lussier RN. Selecting qualified candidates through effective interviewing. Clinical Laboratory Management Review 1995; 9(4): 267–275.
10. Ragan DD. Sexual harassment: know the facts. Medical Laboratory Observer 1993; 25(3): 26–30.
11. Salodof J. Employing persons with learning disabilities: a handbook for employers, trainers, and supervisors. International Center for the Disabled, 1993.
12. Schaupp DL, Parsons BL. Employee-involvement work groups. *In* Snyder JR, Senhauser DA, eds. Administration and Supervision in Laboratory Medicine. 2nd ed. Philadelphia, JB Lippincott, 1989.
13. Thomas RR. From affirmative action to affirming diversity. Harvard Business Review 1990; 68(2): 107–117.
14. Varnadoe L. Requesting additional staff: a model for the generalist supervisor. Tech Sample®. Generalist No. G-11. Chicago, ASCP, 1995.

APPENDIX **16–A**

Federal Government Legislation Related to Hiring Practices

- 1963 *Equal Pay Act*
  Prohibits employers from paying different wages for work requiring similar skills, abilities, experience, and responsibility.
- 1964 *Title VII of the Civil Rights Act*
  Prohibits discrimination on the basis of race, religion, sex, and national origin against applicants or employees relating to their work.
- 1967 *Age Discrimination Act*
  Prohibits discrimination on the basis of age (individuals over 40 years of age).
- 1968–69 *Affirmative Action (executive order)*
  Call for equal opportunities for applicants and employees, in particular employees with federal government contracts.
- 1972 *Title VII (32.01, 32.02, 32.03) Amendments: Equal Opportunity Act*
  Prohibits employers from depriving or adversely affecting employment opportunities for employees based on race, religion, sex, and national origin.
- 1978 *Title VII (32.04) Amendment: Pregnancy Discrimination Act*
  Prohibits employers from depriving or adversely affecting employment opportunities for female employees based on pregnancy and maternity status.
- 1986 *Immigration Reform and Control Act*
  Prohibits discrimination in recruiting, hiring, or as an employee on the basis of lawfully documented alien status.
- 1990 *Title I, The Americans with Disabilities Act*
  Prohibits discrimination against applicants and employees based on any disability(-ies) they might have.

Additional Title VII Amendments include 32.05, which obligates employers to see that all employees, supervisors included, do not engage in any unlawful sexual harassment; 32.06 prohibits discrimination based on gender, and 32.07 requires equal pay for similar work performed by men and women.

17

Rules and Regulations: Compliance

OBJECTIVES

Upon completion of this chapter, the reader should be able to:

- State, with explanation, three reasons for regulation and accreditation of health care facilities and laboratories.
- Describe similarities and differences of required versus voluntary programs for laboratories to operate and cite at least four examples of agencies and their purposes.
- Describe the responsibilities of managers and supervisors to employees regarding laboratory regulatory and legal activities.
- Perform a "mock-inspection" of a laboratory; discuss the findings and possible solutions to any deficiencies that have been identified.

KEY WORDS

laws	certification
regulations	standards
licensure	CLIA '88
accreditation	compliance

Introduction

It is thought that *good* performance by health care personnel is more likely to result in *good* outcomes for patients. Advocates for patients' rights contend that legislative requirements and standards, for example, Good Manufacturing Practices (GMP), demonstrate to the public such performance.

For several decades, public demand for readily available high-quality health care at reasonable cost has resulted in increased and expanded legislation. Legal, regulatory, and legislative activities have impact on health care services and economics. Federal, state, and local governments along with nonprofit private or professional agencies control and monitor health care services under these pressures. In certain situations, international regulations have jurisdiction over (US) laboratory services. Also, accountability for medical diagnosis and treatment, and laboratory services in particular, must be documented. This includes specifying the medical necessity of laboratory tests ordered and billed (which is strictly defined in Medicare regulations).

Regulations consist of laws, rules, and standards of practice (SOPs) instituted to protect the public (patients, their families and physicians) from illegal and unethical medical practices. Laboratory owners and managers must be able to provide information, on request, that the laboratory work performed is legitimate, charged and paid for appropriately, and recorded correctly. At this time, laboratory tests must be ordered by a patient's physician. Therefore, a laboratory can perform *only those procedures that have been requested.* Fees charged for the tests must be fair and, in most situations, billed according to a published schedule: for example, common procedure terminology (CPT) codes. Data of test analyses must be held (stored) for a designated period of time, be legitimate when compared with reported results, and be available if requested by inspectors.

The subject of regulation has become quite complex. Several aspects of legal management of laboratory facilities will be presented in this chapter: licensure, accreditation, certification, and registration. Only the basics of these topics will be addressed.

Regulation of Laboratories and Personnel

Previously, hospitals, health-care facilities, and laboratories that received payment for services from any government-funded medical coverage program were required by law to be identified and inspected before authorization to continue business. Additional requirements came from interstate commerce laws over laboratories accepting specimens from other states and individual state and city laws over laboratories residing or operating within geographic boundaries.

Since 1988, strong public and media concern regarding the quality of laboratory services and accuracy of test results forced the mandate that *all* clinical laboratories in the United States as *required* by federal regulation be identified and approved in order to receive authorization to operate. This law, the 1988 Clinical Laboratory Improvement Amendments (CLIA '88), supersedes previous regulations. (See the Laws, Appendix 17–B at end of this chapter.)

A clinical laboratory, in the HCFA final rule of August 14, 1995, is described as follows:

> An entity furnishing biological, microbiological, serological, chemical, immunohematological, hematological, biophysical, cytological, pathological, or other examination of materials derived from the human body for the purpose of providing information for the diagnosis, prevention, or treatment of any disease or impairment of, or the assessment of the health of, human beings. These examinations include procedures to determine, measure, or otherwise describe the presence or absence of various substances or organisms in the body. Entities only collecting or preparing specimens (or both) or only serving as a mailing service and not performing testing are not considered laboratories.

LAWS AND REGULATIONS

Laws are passed by the United States Congress (House of Representatives and Senate) with approval by the President of the United States. Regulations and rules are developed to implement laws by appropriate government agencies such as Department of Health and Human Services (DHHS), Health Care Financing Administration (HCFA), Centers for Disease Control and Prevention (CDC), Occupational Health and Safety Administration (OSHA), and Federal Drug Administration (FDA) (Fig. 17–1). These agencies also become responsible for overseeing compliance.

All laboratories participating in federal and state reimbursement programs, such as Medicare and Medicaid, must be registered with HCFA. These laboratories are subject to inspection to ensure that their operations meet or exceed standards. After passing inspection, a registered laboratory can be issued a Certificate of Accreditation by HCFA and *licensed* by the CDC. Laboratories providing special services, such as transfusion medicine services (blood banks) or drug testing, must undergo additional inspections to be licensed by authorized agencies such as FDA and the National Institute for Drug Abuse (NIDA), respectively.

Responsibilities of laboratory owners and managers include knowledge of the laws, rules and regulations, compliance requirements, terms of inspections, and renewal criteria (time intervals). They must stay current, especially regarding rules that have been written. Recent regulations affecting laboratories have been changed because of the views and arguments presented

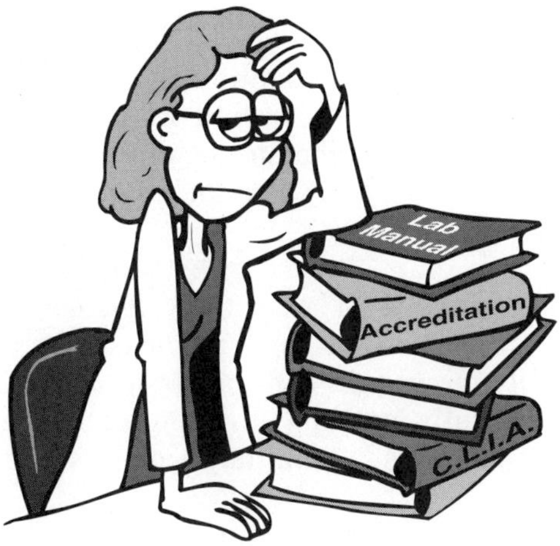

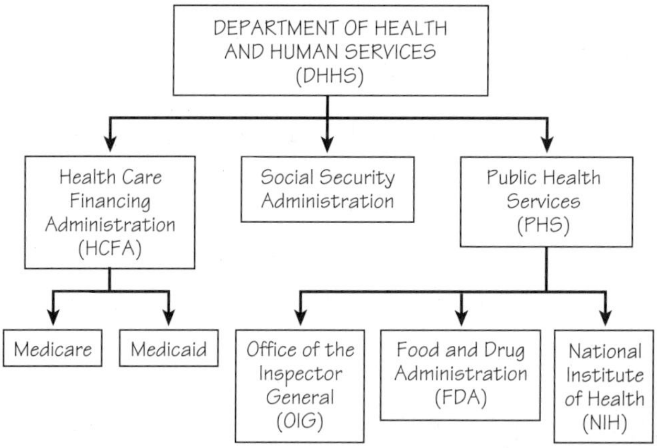

Figure 17–1 Federal agencies.

in the thousands of letters received by HCFA (during the 60-day comment period).

Additional responsibilities require managers to educate employees and document (learning) activities of the knowledge and skills they acquire. What they can do must match with their work assignments and expected performance for compliance with the law. In some situations, education of customers (patients and physicians) must be planned, carried out, and documented also.

In addition to fulfilling legal requirements just to operate, laboratories must also comply with safety and labor laws. (See Chapter 16; List of Agencies and Associations, Laws, appendices 17–A and 17–B at the end of this chapter.)

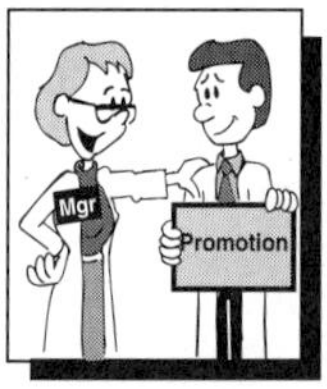

Activity 1: Federal Law Notification

For an area of interest specified by an instructor or supervisor, develop a plan (outline) that you, if you were the manager or supervisor, would follow to communicate and educate employees regarding a newly published federal law and its corresponding regulations.

Registration, Licensure, and Certification

Basically, *registration* means being identified on a list. This can be a legal requirement for a business, facility or individual to operate/work. It can also be a professional listing of laboratories or individuals meeting certain qualifications. Standards and criteria are not necessarily required to be met. A fee may or may not be levied.

Licensure or practice control indicates that a business, facility or individual meets entry level standards in order to do business or perform work or provide services as approved by a government agency, usually at the state level. This refers to public recognition of professionalism. Renewing a license usually consists of annually sending in appropriate records assuring that standards have been maintained. Remittance of fees, if required, would be included.

Certification is a process of title control that laboratorians, among many health care personnel, are offered. They voluntarily seek certification. Usual process is done by laboratory-related associations who set standards for safe and ethical practice of the profession. First, meeting preestablished qualifications of academic, clinical training, and/or experience of the individual is determined. Then passing a written and/or practical examination is required. Certified laboratorians include initials of the profession, professional category, and agency after their names to show as their credentials. Recognition establishes competence or excellence in practice. In the absence of (state) licensure of laboratory professionals, managers often maintain certification of employees as the standard of practice.

Laboratories, on the other hand, may also receive certification to perform tests. When HCFA awards a "Certificate of Accreditation," the tests which the laboratory is approved to perform are recorded.

ACCREDITATION

In addition to fulfilling laws and meeting required regulations mandated by governments, laboratories may choose to subscribe to *voluntary* programs. Standards, many of which are more strict than governmental ones, are developed by national agencies for laboratories to follow. (JCAHO, CAP and COLA represent nonprofit, and private or professional agencies.) These are the guidelines for evaluation and inspection of laboratories. Once a laboratory is recognized to meet these standards, it is considered *accredited.*

Accreditation, the public recognition of an institutional program or activity meeting certain predetermined standards through an evaluation and approval process, offers assurance of quality. Usually this is a voluntary, self-regulatory peer review process. The National Accrediting Agency for Clinical Laboratory Sciences (NAACLS) accredits training programs: MT/CLS, MLT/CLT, HTL, HT; the College of American Pathologists (CAP) accredits laboratories.

Establishing a new program warrants *initial* accreditation. Partial compliance or missing minor pieces might result in *probation. Full* accreditation ranges from 2 to 7 years (depending upon the program and the agency). All accreditation awards are subject to ongoing compliance to the standards. If at any time noncompliance is reported or suspected, the agency can demand a review of documents or inspect without forwarning. If findings warrant it, accreditation can be revoked or reduced (see the section on Compliance in this chapter).

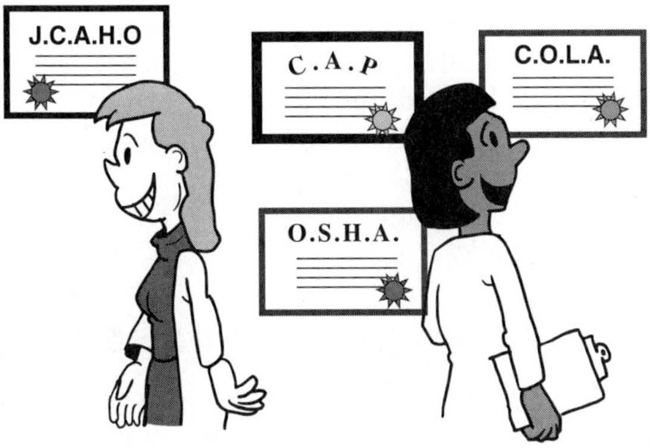

ORGANIZATIONS HOLDING *DEEMED STATUS* FROM HCFA
• American Association of Blood Banks (AABB)
• American Osteopathic Association (AOA)
• American Society for Histocompatibility and Immunogenetics (ASHI)
• College of American Pathologists (CAP)
• Commission on Official Laboratory Accreditation (COLA)
• Joint Commission on Accreditation of Healthcare Organizations (JCAHO)
• New York State
• Oregon State
• Washington State
Private, nonprofit organizations or state agencies as of August 1996.

Prior to CLIA'88, only hospital laboratories were accredited by CAP or JCAHO. HCFA has authorized, by granting *deemed status,* several agencies and states to inspect and accredit laboratories which then is used for federal licensure (see the boxed area).

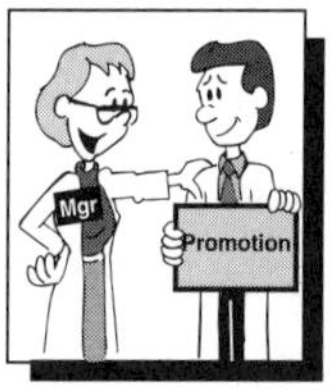

Activity 2: Reasons for Regulation and Accreditation

Discuss (at least three) reasons for regulation and accreditation of health care facilities and laboratories. Explain specific benefits to the public as customers, i.e., patients.

Regulatory Processes

Managers can acquire information regarding the necessary standards and criteria from an agency. The regulatory process begins with registration when an application is made to the agency (or agencies). Next, the manager submits documents for review, after which there is an inspection of the (laboratory) site or facility. All documents and inspection reports are reviewed by the agency's board or administration. Finally, approval is granted with corresponding licensure and/or certification.

Deficiencies or failure to fulfill standards and criteria result in denial of approval to operate. The laboratory owners, directors, and managers can respond with an appeal, challenge, or rebuttal. They may obtain probation until the appeal is addressed.

SURVEYS, SELF-ASSESSMENT AND INSPECTIONS

Several benefits can be gained through self-assessments or self-studies as preliminary steps to inspection. Laboratory personnel, while preparing and organizing materials, should use "self-critique" processes to identify deficiencies or infractions. These can be corrected before the on-site inspection. Periodic reports, between inspections, may be required to detail the laboratory's compliance to standards. Examples from records show the necessary evidence of the laboratory's (self) evaluation and improvements.

The method of inspection depends on the type of laboratory or health care organization, such as hospital, physician office laboratories (POLs), or commercial, as does the type of business operation: for example, inpatient specimens, reference testing of specimens from multiple states or countries, or drug testing. Certain agencies may send one or more inspectors (these employees are often medical technologists/laboratory scientists), whereas other agencies will send a team of "volunteers" from another accredited laboratory. Some inspections are scheduled well in advance (accreditation agencies) and others can be unannounced (government agencies).

Managers should never be surprised by the questions asked or the documents requested for review. Standards and accompanying checklists are provided from agencies with time allowed for compliance practices to be implemented. Actually conducting pre-inspection dress rehearsals or mock visits reduces anxiety for laboratory personnel. Employee volunteers can serve as "inspection teams" and use the checklists provided by the agency. Planning and organizing for the real inspection takes time and cannot be put off until the last minute. Files of personnel training and continuing education, procedure manuals reviews and updates, and method validation records, quality assurance and control records, and patient results verification are examples of documents that inspectors will want to see. Regular review and maintenance of the required documents is essential to a smooth and successful inspection.

When inspectors arrive, managers should extend several courtesies to them: provide a space as needed and possibly refreshments, for their use as they review documents and interview employees. Respond to their requests for information and materials as efficiently as possible. Information should explain materials that are in transition to final form. Notify all employees and officials in the laboratory that an inspection is in progress. Intent to comply, although not the same as compliance, is better than lack of knowing the standard or negligence, and employees might be asked questions regarding their knowledge of laboratory operations and standards. Providing a map of the general areas (laboratories) and names of key personnel is also helpful. Be helpful when asked and under no circumstance obstruct or prohibit contact with employees if this is chosen by inspectors. Be readily but discreetly available (even if by beeper).

Activity 3: Inspection for Accreditation

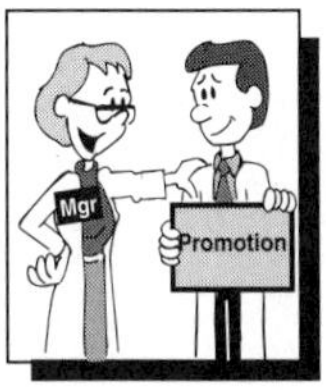

Using the CAP questions, in the boxed area on the next page, along with additional resources provided by the instructor or supervisor, plan an inspection of one laboratory section. Describe a policy and procedures to address each question (usually one policy with several procedures for each question). Identify any examples, records, or documents that an inspector might want to review. When policies are violated, what type of penality or penalities should be levied?

CAP QUESTIONS FOR INSPECTION OF LABORATORIES: ABBREVIATED LIST

General Laboratory

- Has the laboratory documented a system for determining the accuracy and reliability of analytic results on patient samples for which no external proficiency testing program is offered?
- Does the laboratory have a policy requiring oral requests for patient testing to be followed by an attempt to obtain written or electronic authorization within 30 days?
- Has the laboratory defined turnaround time for each of its tests, and does it have a policy for notifying the requester when testing is delayed?
- If the laboratory changes its analytic methodology so that test results or their interpretation may be significantly different, is the change explained to clients?
- Does the laboratory have a system documenting that all analysts are knowledgeable about the contents of procedure manuals relevant to the scope of their testing activities?
- Are reference (normal) ranges established or verified by the laboratory for the population being tested?
- Is there evidence of corrective action taken if acceptable temperature ranges for refrigerators and/or freezers are exceeded, including evaluation of contents for adverse effects?

Alternative

For laboratories that qualify, the option to circumvent an on-site visit and respond to a written questionnaire is granted. These laboratories must have demonstrated good performance from previous on-site inspections. Documents and examples of records might be requested with the questionnaire.

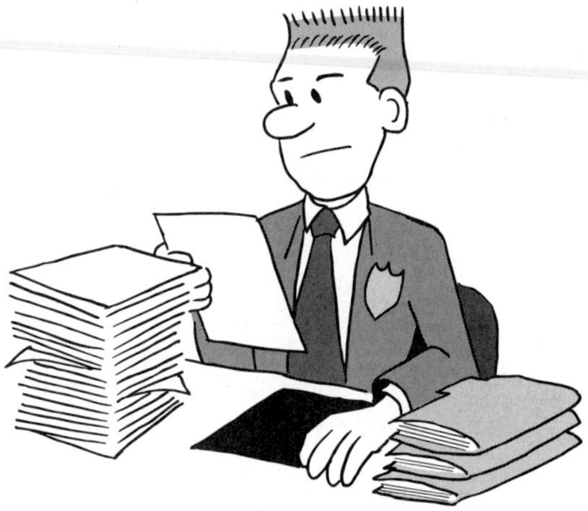

CLIA '88 allows use of the Alternate Quality Assessment Survey (AQAS) in lieu of biennial inspections. Laboratories with demonstrated good performance from the previous on-site inspections may qualify. The 1996 AQAS consisted of 45 questions and was due within 15 days of receipt.

Exemption may be granted to certain laboratories (excused) from required participation with federal laws if another agency oversees compliance with more stringent standards. One example is the State of New York, which imposes significantly more stringent standards than the CLIA regulations for all laboratories except POLs: safety, laboratory information systems (LIS), proficiency testing for forensic testing, and requirements for paternity testing and workplace drug testing.

REGULATIONS AND RULES

Four major concerns that can affect the quality of laboratory services are specified in the regulations and rules for laboratories. One concern covers categorizing tests according to ease or difficulty of performance. A second concern addresses minimum standards for personnel (education and training) performing different groups of tests. The third concern considers demonstration of proficiency by the laboratory, and the fourth concern addresses quality assurance and improvement. Only an introduction to each regulation is presented here.

Test Complexity

Clinical laboratory tests must be categorized according to HCFA regulations (Table 17–1). Excerpts from the CLIA '88 regulations follow (see Laws, Appendix 17–B). *Waived tests* are "simple laboratory examinations and procedures" that compose about 1% of all tests done. *Physician-performed microscopic procedures* (PPMP) make up a new category in which less than 1% of all laboratory tests are performed. *Moderately complex tests,* about 75% of all testing, involves "a reasonable risk of harm to a patient if the test is performed incorrectly; the risk of erroneous result is present but is minimized because testing methodologies are not complex. Their interpretation requires a moderate level of independent judgment, and interpretation of test results involves knowledge of a limited number of factors that can influence the results." *Highly complex tests,* about 24% of all testing, consist of those tests in which there is "generally a substantial risk of erroneous results because testing methodologies are complex. Test interpretation requires independent judgment and a comprehensive understanding of the method, instrumentation, physiology, interpretation of data, and clinical significance of the result; interpretation of test results requires knowledge of a number of factors that can influence tests results; and training is required prior to performing tests."

As of 1995 the CDC became officially responsible for complexity categorization of clinical tests under CLIA '88.

Proficiency Testing

All licensure and accreditation criteria require laboratories to subscribe to a proficiency testing (PT) program with an external agency and "participate *successfully.*"[2] Regulations stipulate the frequency, protocol to be followed, and consequences for failure. PT is required only for the primary test system

Table 17–1
CATEGORIES OF TEST SYSTEMS ACCORDING TO CLIA '88

Waived (1%)	Physician-Performed Microscopic Procedures (<1%)	Moderately Complex 75%	Highly Complex 24%
Requirements: Follow manufacturer's instructions; good lab practice.		***Requirements:*** QC, QA, PT, PTM; limited personnel standards	***Requirements:*** QC, QA, PT, PTM; stringent personnel standards
Three criteria: 1. Approved by FDA for home use 2. Methods are so simple and accurate; likelihood of erroneous results negligible 3. Poses no reasonable risk of patient harm if performed incorrectly		***Seven criteria:*** 1. Degree of knowledge needed to perform the test 2. Training and experience required 3. Complexity of reagent materials and preparations 4. Characteristics of operational steps 5. Characteristics and availability of calibration, quality control, and proficiency testing materials 6. Trouble shooting and maintenance required 7. Degree of interpretation and judgment required in the testing process	
Examples: (There were 10 tests in early 1996) • Urine dipstick, nonautomated • Visual urine pregnancy tests • Erythrocyte sedimentation rate, nonautomated • Hemoglobin by copper sulfate method, nonautomated • Fecal occult blood • Spun microhematocrit • Blood glucose (home use devices) • Cholesterol, AccuMeter	***Examples:*** • Gram stains • KOH preparations • Pinworm exams • Postcoital exams • Urine sediments • Vaginal wet-mount preparations • Nasal smears for presence of granulocytes	***Examples:*** *Bacteriology:* primary culture inoculation; urine culture; aerobic organism isolation and identification *Virology and Immunology:* manual procedures with limited steps *Chemistry:* Blood gas analyses that do not require operator intervention; osmolality *Urinalysis:* microscopic analysis of urinary sediment *Hematology:* automated procedures without differentials; manual hematology or coagulation procedures with limited steps and with limited sample or reagent preparation	***Examples:*** *Cytology:* all procedures *Bacteriology:* aerobic and anaerobic organisms; semi-automated bacterial identification; semi-automated susceptibility testing; all serotyping *Virology:* isolation and identification techniques *Immunology:* complement fixation; gel-based immunochemical procedures; Western blot; hemagglutination; RIA *Chemistry:* manual methods of multiple steps; chromatography; electrophoresis and densitometry; blood gas analyses; automated procedures requiring extensive operator intervention *Hematology:* reticulocyte counts; hemoglobin electrophoresis; manual white-cell differential counts; flow cytometry; manual platelet counts *Immunohematology:* compatibility testing; unexpected antibody identification *Other:* semen analysis (quantitative)

QC = Quality Control
QA = Quality Assurance
PT = Proficiency Testing
PTM = Patient Test Management

(assay) for patient specimen testing used in a lab (in other words, only the assay used the most often for an analyte rather than all of the assays performed in the lab for the same analyte and not those assays used for research). PT programs send, according to a schedule, "unknown" samples to be handled, processes, and analyzed in the same manner as patients' samples. Laboratories requesting certification for many tests, must be enrolled in approved PT program(s) for each test or subspeciality within that particular laboratory.

Results are compared among participating laboratories and reports inform laboratory managers whether or not their laboratories demonstrate acceptable performance (proficiency). Consecutive failures of not obtaining and reporting answers comparable with other laboratories may cause the laboratory to suffer suspension or loss of their license and closure. (Rigorous decisions such as these depend on the PT program and the analysis.) Some laboratory managers develop their own programs of internal PT in additional to the external ones. They seek to assess the strengths and weaknesses of their testing systems and to evaluate consistency of performance among technical personnel and the various methods used within the same laboratory section.[3]

Personnel Standards

CLIA '88 requires clinical laboratories to consider for their employees the "competency, training, experience, job performance, and education and which qualifications shall, as appropriate, be different on the basis of the type of examinations and procedures being performed by the laboratories and the risk and consequences or erroneous results associated with such examinations and procedures." This translates into no requirements to perform *waived tests* but (some) education and training to perform *moderately complex tests,* and more or advanced education and training to perform *highly complex tests* (Fig. 17–2).

Competence assessment is an annual requirement for testing personnel. This determines that their knowledge of and technical abilities to perform assigned tests meet the laboratory's acceptable criteria. Institutional and departmental policies and procedures to be covered include general information; fire, safety, and disaster information; infection control information; personnel information; the quality improvement plan; and procedure and reference manuals. Employees (and students) need not memorize all this information except for the information critical or directly applicable to their current work. They need to know where to find the information, how to use the manuals, and how to interpret and apply policies and procedures to their immediate work, (Manuals and information must be readily accessible.) Their actions should reflect their training in all emergencies.

Quality Assurance

A plan to ensure ongoing and overall quality work and results necessitates placing monitors and evaluation tools at the appropriate stages of the total testing operation. The *preanalytic* stage includes patient test management, personnel information (job descriptions, responsibilities, and duties), and personnel competence. The *analytic* stage includes QC, proficiency testing, test and method comparisons, test calibrations and verifications, and test results. The *postanalytic* stage includes clinical criteria and relevance, complaints and communications, staff review, and records/documentation.

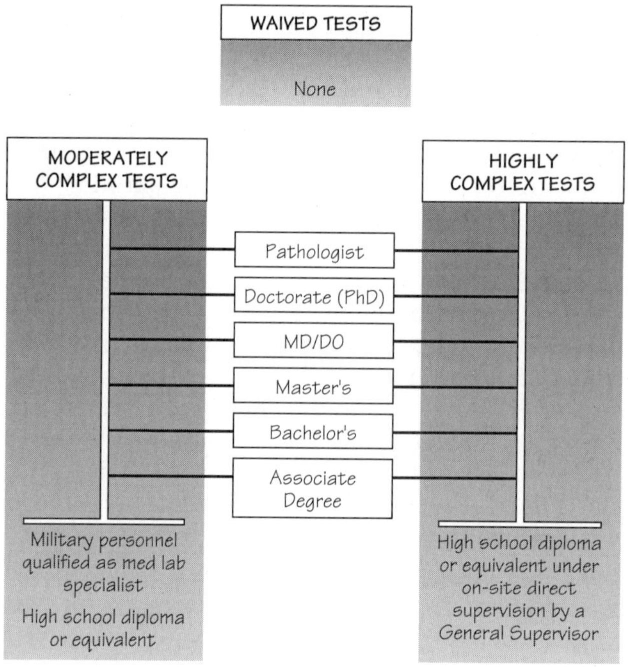

Note: Individuals who qualified under final March 14, 1990 rules will continue to qualify under CLIA '88. (493.1461,p.7175)

Figure 17–2 Testing personnel standards according to CLIA '88.

Regular attention to identify trends, unique incidents that are valid, and underlying problems masked by acceptable results will reduce and might even prevent serious quality issues. When a problem *at any stage* is suspected or identified, the quality assurance plan should be implemented to prevent or correct it. Employees should be able to rectify situations and problems within their work area. Documentation of action should be reviewed monthly.

Meeting and Complying With Standards

Adhering to or following the established standards, regulations, and rules (called *compliance*), is expected in order for an individual/organization to hold and maintain licensure, accreditation, and/or certification. In most circumstances, variations, such as a laboratory's own policies that are considered to be less strict, are not condoned or accepted. Occasionally, a laboratory can request an exception such as using a "home-brew" test method when no other method for that (rare) analyte exists. Reciprocity of licenses rarely exists for laboratorians.

When found to be noncompliant or negligent, organizations may be fined and/or suspended or shut down. The reprimand depends on the type and extent of violation. The fines can amount to thousands of dollars and, in cases of serious violations, loss of authorization to conduct business for months or years. HCFA, for example, "can propose a range of sanctions . . . from directed plans of correction to revocation of . . . certification."[4]

Managers are obliged to educate and inform employees. If employees then

QUESTIONS AN INSPECTOR MIGHT ASK YOU

1. What is the *mission* of your organization? How do you apply the mission to your area?
2. What *inservices and (continuing) educational programs* have you attended in the last year?
3. A *fire* occurs in the STAT Chemistry laboratory at 7:30 A.M. What would you do?
4. What is a *Material Safety Data Sheet* (MSDS) and where would you go to get one?
5. How do you ensure *patient confidentiality* in your work area?
6. What department do you call to report *faulty equipment* that is *NOT* used for patient care? What is the telephone number?
7. Where is a *fire alarm pull station* nearest your work area?
8. How do you handle specimens from patients with *tuberculosis?*

do not follow policies and procedures and a problem results, reprimands should be carried out. Likewise, individuals who are negligent in their work and do not comply with performance standards of their (professional) licensure may also be reprimanded publicly or fined or lose their authorization to work by the appropriate agency.

Laboratory managers should become involved with developing compliance plans for their institutions. Components of compliance plans should include employee conduct rules such as Code of Conduct regarding legal standards; who is responsible to supervise compliance; appropriate delegation of authority; effective communication; effective training; monitors; enforcement and discipline; and corrective action.[5] Managers should frequently address conduct and compliance with employees. An investigation by federal agencies into any alleged problem frequently occurs from a *qui tam* (whistleblower) suit by a current or former employee.

Activity 4: Inspection Questions

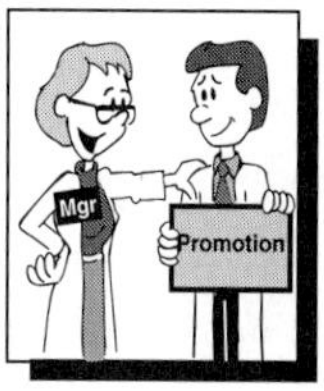

As pairs or teams, one person "role plays" an employee and a second "role plays" as an inspector. Use the questions presented in the boxed area and additional information, as needed from the instructor or supervisor, to conduct an interview by the inspector of an employee. Identify the law or regulation to which each applies. What responses would you give relative to your current school or work situation?

Legal Issues in the Laboratory

Managers and laboratorians must acknowledge their responsibilities according to legal and professional standards and codes. Two important issues often arise that confuse personnel: patient confidentiality and record storage.

Patients have a right to their own health care or hospitalization information, including laboratory test results, according to the Code of Federal Regulations, 493.1109(e).[6] To address situations in which patients request their own (or a family member's) information, managers must develop policies regarding the release of any information in order to ensure patient confidentiality. Equally important is to monitor the casual observation by an "outsider" that might occur when a laboratorian, phlebotomist, or clerk is using the computer to access specimens or print information, data sheets, or discard files without shredding them.

Minimum requirements are stated by CLIA '88 regulations for retention of laboratory records and materials. Stricter recommendations by the CAP were recently announced. These recommendations suggest retaining materials for a longer period of time than specified when such would be appropriate for educational or quality improvement needs . . . (and) when patient care needs so warrant.[7] State regulations may exceed CLIA '88 specifications and should be reviewed carefully before the laboratory establishes its own policy.

Managers must also develop policies regarding other issues: medical waste (especially infectious substances), latex allergies to gloves, use and reuse of medical devices, sexual harassment, violence in health care, needlestick injuries, and fraud (billing and receiving payment).

Summary

Managers of laboratories or health care facilities offering multiple discipline services face constantly changing complex problems regarding legalities, personnel, customers, and work environments. Inspections that previously addressed existence of quality assurance (QA) programs, covering multiple func-

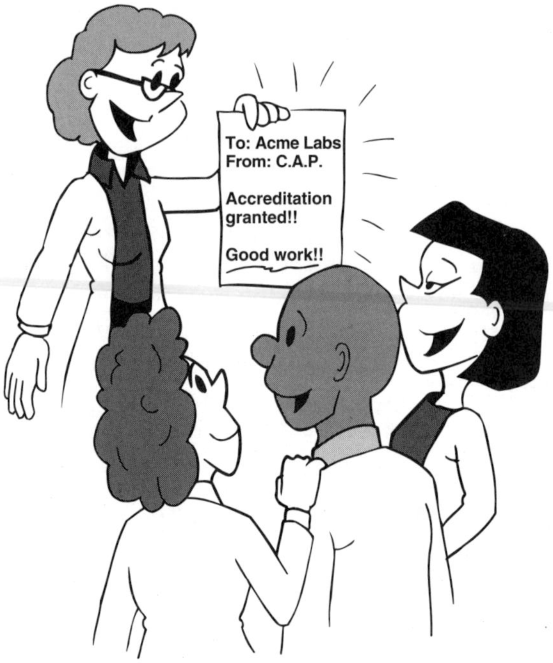

tions of health care facilities, such as management, technical issues, and quality control, are being changed to address improvements and effectiveness of QA programs in addition.[8] The responsibility for (employees and customers) action begins with managers who must educate, train, oversee, and require agreement and compliance to accomplish the work.

It is not a question of satisfactory performance but delivering consistent exceptional service. Everyone is responsible, including the patient. Breaking the law is serious, and laboratorians must be careful to not do so.

Review Questions

1. Which of the following agencies advocate *voluntary* standards for laboratories?
   a. HCFA
   b. JCAHO
   c. OSHA
   d. CDC
2. Describe the importance of legal, regulatory, and legislative control of health care to the public.
3. Of the following documents, which ones are appropriate for a CLIA inspector to review?
   a. The salary scale for certified laboratorians.
   b. The lecture schedule for the School of Medical Technology.
   c. The competency program for the clinical chemistry laboratory.
   d. The result data from 18 months previously.
   e. Training schedules for fire safety and medical waste management.
4. The public may respond to federal regulations during the "comment period." To which of the following agencies would they address their written comments?
   a. OSHA
   b. JCAHO
   c. HCFA
   d. CAP
   e. COLA

See p. 411 for answers.

References

1. *The Federal Register: What It Is and How to Use It.* Washington, DC, Office of the Federal Register, 1992.
2. Nichter EA. PT surveys: Monitoring corrective action. Medical Laboratory Observer 1994; 26(1): 49–51.
3. Ferrence-Ramirez NE, Procopio NA. Internal proficiency testing for hematology. Medical Laboratory Observer 1992; 24(12): 43–48.
4. Hudson T. Laboratory regulations create new opportunities for hospitals. (In Law column.) Hospitals 1992; Sep: 5:55.
5. Boothe JF, Korns JH. Clinical laboratories should have compliance plans in place. Management Briefs 1996; 18(18–19): 1,10–11.
6. Klosinski DD. Releasing patient information. (In Q&A.) Laboratory Medicine 1996; 27(8): 506.
7. College of American Pathologists Fall National Meeting. Government affairs update seminar. San Diego, Sept 1996.
8. Auxter S. CLIA '88 deemed organizations implement new strategies for '95. Clinical Laboratory News 1995; 21(3): 12.
9. Managing Laboratory Personnel. The CLIA and OSHA Manual. New York, Thompson Publishing Group, Inc., 1995; 2(10): 4.

Suggested Reading and Resources

1. Clinical Laboratory Management Review Journal; Management Briefs newsletter. Published by Clinical Laboratory Managers Association., 9 Old Lincoln Highway, Suite 201, Malvern, PA 19355-2135. 610/647-8970.
2. Gore MJ: A walking tour of Washington: How laws are implemented through the regulatory process. Clinical Laboratory Science 1992; 5(3): 133–136.
3. National Intelligence Report. (ISSN 0270-6768) Washington G-2 Reports, L.L.C., 1111 14th St., NW, Suite 500, Washington DC 20005-5663. 202/289-4062. Dennis W. Weissman, publisher.
4. McNett CL. Rocky road for new OSHA rules. Laboratory Medicine 1992; 23(10):641–642.
5. Nevalainen DE, Lloyd HL. ISO 9000 quality standards: a model for blood banking? Transfusion 1995; 34(6): 521–52.
6. Passey RB: How to read the federal register and other CLIA-related documents. Medical Laboratory Observer 1992; 24(10): 47–52.

APPENDIX **17–A**

List of Agencies and Associations

PUBLICATIONS AND SUGGESTED READINGS

1. **American Association of Blood Banks** (AABB), Bethesda, MD. A nonprofit professional organization of members, individuals, and entities: determines standards for operations of blood banks/transfusion services.

- The Quality Program, 1994
- Nevalainen DE, Gallery MF. Applying Self-Assessment and Process Analysis to Create a Quality System, 1995.

2. **American Hospital Association** (AHA), AHA Publishing, Inc., Chicago, IL.

- Gift RG, Mosel D. Benchmarking in Health Care: A Collaborative Approach, 1994.
- Leebov W, Scott G. Service Quality Improvement: The Customer Satisfaction Strategy for Health Care, 1993.
- Trotter JP. The Quest for Cost-Effectiveness in Health Care: Achieving Clinical Excellence While Controlling Costs, 1995.

3. **Centers for Disease Control and Prevention** (CDC), 4770 Buford Highway, NE, Atlanta, GA 30341-3724. CDC's primary operation is to address disease trends and monitor strategies for prevention. It is a federal agency authorized by DHHS and HCFA to interpret and implement regulations and practices for laboratories. It appoints representatives to CLIAC, a group of professionals who recommend regulations to CDC and HCFA. Web site: http://www.cdc.gov

4. **College of American Pathologists** (CAP), Northfield, IL. CAP is an agency providing standards for laboratory operations; subscribers participate in peer-review on-site inspections. Laboratories determined to comply with standards are accredited by CAP. More importantly, accreditation by CAP, which has been granted *deemed status,* is accepted by JCAHO and HCFA so that no additional inspections are required. CAP uses a peer-review system of inspection by one team visiting one laboratory that likewise provides a similar team to inspect another. CAP surveys more than 4900 laboratories.

5. **Commission on Office Laboratory Accreditation** (COLA). 800/298-8044. An independent agency accrediting approximately 7,500 physician-office laboratories (POLs), COLA promotes education by developing informa-

tion fact sheets to help people understand why regulations are necessary, to comply with them, and to develop good laboratory practices.

6. **Department of Public Health** (DPH), individual states. DPH is usually the state agency that develops rules and regulations to implement a state's laws. Some DPH agencies are changing their names to Department of Community Health.

7. **Food and Drug Administration** (FDA). FDA is a federal government agency responsible for approving and authorizing products intended for human consumption: inspects transfusion medicine (immunohematology, blood bank) facilities and services, as (donor) blood and components are consumable products. Web site: http://www.fda.gov

- Current Good Manufacturing Practice for Blood and Blood Components. CFR21, Part 606. April 1992.
- Center for Biologics Evaluation and Research. Guideline for Quality Assurance in Blood Establishments. Rockville, Md, July 11, 1995.

8. **Health Care Financing Administration** (HCFA). HCFA is the federal government agency responsible for developing rules and regulations that carry out laws related to health: issues Certificate of Accreditation to laboratories complying with CLIA '88 or other statutes. Web site: http://www.hcfa.gov

9. **International Organization for Standardization** (ISO), Geneva, Switzerland.

- ISO Standards Compendium. ISO 9000 Quality Management. 6th edition.

10. **Joint Commission on Accreditation of Health Care Organizations** (JCAHO), Oakbrook Terrace, IL. First offering accreditation of hospitals in 1953; any facility providing health care services can now be accredited by JACHO, which is accepted by HCFA so that no additional inspections are required. JACHO surveys (inspects) more than 4000 organizations annually (of these, approximately 2600 offer laboratory services). JCAHO recognizes CAP and COLA accreditations. In 1998, JCAHO will include OSHA's safety standards in their laboratory inspections. Web site: http://www.jcaho.org

- Accreditation Manual for Hospitals (AMH), 1996.
- Accreditation Manual for Pathology and Clinical Laboratories Services, 2nd ed, 1996.
- A Guide to Establishing Programs for Assessing Outcomes in Clinical Settings, 1994.
- Framework for Improving Performance: From Principles to Practice, 1994.
- Implementing Quality Improvement Principles: A Hospital Leader's Guide, 1993.
- Performance Improvement in Plant, Technology, and Safety Management. PTSM series, 1994.
- Understanding the Patient's Perspective: An Important Voice in Performance Improvement, 1994.

11. **NCCLS** (formerly National Committee for Clinical Laboratory Standards), 940 West Valley Road, Suite 1400, Wayne, PA 19087.

- Clinical Laboratory Technical Procedure Manuals, 2nd ed. Approved Guideline, GP2-A2 (ISBN 1-56238-156-3).
- Training Verification for Laboratory Personnel. Proposed Guideline, GP21-P (1994).

12. **National Institute on Drug Abuse** (NIDA). NIDA certifies laboratories performing drug testing.

13. **National Technical Information Services,** US Department of Commerce, 5285 Port Royal Road, Springfield, VA 22161. Survey procedures and interpretive guidelines for laboratories and laboratory services. PB92-146174.

14. **Occupational Safety and Health Administration** (OSHA), U.S. Department of Labor, 200 Constitution Avenue, NW, Washington, DC 20210; 202/219-8151. (OSHA also maintains regional and state offices.) OSHA develops regulations and provides detailed guidance to health care organizations regarding health care worker safety requirements and establishes the minimum legal standards that organizations must meet. In July 1996, OSHA provided a "Quick Fix" abatement incentive program of penalty reduction if an inspector discovers a violation, compliance directive CPL 2.112. Web site: http://www.osha.gov/

APPENDIX **17–B**

Laws

FEDERAL GOVERNMENT LEGISLATION RELATED TO MEDICAL PRACTICE

Laws are codified in the *United States Code.* Rules and regulations are published in the *Code of Federal Register.* Documents are available in designated libraries, Regional Federal Dispositories; some local colleges, universities or law libraries; US Government Printing Office, 202/783-3238; or the Internet via GPO Access, free, http://www.access.gpo.gov/su_docs/ or Regulatory Affairs Information, free, http://www.medmarket.com/tenants/rainfo/rainfo.htm

- **Medicare, PL 89-97,** 1965, and **Medicaid.** Title XVIII and XIX of the Social Security Act. This law was enacted to provide payment for medical care. Standards of patient care to be followed by hospitals for reimbursement of medical services. The Health Care Financing Administration (HCFA) is responsible for administration of the Medicare program.
- **Clinical Laboratory Improvement Act,** 1967 and **Amendments,** 1988. (CLIA '67 and CLIA '88). CLIA '88 Amendments to Public Law 100-578, 42 U.S.C. Sec 263a *et seq.* were passed to ensure that clinical laboratories accurately test samples of materials derived from the human body. The act authorizes the secretary of the Department of Health and Human Services (DHHS) to promulgate standards. See Regulations in the *Federal Register* Title 42, Public Health, Part 493, HSQ-176, Vol. 57, No. 40, Friday, February 28, 1992, pp. 7001–7288. Revised every October 1.
- **Occupational Safety and Health Act (OSHA).** See *Federal Register* Title 29, Labor. First separate standard in 1986 targeted health care for occupational exposure to toxic substances in the laboratory: chemical hygiene plan, and a separate hazard communication program. In 1989, initial standard to regulate exposure to blood-borne pathogens (Final rule, December 6, 1991). Other recent standards include permissible exposure limits (PELs) for toxic substances such as acrylamide, paraffin wax fumes, formaldehyde, and occupational exposure to tuberculosis. Revised every July 1.
- **Stark I, 1989 and Stark II, 1993.** Legislation written by Rep. Fortney "Pete" Stark (D. California). "If a physician or a member of a physician's immediate family has a financial relationship with an entity, the physician may not make referrals to the entity for the furnishing of clinical laboratory services under the Medicare program, except under specified circumstances."[9]

18

Managing Finances

OBJECTIVES

Upon completion of this chapter, the reader should be able to:

- Define financial and accounting terms commonly used in laboratory fiscal management.
- Identify revenue sources for laboratories and explain challenges managers face in obtaining these revenues.
- Describe costs within specific categories and explain how each is used in calculating total expense, cost per test, and break-even numbers.
- Compare and contrast cost containment strategies, specifically those that would increase revenues and reduce expenses.

KEY WORDS

finance
budget
revenue
reimbursement
operating expense
capital costs
cost management
break-even analysis

Introduction

News reports inform Americans daily that their health care costs too much. It is nearly 14% of the gross national product (GNP), more than three times the amount spent on defense, and more than twice the amount spent on education. Medicare, the federal government program, covered 37 million elderly and disabled Americans at a cost of $200 billion in 1996. In spite of these figures, estimates report that 37 million Americans (more than 14%) have no health care coverage and that 22 million Americans (more than 8%) have inadequate health care coverage. (Percentages were based on 1990 US Census of 260 million Americans.) Health care concerns include finances, delivery, and accessibility. These concerns have entered the domains of politics, business, society, and economics. Few definitive conclusions have emerged thus far into the late 1990s.

Since 1982 when the Tax Equity and Fiscal Responsibility Act (TEFRA) was enacted, laboratories have been thrust into cost center status. Although no longer holding reputations as profit centers, laboratories are recognized for generated revenues, especially if operating for-profit. In today's economic climate, management by controlling and containing costs has emerged as a hefty challenge for owners, managers, and employees. It is not only a matter of spending less but also of maintaining quality, improving efficiency, and increasing volume of services, all for fewer dollars (revenue).

In this chapter, the most basic concepts and applications are introduced with the intent that readers will be able to grasp the importance and the relevance of accounting methods, budgeting processes, and cost-management strategies. One of the most important finance issues relates to documenting exchange of money for services and/or products. A laboratory "sells" services and "buys" labor, supplies and materials, equipment, and instruments in order to provide its services. Proof of revenues received for services provided must be accurate and complete. Proof of payments as costs for purchase of labor or supplies must be equally accurate and complete. Legal, legislative, and ethical practices must be strictly followed for government reports: for example, filing tax returns, securing exemptions or fulfilling licensure requirements, and operating according to professional codes of conduct.

Basic Finance Principles

Preparing annual reports provides information regarding past and present activities, finances, and achievements. Whether or not a laboratory is privately or publicly owned, strong interests always surface regarding viability and profitability. One question focuses on these concerns: Is the laboratory capable of paying its own way, that is, generating revenue to cover its costs for services and/or products rendered?

Financial reports can be used to predict future and cohesive plans of action to influence future activities. These plans of action might be to reduce operating costs, identify and target high-profit margin markets, drop a service that is not profitable, leave a market if competition becomes too strong,

---

NOTE: In this chapter, the words "laboratory" and "laboratories" are used for brevity, but in most instances, health care or medical organizations and companies, hospitals, or private facilities could be substituted.

Table 18–1
FACTORS INFLUENCING BUSINESSES

Rising costs • salaries (the single greatest cost) • supplies • equipment Declining reimbursement Increasing competition Increasing government regulation	Increasing managed care Changing (clinical) utilization trends Changing workplace environments (place and space) Uncertain future Mergers, buyouts, and acquisitions

develop new products, offer new tests, and shift capital into new areas. Financial matters related to operating a laboratory involve many factors similar to those encountered by any business (Table 18–1).

Three key worksheets demonstrate activities related to revenue and expenses as financial transactions. As computer-generated spreadsheets, these worksheets enable managers to plan and control operations. Managers may decide to change activities based on loss of revenue or increase in expenses. These worksheets serve as legal records for owners and investors, the Internal Revenue Service (IRS), or the Securities and Exchange Commission (SEC).

An income/expense statement, showing profits and losses (P&L), depicts accumulated financial transactions of a laboratory or one of its sections over consecutive periods of time (month, quarter, or year). Net revenues from sales and/or services performed and expenses (operating, marketing, general, and administration) are summarized according to differences, either as net profit or net loss. The formula appears as "revenues − expenses = net income" or "$$ in − $$ out = $$ income."

A balance sheet shows the financial position of a laboratory at a given point in time. In Table 18–2, several items are listed that should be identified on a balance sheet either as assets or resources and as liabilities or financial obligations. The dollar amounts (value) of assets such as cash, potential revenue such as receivables, or holdings such as inventory, are tabulated. The dollar amounts (value) of liabilities such as (open) accounts that would come due for payment, salaries that are to be paid, and loans are tabulated. Assets minus liabilities produce the equity or net worth in dollars of the organization.

Cash-flow statements reflect net in-flows and out-flows of cash during a specified period. Cash flow is commonly presented in the form of reconciliation of net income or loss for a period (from income statement) to the net change during that period, that is, the difference between the amount of cash

Table 18–2
BALANCE SHEET ITEMS

Current Assets	Current Liabilities
Cash Patient receivables Inventory	Accounts payable Accrued salaries
Property and Equipment	**Long-term Obligations**
Land Building Equipment & instruments	Bonds payable Loans

Table 18–3
COMPARISON OF ACCOUNTING METHODS

	Cash Method	Accrual Method
Expense for a Test Procedure		
January: received item		January
February: invoiced		
March: paid	March	
Revenue from Same Test Procedure		
April: performed		April
May: billed		
June: collected	June	

reflected on the balance sheet at the beginning of the period and at the end of the period. There are three components of the cash flow statement: net cash flows from operating activities, net cash flows from investing activities (including purchase of property and equipment), and net cash flows from financing activities (including net borrowing and repayment, stock issuances, and payment of dividends).

Accrual accounting methods show how much money will be received for services and/or products and how much money will be spent to provide them. This is the preferred method as it represents all income and expenses at the time of performance, delivery, or consumption of services and/or products. Cash accounting methods that show money only when it is received and when it is paid out do not reflect when services and/or products were actually performed, delivered, or consumed. In Table 18–3, an example compares these two methods.

Other annually tabulated financial and activity information of interest to managers and supervisors includes test volumes per laboratory section (census of tests performed), supplies and/or materials and labor costs, cost per test, and workload and/or productivity. Expenses, such as depreciation for equipment, are subtracted at the end of each of the lifetime years. Each item of information would be compared with the previous year's statistics. Unfortunately for health care organizations, charges issued and dollars collected are rarely identical.

Budgets

A budget is the financial plan derived from estimating revenues and expenses. This budgeting process is most often done annually. Activities and work are then planned that align with each item listed in both categories (revenues and expenses). The budgeting process should take into consideration new programs identified in strategic planning. Information necessary to determine budgets incorporates test costs, workload statistics, estimates of revenues and its sources, capital equipment costs (initial, life expectancy, and yearly depreciation fees), operating expenses, and labor costs.

Traditional budgets present desired percentages of growth and/or profit and cost-control or reduction as targets over previous periods of time. Percentages may be established as "fixed," proposing 5% to be achieved monthly,

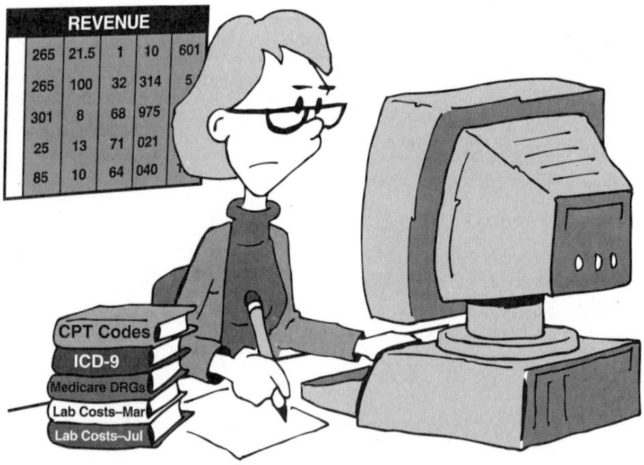

quarterly, and definitely by the end of the year or "incremental," proposing 2% for the first quarter, 4% for the second quarter, 6% for the third quarter, and 8% for the fourth quarter. Zero-based budgets represent another budgeting technique often employed by professional societies. This budget stems from planned objectives and activities for a given period of time or fiscal year and is based on the assumption that there is no money available from previously earned revenue. The idea is that expenses will not exceed revenues during the designated time period.

REVENUE

At present, revenues are received through several different reimbursement methods. Government programs, such as Medicare and Medicaid, reimburse based on fixed averaged rates of cost assigned to the patient's diagnosis for a given event of care. This method of determining the amount to be paid before the costs are incurred is called the *prospective payment system* (PPS). For example, a hospital patient may undergo an appendectomy for which the hospital receives $3300 from Medicare. This is the fee paid to the hospital, regardless of the number of laboratory tests, such as CBCs, or other inpatient hospital services performed or the costs incurred by the hospital in order to perform this procedure.

Other reimbursement methods also depend on predetermined fees identified in contractual arrangements or "plans" between health care providers and privately sponsored programs such as Blue Cross/Blue Shield or specific health maintenance organizations (HMOs). Depending on the arrangements, patients in these programs may be expected to go to only designated laboratories (hospitals and physicians). Third-party payers "contract" to pay on a cost, a cost-plus, or even a less than cost basis rather than on a price basis. Most fee schedules refer to the ICD-9-CM system* and Diagnostic Related Groups (DRGs) to denote why a patient was treated and Current Procedural Terminology (CPT) codes from the American Medical Association to determine how the patient was treated.[1] By coding tests, a standardized value or "price" can be assigned before accepting the contract and member patients.

In each method, the fees for doing business may differ with several fee

---

*ICD-9 connotes the 9th edition published in 1977 of the World Health Organization (WHO) statistical listing, called the *International Classification of Diseases*.

schedules instituted by one laboratory. For patients covered by Medicare, reimbursement is fixed according to one of the more than 400 DRGs. For patients covered by a contract or plan through their employer or other group, fees for designated services may be discounted based on anticipated volumes but certain special testing may not be included. Managed care agreements negotiated between large primary care providers and laboratories may be based on capitation, which is a set per member per month dollar amount.

Rarely, patients who are not otherwise covered may pay their own incurred costs. For patients who pay their own costs, negotiating to reduce fees may not be available but cash payments often will be discounted.

If the laboratory is a department of a larger organization, specific revenues are allocated and appear "on the books" to the laboratory as well as other departments. Recall that if accrual accounting methods are used, revenues will be listed in the month the services were provided rather than when they are paid for. Eventually discounts, disallowances, and other assessments will be subtracted from the total revenues. Figure 18–1 shows estimated revenue sources for a hospital laboratory.

OPERATING COSTS

An example of averaged disbursements of laboratory funds is shown in Figure 18–2. Although not considered a part of the operating costs, capital disbursements are included here only as a part of total expenditures. Payroll and related personnel expenses compose more than half of all the expenses.

Operating costs refer to those expenses incurred or cash paid out during day-to-day activity or work as "something" that is consumed: for example, payroll, reagents, supplies, or paper. Cash or credit buys this "something," which is used during the work process and, when gone, must be purchased again in order to perform further work. These costs can be assigned to several categories to determine where expenses exceed the budget or are less than predicted in the budget. One category separates costs as either *direct* or *indirect.* Another category separates costs as either *fixed* or *variable.* A third category separates costs as either *controllable* or *noncontrollable.*

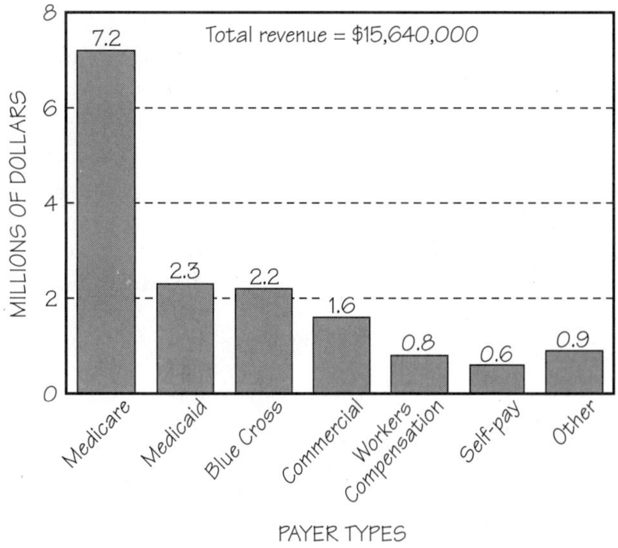

Figure 18–1 Estimated payer revenues.

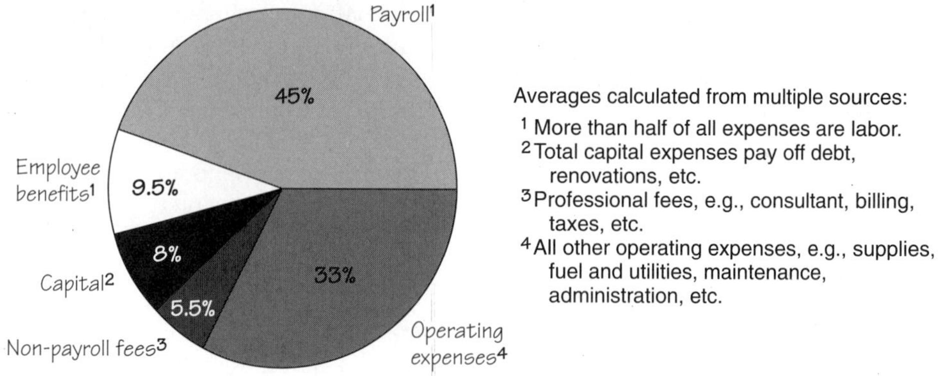

Figure 18–2 Disbursement of laboratory funds.

Direct costs are those that can be identified or traced to specific work done. Direct costs can be supplies and/or material or labor. Supply and/or material costs are considered an integral part of the finished product and can be traced to specific physical units: for example, to microbiology for culture media, reagents, and glassware. Examples of labor costs include the wages paid and benefits provided to technologists and technicians who actually perform the tests. Indirect costs consist of overhead and represent those expenses somewhat associated with the activity or work but not incurred in producing tests. These costs can also be supplies and/or materials, labor, or other expenses. Called "overhead," these necessary materials include utilities, paper, soap and bleach, and computer software. These consumables are not easily traced to a particular test or activity. Indirect labor expenses include phlebotomy, janitor or environmental services, administrative, clerical, courier, and support personnel such as those working on the information and communication systems. Other indirect expenses include depreciation and maintenance of instruments, taxes, and rent.

Fixed costs remain constant per month regardless of volume of work done. These costs do not change in their total amount over a given period of time or for the activity or work. For example, fire insurance on equipment remains constant even if volume of tests rises or decreases during a 6-month period. The depreciation of a specific instrument, although predicted for several years, does not change either. The fixed "cost per test" will go down as the volume of tests goes up.[2]

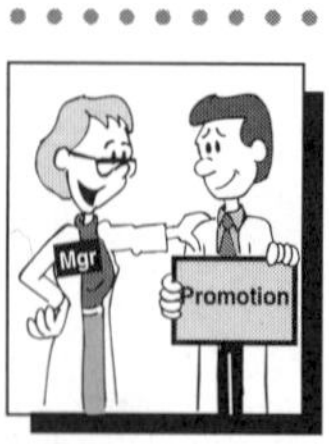

Activity 1: Calculate Costs Per Test

1. The monthly depreciation cost of an analyzer is $150.00. Calculate this fixed cost per test for the following number of reportable tests per month:

Number of Tests	**10**	**100**	**1000**
Fixed cost per test	$ ____	$ ____	$ ____

2. The cost of a reagent to run one test is $0.17. Calculate the variable costs of this reagent for the following number of tests run:

Number of Tests	**10**	**100**	**1000**
Variable cost per test	$ ____	$ ____	$ ____

See Activity Discussion 1 at the end of this chapter.

Variable costs, on the other hand, change proportionately to the volume of work done or tests performed. These costs are uniform on a per-unit basis but fluctuate according to changes in the related volume of activity; this may or may not be directly proportional to the volume increase or decrease. Reagents used in a particular test is one example. The total cost of reagents would rise as number of tests increases: that is, it takes more reagent to run more tests even though the cost per test remains the same (constant) and in this case is directly proportional.

Activity 2: Calculate Total Costs Per Test

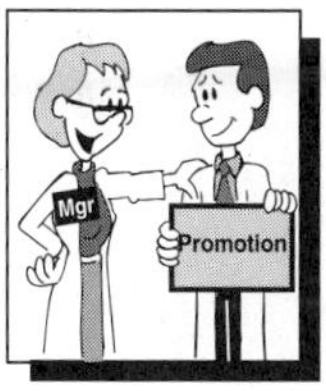

Calculate total costs of performing tests and total cost per test:

Number of Tests	**100**	**200**	**400**
Total variable cost	$ 500	$1000	$2000
Total fixed cost	$ 500	$ 500	$ 500
TOTAL COSTS	$____	$____	$____
Variable cost per test	$ 5.00	$ 5.00	$ 5.00
Fixed cost per test	$ 5.00	$ 2.50	$ 1.25
TOTAL COST PER TEST	$____	$____	$____

See Activity Discussion 2 at the end of this chapter.

Costs also considered either controllable or noncontrollable depend on the time period and level of responsibility. Time periods are either designated short, for 6 months and less, or long, which exceed 6 months. Level of responsibility indicates whether it is the owner, director, manager, supervisor, or technical staff. Controllable costs can be directly regulated for both short or long periods. Normally, for 6 months or less, only variable costs are controllable no matter what the level of responsibility. Costs, such as taxes and rent, for long periods can be controlled only at the owner or director level. Many controllable costs are negotiated on the basis of volume. Other costs are specified, such as taxes by external agencies, but can be reduced or diverted by astute financial planning. Noncontrollable costs include taxes and rent either for short or long times and are outside the realm of control for supervisors. Depreciation of instruments may not be controlled by a supervisor either because this calculation is based on cost of the instrument and method of payment.

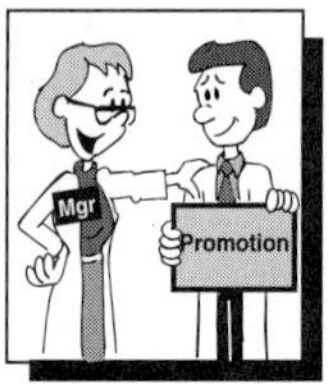

Activity 3: Determining Cost Types and Impact of Change on Costs

Categorize each of the following costs as either direct or indirect and fixed or variable. Describe what effect, if any, a 10% increase and a 10% decrease in the volume of work would have on these costs for 1 month.

	Direct/Indirect		Fixed/Variable		10% Inc/10% Dec	
Reagents, automated CBC						
Glass slides, blood cell differentials						
Manager's salary						
Medical technologist's salary						
Depreciation, hematology analyzer						
Overhead charges, laboratory space						
Electric and water utilities						
Laboratory information system (LIS)						

See Activity Discussion 3 at the end of this chapter.

CAPITAL COSTS

Capital equipment refers to items, usually equipment or instruments, that cost more than $500 with a technological working life greater than 1 year. Capital costs represent an investment in "tangibles that are not consumed" in order to perform activities related to the work of the organization: for example, computers, buildings, and property.

Depreciation of capital equipment owned by nonprofit hospitals occurs over a 10-year period as required by the federal government. Equipment purchased with a technological life of 12 years would be written off as an expense at one-half the cost of that equipment at the end of each of the 12 years. A vendor may issue a written statement that the technical life of a specific type of equipment is shorter, a statement that the government may accept, and allow depreciation to be expensed off for the shorter time.

Using alternative financing methods besides paying the total amount in cash for outright purchase of expensive equipment and instruments requires comprehensive planning, negotiation skills, and an accurate perception of future needs. Several examples of creative "buying" include installment payments to purchase, rent-to-own, lease for shorter period of time than technological life, combination of rental or lease with purchase of reagents, lease or purchase with periodic upgrades included, and purchase or lease with inclusion of other essential equipment such as a PC, refrigerator, or centrifuge that could also be used in performing other tests. Training is almost always included in the total cost but can be addressed as possible cost savings. Vendors desire to work with managers, pathologists, bioscientists, and technologists to achieve sales and place their instruments in reputable laboratories. They may also subsidize facilities' renovation costs if their instruments have specific requirements such as dedicated electrical lines, deionized water sources, and different cabinet height.

Medical equipment manufacturers rarely publicize costs or sale prices of instruments. Likewise, customers adhere to similar conventions of not revealing prices given to them from manufacturers to the manufacturer's competitors in order to obtain the lowest prices. Decisions of which equipment or instrument to purchase must be made primarily based on needs driven by the services to be provided. Final decisions rest with the laboratory management to select instruments that will perform optimally in the specified laboratory worksettings and meet their customers' needs. These sale practices differ from those used by automobile dealers selling or leasing cars and real estate agents selling or renting homes of comparable worth (to many pieces of medical equipment and instruments).

Reasons why an instrument should be replaced or upgraded require close scrutiny. Almost all decisions about new technology relate to cost management.

THESE QUESTIONS ASSIST MANAGERS IN THE INSTRUMENT ACQUISITION PROCESS[3]

- Will operating costs be reduced (for reagents, supplies, utilities)?
- Will maintenance time and service cost be reduced?
- Will less technical personnel time be required?
- Will more tests be available (offered)?
- Can workstations be consolidated?
- Will service and support be improved?
- Will turnaround time be shortened?
- Is new technology more precise and accurate?
- Is specimen volume reduced?
- Can unusual specimens, such as fluids, be analyzed?
- Can daily through-put be increased (increase test frequency)?
- What value will be gained for additional investment?

Cost Management

Legislators tackle the Medicare cost issue with each new session of Congress. (This was attempted in 1995 and 1997.) Companies and their employees, groups and their members, and even individuals seek health care coverage providing choice, cost savings, and accessibility. Pressures have increased on health care administrators to respond. They place equivalent pressures on the department managers and employees to rise to this challenge.

Laboratory managers, comfortable with statistical analysis, began acquiring financial acumen as their responsibilities and challenges grew. Employee participation has become important for changing methods and work patterns to increase efficiency and effectiveness of work. Several processes, such as cost analysis, cost accounting, and cost containment, essentially produce the necessary data for analysis and strategies to offset these challenges.

Cost management systems provide continual mechanisms to plan, monitor, and control operations and costs of discrete services. A balance must be produced among profitability, quality of patient services, and the mission of the organization.[4] Cost management information will enable managers to perform their work, in the conceptual domain, with validity from statistical assessments.

COST ANALYSIS

Determining the actual cost of performing a test in the laboratory entails time and attention to many details. Expenses incurred in performing tests can be assigned to one of four general categories consisting of supplies and/or materials (called disposables or consumables), equipment and instruments, labor (personnel), and administration (Table 18–4). Cost information must be generated in order to determine the "price" of a test (Fig. 18–3).

TEST COST ANALYSIS FORM

Prepared by ____________

ANALYTE ____________ Date ____________

Direct costs: Wages

Technical – pay at $____/min ____________

Collections and handling ____________

Materials

Reagents ____________

Controls and references ____________

Disposables ____________

Instrument

Maintenance ____________

Depreciation ____________

Miscellaneous costs ____________

TOTAL DIRECT COSTS ____________

Indirect costs: (____% of direct costs) ____________

TOTAL DIRECT AND INDIRECT COSTS ____________

Laboratory administration costs:
(____% of direct and indirect costs) ____________

TOTAL COSTS ____________

Proposed charge ____________

Current charge ____________

Figure 18–3 Test cost analysis form.

Table 18–4
LABORATORY OPERATING EXPENSES

Supplies: 29.6%	Reagents and controls
	Pipettes
	Gauze, tissue wipes, alcohol swabs
	Oxygen and gases
	Plastic trays and containers
Instrumentation: 10%	Equipment
	Service and repair contracts
	Depreciation
	Maintenance contracts
Labor: 44.8%	Salaries
	Shift differential
	Overtime pay
	FICA
	Benefits: Medical, life insurance; pension plan
Administration: 15.6%	Paper, forms, and labels
	Postage
	Telephone
	Printing
	Transportation, freight, delivery charges
	Cleaning supplies
	Dues, subscriptions, continuing education
	Computer software
	Protective coats/gowns, gloves, eye shields
	Computer maintenance

Percentages adapted from Hanford.[5] Recently, P. Thomas Hirsch, a reference laboratory company president, reported his "Hirsch rule of thumb" for costs of revenues: personnel about 40%, supplies about 15%, and other expenses less than 30%.[6]

Activity 4: Factors Influencing Costs

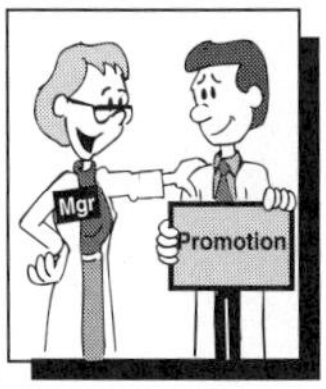

For each category of operating expenses, discuss how factors associated with items listed in Table 18–4 could force costs to increase.

See Activity Discussion 4 at the end of this chapter.

Cost analysis for all tests should be calculated before implementing a test and periodically, especially if any changes occur in the factors influencing costs. Several beneficial applications of the information from cost analysis are shown in Table 18–5.

Cost Per Test

This process has expanded into current concepts of calculating the costs of production. Calculating the cost per test as supplies and reagents only became inadequate. Calculating the cost per patient that included supplies, reagents, billables and unbillables, and labor was more beneficial. Calculating the costs of production includes supplies, labor, instrumentation, and administration.

The rule of 80/20, the Pareto principle, applies here also in that 20% of

Table 18–5
COST ANALYSIS INFORMATION APPLICATIONS

- Determine minimal number of samples needed to be run at a time (batch) in order to break even or make a profit.
- Determine how often or even when batch or groups of tests should be run (testing frequency).
- Assess whether or not to add a new test or delete current one.
- Determine where test will be performed: in-house or sent out.
- Determine which method/instrument is the most cost efficient for analysis.
- Determine price of test in order to break even or make a profit.
- Obtain additional information in developing department objectives.
- Identify responsibility for supervisors' performance appraisal.

laboratory tests generate 80% of volume and revenue, seen predominantly as chemistry tests in most laboratories (Table 18–6).

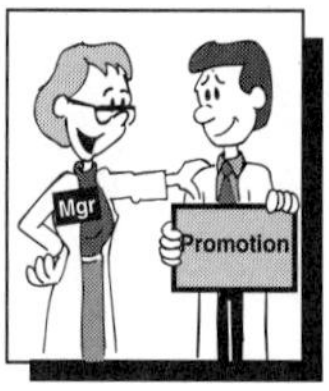

Activity 5: Test Production* and Revenue Calculations

1. Data collected in a hospital laboratory indicated costs to perform one glucose test were $0.27 for instrumentation, $0.42 for administration, $0.80 for supplies, and $1.21 for labor. Fill in the chart below using the information provided in Table 18–6 and calculate revenue, expenses, and profits.

   Revenue per test: Annual revenue/Annual number of tests = __________

   Cost per test:
   Instrumentation + Administration + Supplies + Labor = __________

   Profit: Revenue per test − cost per test = __________

   Annual profit/loss:
   Profit/loss per test × annual number of tests = __________

2. Data collected in a hospital laboratory indicated costs to perform one alcohol test were $0.54 for instrumentation, $0.42 for administration, $1.80 for supplies, and $3.96 for labor. Fill in the chart below using the information provided in Table 18–6 and calculate revenue, expenses, and profits.

   Revenue per test: Annual revenue/Annual number of tests = __________

   Cost per test:
   Instrumentation + Administration + Supplies + Labor = __________

   Profit: Revenue per test − cost per test = __________

   Annual profit/loss:
   Profit/loss per test × annual number of tests = __________

---

*Both variable and fixed costs have already been allocated on a per test basis based on an annual test volume of 15,000.

Note: calculations in Activity 2 differ from these because variable and fixed costs were based on daily numbers of tests rather than an annual total number.

3. Total annual profit/loss:
   Profit/loss per test × annual number of tests = ____________
   (glucose $ + alcohol $).

See Activity Discussion 5 at the end of this chapter.

Activity 6: Performance of Glucose Testing in a Hospital Setting

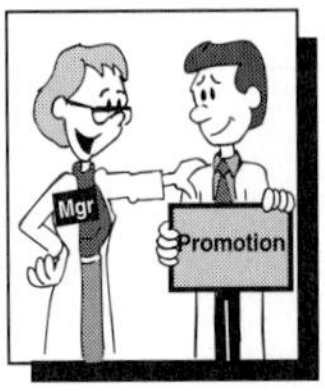

Review materials regarding glucose methods and instrumentation learned in other courses: for example, clinical chemistry or from the instructor or a supervisor. Compare use of methods and instruments for various patients and various sites within the hospital. Explain why the number of glucose tests might be as high as reported in Table 18–6. Discuss the financial impact (profit/loss) of offering several methods by one laboratory facility; include in the discussion the cost of personnel who might perform these glucose procedures.

If test volumes are low, costs are often perceived as high. The corollary is that when test volumes are high, costs are low. Reasons appear to stem from the following factors: (1) more tests are done in one run or batch, (2) quality control is performed for the run or batch, (3) reagents and consumables may be purchased in volume at a cost savings, (4) labor capacity already exists and can be efficient, (5) the instruments already exist for any number of runs or batches, and (6) administration costs exist regardless of the test volume. Activity 5 and Activity 6 demonstrate the Pareto principle very well, because alcohol tests constitute 2% of the test volume and do not generate sufficient revenue per test expense (Table 18–7).

Table 18–6
CHEMISTRY TEST VOLUMES AND REVENUES*

Test	Volume	%	Revenue	%
Chemistry profile	25,000	29	2,300,000	41
Electrolytes	6000	7	900,000	16
Blood gases	3500	4	525,000	9
Glucose	15,000	17.5	255,000	5
Amylase, serum	3500	4	180,000	3.2
Creatine phosphokinase (CPK)	4500	5	161,000	2.8
Alcohol, blood	1800	2	99,000	1.7
CKMB	2200	3	191,000	3.3
All others, approx 140 tests	24,500	28.5	1,030,000	18
TOTALS for 150 tests	86,000†		5,641,000‡	

*Highest per year either by volume or revenue.
†Approximately 50% of all laboratory tests performed in-house/on-site.
‡Approximately 30% of total laboratory revenues.
Percentages are rounded to nearest significant number and do not necessarily total 100%.

Table 18–7
COMPARISON OF HIGH- AND LOW-VOLUME TESTS

Test Comparisons	Glucose	Alcohol
Specimen collection	Easy	Difficult, requires paperwork
Specimen handling	Easy	Difficult, requires documentation of who handles it
Specimen processing	Easy	Difficult, must be isolated from other specimens
Analysis	Easy	Always STAT
Instrumentation	Several	One dedicated in one location in facility
Methods	Variety	One special method
Test frequency	Can be batched	Usually one at a time, off-shifts most frequently
Patient source	Variety	Usually Emergency Center (EC)
Result validation	Easy, can be repeated on same or another specimen; compare with previous results; patient may be known to have diabetes	Difficult, must be repeated on same specimen; contamination must be avoided
Result reporting	Easy, reference ranges well established for gender and age	Difficult, narrow range; for legal purposes
Legal responsibility	Accuracy expected	High level of patient confidentiality required; can be subpoenaed to testify in court

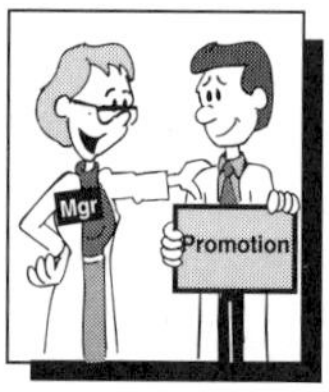

Activity 7: Decisions on Test Offerings

Consider the information presented in Table 18–7. Discuss the reasons why alcohol tests should be performed in the laboratory given the fact that expenses exceed revenues in order to perform these tests. Given the materials learned thus far, what recommendations could be made in order to improve test costs for both glucose and alcohol testing?

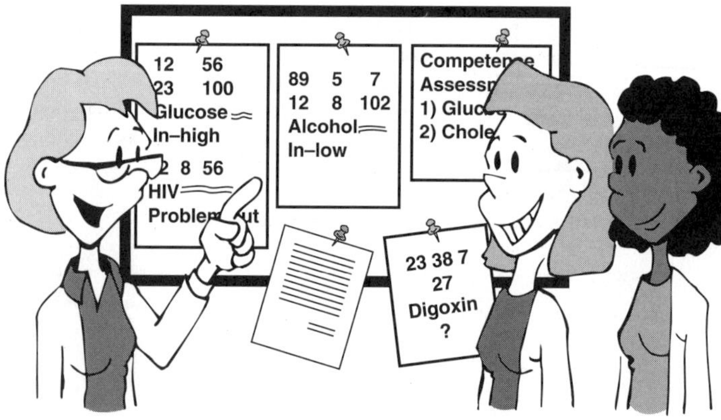

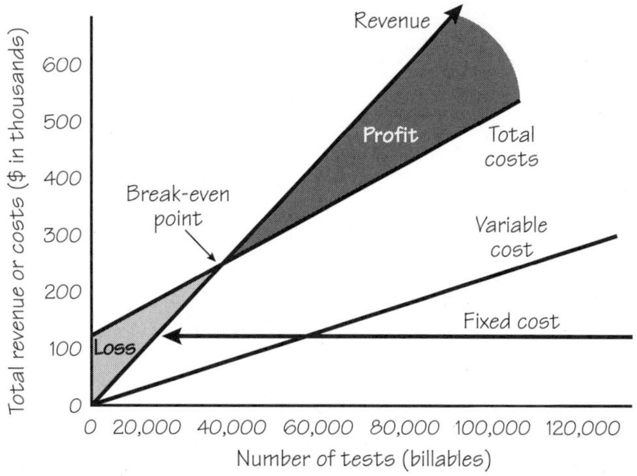

Figure 18–4 Break-even analysis.

Break-even Analysis

Break-even analysis[3, 7] determines the level of activity at which revenues equal expenses—that is, profit equals zero—or exceed expenses and net income is earned. Analysis of data and costs to determine the break-even point can ascertain the number of units needed to be sold or tests to be done, the dollar amount needed to be obtained through sales, and the price per test in order to make a profit and not suffer any losses (Fig. 18–4). If one uses price per test as revenue and costs information in the basic formula, the minimum number of tests to break even financially can be calculated (Fig. 18–5).

Necessary calculations for break-even analysis (BE) are:

- Variable costs (VC)
- Fixed costs (FC)
- Test price (TP)
- Test volume (TV)
- Total cost (TC = [VC x TV] + FC)
- Total revenue (TR = TP x TV)
- Contribution margin (CM = TP – VC)
- Contribution margin% (CM% = CM / TP)
- Profit margin% (PM% = [TR – TC] / TC)

$$\text{BE test volume} = \frac{\text{annual fixed costs}}{[\text{test price} - \text{variable costs}]} \quad \textbf{OR} \quad TV = FC / [TP - VC]$$

$$\text{BE minimum price per test} = \frac{\text{annual fixed costs}}{\text{test volume}} + \text{variable costs} \quad \textbf{OR} \quad TP = [FC / TV] + VC$$

$$\text{BE minimum revenue} = \frac{\text{annual fixed costs}}{[\text{test price} - \text{variable costs}] / \text{test price}} \quad \textbf{OR} \quad TR = FC / CM\%$$

Figure 18–5 Break-even analysis form.

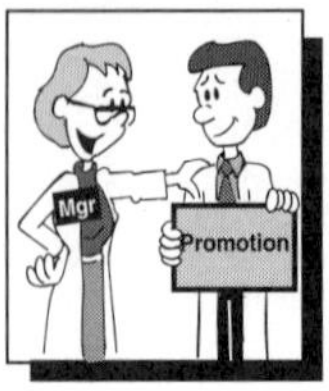

Activity 8: Break-even Analysis for Alcohol

Using the information provided in Activity 5 and Figure 18–5, calculate what the minimum number of alcohol tests performed annually should be to break even financially. Discuss strategies that a laboratory manager might use to (1) increase number of tests performed and (2) reduce variable costs in order to break even or make a profit.

See Activity Discussion 6 at the end of this chapter.

COST ACCOUNTING

Cost accounting systems[8] identify and study costs associated with performing a test. Specific information enables managers to prepare budgets; decide which tests to implement, drop, or send out; monitor procedure (method and instrumentation) effectiveness; and evaluate charges and prices. Revenues and expenses can be tracked more easily. From available information, standards can be set to determine appropriate use of resources. Staff and instrument productivity can be defined and measured. Also, use of resources can be analyzed according to specific DRG categories.

Differences exist between financial accounting and cost accounting. Financial accounting serves external purposes, in particular for tax authorities, regulatory agencies, the public (as consumers), creditors, and others who would certify the laboratory's "fairness" and legitimacy of operation. These systems usually follow rigid, universally accepted rules. Cost accounting focuses on internal transactions or management purposes. Methods most often used include (1) technical estimates usually based on previous information; (2) industrial engineered standards, time-consuming to produce, but highly accurate and including personal, fatigue, and delay time within the standards; and (3) relative value units (RVUs) from professional organizations that provide independent measures of resource consumption.

Cost accounting is conducted like other types of analysis: collect data/costs, identify and categorize costs, and allocate costs to laboratory sections, departments, or divisions. Clearly, in this process, labor and supplies/materials should be designated as *preanalytic, analytic,* and *postanalytic* for further justification and plan and control of operations. Unusual information regarding costs and calculations, such as service contracts and reagent rentals, should be presented for review to managers and/or owners.

COST CONTAINMENT

Cost containment strategies primarily focus on methods of reducing cash outflow or expenses[9, 10] (Table 18–8). (Cost management strategies address increasing revenues.) Enhancing quality, as a secondary focus, ranks as another important issue not only in processes but also in results (or outcomes) that managers and pathologists desire to maintain and improve whenever feasible.

Several strategies can be implemented that apply to the work environment, to the job itself, and to personnel. One successful strategy for the work environment has been to centralize selected services. Centralized purchasing can control expenditures through coordinated group purchasing for volume

Table 18–8
GOALS AND BENEFITS OF COST ACCOUNTING

1. Identify test numbers and costs to assess prices.
2. Determine costs involved in production/work for preparing budgets, controlling and monitoring resource consumption, assessing needed technology, and planning changes.
3. Assess financial status periodically: compare with competitors; negotiate fees and contracts based on substantiated information.
4. Improve productivity: maintain quality, on-time performance, clinical relevance, throughput, and flexibility.
5. Financially manage the value and time invested in test performance and services.

Data from Castañeda-Méndez K. Time to change. Advance/Laboratory 1995; 4(8): 20–27.

buying. Occasionally, difficulties arise if individual preferences for a particular brand or item type have been tolerated. Compromising on the type of supplies, equipment, and even instrument service (but not on quality) becomes necessary for this to work. Stock can be shared when levels of use change.

Centralization of jobs and/or work can occur through realignment into one large center or more sites dedicated to similar tasks. The choice of either one or both depends on services offered and commitment to customers. In a large hospital with a reference laboratory service, automation and robotics may determine both a centralized hematology laboratory section with instrumentation and two or three dedicated laboratory sites such as a cancer center, open heart surgery suites, and a presurgical testing area. In a commercial laboratory, only one centralized laboratory may exist. In an outpatient setting, limited procedures for point-of-care (POC) testing may exist, with all other specimens being transported to a central off-site laboratory.

Another strategy addresses eliminating unnecessary testing. Techniques that improve turnaround times and accuracy in reporting results can prevent additional ordering of tests. Advocates of algorithmic testing recommend testing protocols for specified analytes, including authorization to perform follow-up testing.

Cost savings can also be derived through employee retention, retraining/crosstraining, and creative wage and benefits programs.[11, 12] Administrators and managers should ferret out strategies to corral the costs for recruitment and training of new employees into benefits and incentives for experienced employees to stay. When pay is cut or not increased, morale, productivity, and efficiency will drop. Managers should strive to prevent these problems, which can evolve into costly situations.

Many employees entering the job market today seek benefits rather than high taxable incomes (Table 18–9). With the average of one-third of labor costs paid into benefits, providing more (optional benefits) through choices can be done for less (money). Creatively designing "cafeteria-style" benefit programs will entice a broad range of employees with differing needs and interests. Recent trends produce programs with greater individual and family selection opportunities and costs shared by both employer and employee.

Several job-related benefits that have strong appeal and produce cost savings in the long term promote safety and satisfied experienced employees who like what they do. Safety programs with superior provisions and training are by far less costly than workers' compensations and medical leaves. Desirable job-related benefits consist of pleasant working conditions, good modern equipment, adequate staffing, overtime available occasionally but not re-

Table 18–9
EMPLOYEE BENEFITS WITH OPTIONAL CHOICES

- Earned time off*: vacation
- Other scheduled time off*: holidays
- Sick time OR part of earned time off as personal,* variable such as one emergency call-in day, or "bank" with unused paid off
- Medical, maternity, or family† leave pay coverage
- Health, disability, accident insurance: choice of plans or even organization's own program
- Program to set aside money before taxes for medical expenses not covered by insurance
- Life insurance; deferred income: annuities
- Discounts on services: pharmacy, supplies, diapers for employees' babies, meals
- Child care
- Tuition reimbursement‡
- Dental and/or optical care coverage
- Unemployment protection
- Liability protection
- Retirement plan

*When time off is scheduled, staffing can be planned for adequate coverage.

†Certain benefits are mandated by the federal government such as family leave but pay does not have to be included.

‡IRS considers tuition reimbursement monies paid to an employee as taxable income if NOT job related, but if it enhances one's job skills, money paid would be considered "ordinary and necessary" trade or business expense.

quired, continuing education available or supported by fees and time from work, superior safety prevention training provided, and free but secure parking and grounds. Significant costs for safety protection and training have been noted; regulations require wearing gloves and/or eye and face shields.

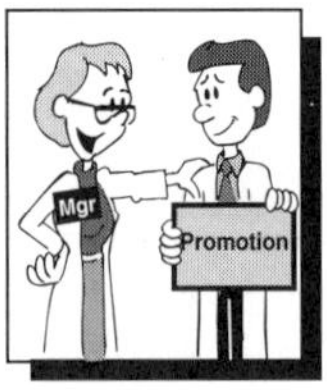

Activity 9: Small Actions for Big Savings

For each of the following situations, describe elementary actions that the class, readers, or laboratory personnel could carry out that would control or reduce costs:

1. Energy consumption or reduction
2. Safety practices including fire and accident prevention, chemical hygiene plans, and universal precautions
3. Personnel punctuality and attendance, theft, and "sink-testing" policies
4. Specimen acceptability standards and checks
5. Test procedure performance: standards/calibration/controls and repetition of tests

See Activity Discussion 7 at the end of this chapter.

The use of cost management strategies helps maintain an organization's viability, creates a proactive management, and involves managers and employees (to a lesser extent) in business decisions and operations.

Summary

The basic financial information and activities presented in this chapter will prepare readers for initial responsibility in certain fiscal management roles. Three major areas were discussed in which novice managers and supervisors, experienced laboratory professionals, and clinical laboratory science students should develop their knowledge and skills. The first area requires using relevant accounting methods in order to assess and subsequently monitor a laboratory's financial status. The second area offers participation in budgeting processes in order to plan and control operations and services by the laboratory for viability and accountability. The third area involves continual attention to developing and implementing cost management strategies to provide the most effective and highest quality services within a highly efficient operation (work) setting.

The financial picture represents only part of overall health (well-being) of a laboratory. Keep in mind many other factors not as easily obtained, measured, or monitored, that are considered to be intangible, and that influence the viability and growth of an organization.

The use of cost management strategies enhances a laboratory's status, creates proactive management, involves managers and even employees in business decisions, and focuses initiatives. Many programs challenge laboratory managers to acquire new and greater knowledge and skills in finance and negotiation. Managers must now incorporate reliable data collection, statistical analysis, and projection strategies into their daily repertoire of functions.

Activity Discussion 1: Calculate Costs Per Test

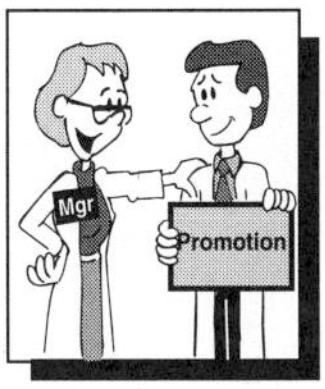

Fixed costs for 10 tests = \$15; for 100 tests = \$1.50; and for 1000 tests = \$0.15.

Variable costs for 10 tests = \$1.70; for 100 tests = \$17; and 1000 tests = \$170.

Activity Discussion 2: Calculate Total Costs Per Test

Number of tests	100	200	400
Total variable cost (VC)	\$500	\$1000	\$2000
Total fixed cost (FC)	\$500	\$500	\$500
TOTAL COSTS = VC + FC	\$1000	\$1500	\$2500
Variable cost per test (VC/No. tests)	\$5.00	\$5.00	\$5.00
Fixed cost per test (FC/No. tests)	\$5.00	\$2.50	\$1.25
TOTAL COST PER TEST (TC/No. tests)	\$10.00	\$7.50	\$6.35

Activity Discussion 3: Determining Cost Types and Impact of Change on Costs

Costs are either fixed or variable and direct or indirect. Describe what effect, if any, a 10% increase and a 10% decrease in the volume of work would have on the costs for one month.*

	Fixed	Variable	10% Increase Effect	10% Decrease Effect
Reagents for automated CBC		X (direct)	Yes	Yes
Glass slides for blood cell differential		X (direct)	Yes	Yes
Manager's salary	X (direct)		No†	No†
MT's salary		X (direct)	Yes‡	Yes‡
Depreciation hematology analyzer	X (direct)		No	No
Overhead charge lab space	X (indirect)		No	No
Electric, water utilities		X (indirect)	Yes	Yes
LIS	X (indirect)		No	No

*In-depth discussions should be facilitated by instructors and experienced managers.
†Possibly affected in long-term by eliminating a position or reducing salary or benefits.
‡May be assigned to perform less/more variety of procedures.

Activity Discussion 4: Factors Influencing Cost Increase

Supplies
- Repeats
- Standards and controls
- Standing order purchasing versus order as needed versus STAT
- Reagent monitoring by automatic sensor within reagent lines on an instrument

Instrumentation
- Capacity or volume per run, runs per shift/24-hour day
- Efficiency
- Nonbillables such as competence assessment, student practice, reference range specimens, controls
- Calibration frequency

Labor
- Staffing mix: MT/CLS and MLT/CLT, day shift and off-shift
- Wage rate (as compared with other laboratories in area)
- Overtime
- Benefits
- Efficiency (or productivity)

Administration
- Excess overhead
- Efficiency
- LIS unsuitable or incapable of fulfilling need
- Inappropriate allocation

Activity Discussion 5: Test Production* and Revenue Calculations

1. Glucose test revenue and costs:

   Revenue per test = \$255,000/15,000 = *\$17.00*

   Cost per test = \$0.27 + \$0.42 + \$0.80 + \$1.21 = *\$2.70*

   Profit/loss = \$17.00 − \$2.70 = *\$14.30*

   Annual profit/(loss) = \$14.30 × 15,000 = *\$214,500*

2. Alcohol test revenue and costs:

   Revenue per test = \$99,000/1,800 = *\$55.00*

   Cost per test = \$12.54 + \$9.25 + \$13.80 + \$23.63 = *\$59.22*

   Profit/loss = \$55.00 − \$59.22 = *(\$4.22)*

   Annual profit/(loss) = (\$4.22) × 1,800 = *(\$7,596.00)*

3. *Total annual profit/(loss):*

   Glucose \$214,500 + Alcohol (\$7,596.00) = *\$206,904.00*

---

*Both variable and fixed costs have already been allocated on a per test basis based on the annual test volume of 15,000.

Activity Discussion 6: Break-even Analysis for Alcohol Tests

Calculations for break-even (BE) analysis are as follows:

Variable costs (VC)	\$13.80 + 23.63 = \$37.43
Total fixed costs (TFC)	\$12.54 + 9.25 = \$21.79 × 1,800 = \$39,222.00
Test price (TP)	\$55.00

$$\text{BE test volume} = \frac{\text{Total fixed costs}}{[\text{Test price} - \text{Variable costs}]} = \frac{\$39{,}222}{\$55.00 - \$37.43}$$

$$= \frac{\$39{,}222}{17.57} = 2232 \text{ tests}$$

Activity Discussion 7: Small Actions for Big Savings

1. Energy consumption/reduction
   - Lower temperature setting for heat/increase for cooling; keep constant when possible
   - Reduce hot water temperature setting
   - Lights: standard is 40 footcandles measured at 30″ above the floor where employees must read printed material when performing work (most are

over 200 footcandles due to fluorescent bulbs); turn off when leaving a room for a long period of time

- Turn off instruments when not used for several hours
- Conserve water by having dripping faucets fixed, using foot pedals, and turning off water when soaping hands
- Install or replace insulation around windows
- Place blinds on windows to cut sun (to lower temperature)
- Recycle or reuse (when appropriate) "glass" disposables instead of plastics (petroleum based)

2. Safety practices including fire and accident prevention, chemical hygiene plans, and universal precautions
   - Training
   - Regular checks of working fire extinguishers, eye wash stations, safety showers
   - Clean out "boom room" and other storage areas
   - Include safety in competence assessment
3. Personnel punctuality and attendance, theft, and "sink-testing" policies
   - Develop policies with penalties that do not tolerate abuse and violation of work-time, workplace, and performance protocols
   - Recognize perfect attendance and punctuality
   - Monitor resource inventory
   - Promote cost savings when employee theft is decreased, not only of others' personal items and money but of laboratory's supplies and equipment, and the like. (Retailers advertise customers' savings when shoplifting is down.)
   - Seek programs to assist employees with behavior and performance problems
4. Specimen acceptability standards and checks
   - Develop, advertise (reference laboratory clients) specimen preferred/minimum requirements
   - Develop policies for rejection and protocols to obtain acceptable replacements
   - Monitor inventory and shelf life of collection equipment and containers (tubes)
   - Perform periodic evaluations of collection equipment to ensure valid results
5. Test procedure performance: standards/calibration/controls and repetition of tests
   - Evaluate manufacturers' protocol for instrument calibration to ensure frequency is acceptable if different from or less often than what is perceived to be necessary

• Develop policies for validation of results and appropriate repeat testing

Review Questions

1. Reimbursement based on fixed averaged rates of cost assigned to the patient's diagnosis for a given event of care is based on
   a. diagnostic related groups.
   b. current procedure terminology.
   c. American Hospital Association codes.
   d. International Classification of Diseases.
2. Which of the following financial accounting methods is preferred for use by laboratory managers?
   a. Profit
   b. Cash
   c. Expense
   d. Historical
   e. Accrual
3. The greatest portion of operating expenses in a laboratory's budget is
   a. supplies/materials.
   b. administration.
   c. purchase of instruments.
   d. salaries.
   e. controls and reagents.
4. Criteria to bring a drug test in-house has been met. How many tests must be performed before a profit is realized if the annual fixed costs are $96,000, the price for the test has been set at $32, and the variable cost is $18.48?
   a. 710
   b. 7100
   c. 3550
   d. 71,000
   e. insufficient information to determine
5. Describe five specific policies or recommendations for laboratory personnel which would control/reduce costs related to (a) using lights, (b) fire prevention, (c) employee attendance, (d) specimen acceptability, and (e) repetition of tests.

See p. 412 for answers.

References

1. Jandreski M. What's what in laboratory finance. Clinical Laboratory News 1996; 22(5): 10–11.
2. Fantus JE. Price yourself into the market. Clinical Laboratory Management Review 1996; 10(6): 1–2.
3. Cook J. Cost-containment challenges met with workstation consolidation. Advance/Laboratory for Administrators 1994; 6(43): 10–11.
4. Johnson TM. More with less. Advance/Laboratory for Administrators 1995; 4(3): 35–36, 38.
5. Hanford W. Finance skills for the non-financial manager. ASCLS Annual Meeting workshop, Anaheim, July 22, 1995.
6. Nace L. Interest renewed in smaller labs. Advance/Laboratory 1995; 4(8): 80.
7. Tirabassi CP. Test evaluation and the break-even analysis. Tech Sample® Management

and Education No. MGM-2. Chicago, ASCP, 1993.
8. National Committee for Clinical Laboratory Standards. Cost accounting in the clinical laboratory: Proposed guidelines. Villanova, Pa, National Committee for Clinical Laboratory Standards 1993. GP11-T: 1, 44, 45, 63.
9. Evans D, Franz DK, Ng VL, et al. Cost Containment in the Laboratory. Denver, Berkeley Scientific Publications, 1995.
10. Castañda-Méndez K. Time to change. Advance/Laboratory 1995; 4(8): 20–27.
11. Snyder JR. Wage and salary administration. *In* Snyder JR, Senhauser DA, eds. Administration and Supervision in Laboratory Medicine, 2nd ed. Philadelphia, JB Lippincott, 1989, p 440.
12. Snyder JR, Bissonette CA. Cost accounting of personnel turnover. Tech Sample® Management and Education No. MGM-3. Chicago, ASCP, 1991.

Suggested Reading

1. Berman HJ, Kukla DF, Weeks LE. The Financial Management of Hospitals. 8th ed. Ann Arbor, Health Administration Press, 1994.
2. Brase DJ, Matysik MK. Laboratory manager's financial handbook: how to speak "finance." Clinical Laboratory Management Review 1992; 6(2): 164–169.
3. Brighman EF. Fundamentals of Financial Management. 5th ed. Chicago, The Dryden Press, 1989.
4. Brown M. Health Care Financial Management. Gaithersburg, Md, Aspen Publications, 1992.
5. Cleverley WO. Essentials of Health Care Finance. 3rd ed. Gaithersburg, Md, Aspen Publications, 1992.
6. Getzen TE. Laboratory manager's financial handbook: what is value? Clinical Laboratory Management Review 1992; 6(3): 237–240.
7. Westgard JO. Strategies for cost-effective quality control. Clinical Laboratory News 1996; 22(10): 8–9.

CHAPTER GLOSSARY

Assets are unexpired costs that are used in future periods of time and applicable to the production of future revenues such as buildings, desks, and centrifuges. **Assets** are resources available to sustain operations and satisfy financial obligations because of cash on hand, or "current," such as net accounts receivable, and so on, that will be expended or converted to cash within one year's time; "noncurrent" is all property and equipment having a useful life of one year or more.

Balance sheet reports financial position at a given point in time: end of month, quarter, year of an organization's assets, liabilities, and equity.

Billable procedures are the actual reported results of physician-ordered tests for which payment should be received by the organization. Examples of testing performed that are NOT considered billable are controls, standards, and repeats to verify results.

Capital assets are those resources with a life of more than 1 year, usually valued at more than $500, which are not bought and sold in the ordinary course of business.

Cash flow statement reflects net inflows and outflows of cash during a period; commonly presented in the form of reconciliation of net income or loss for a period (from the **income statement**) to the net change during that period (the difference between the amount of cash reflected on the balance sheet at the beginning of the period and at the end of the period).

Contribution margin is the difference between the test price and variable costs; it is the amount contributed by each test to cover fixed costs. The contribution margin percentage is the contribution margin/test price and is divided into the annual fixed costs to determine the minimum revenue to break even.

Cost is the monetary valuation of an asset or service that has been obtained by an expenditure of cash or a commitment to make a future expenditure; it is the value of something purchased for cash or on credit.

Cost accounting is the process of identifying all costs incurred and expended by the organization in order to be balanced by generated revenues.

Depreciation is a process by which the costs of assets are expired (reduced) over the expected life of the asset. The longer the asset is owned, the less it is worth. The owner receives years of service from that asset. Depreciation is a way of charging part of the remaining, unexpired costs each year as an expense until the remaining cost is equal to zero or some predetermined salvage value. The loss of value of an item over time may occur through its use or technologic obsolescence. Depreciation is considered a real expense, although it is not a cash expense because it is carried on a laboratory's books as an asset. The IRS gives clear and complete descriptions for acceptable depreciations; tables standardize this financial process.

Expenses are expired costs that have been consumed and from which no measurable benefits will extend beyond the present accounting period: for example, salaries.

Full-time equivalent (FTE) represents a 40-hour work unit or other amount so assigned, such as, 12 hour/day × 3 = 36 hour/week. To calculate the annual salary of 1 FTE @ 40 hours, multiply the hourly rate by 2080 (40 × 52).

Gross margin is the gross revenue less direct expenses. **Gross margin percentage** is the gross margin divided by the gross revenue; this number mirrors controllable expenses.

Gross revenues are the total revenues (after taxes) before expenses (charges × number of tests).

Liabilities are obligations incurred to obtain assets and to sustain operations; either "current," such as accounts payable, accrued payroll costs (including vacation liability), amount of long-term indebtedness payable within 1 year, and other obligations incurred and payable within 1 year, or "noncurrent," all future obligations not due within next 12 months.

Net income is the dollars remaining after all expenses are deducted; this is a laboratory's "profit." **Net income percentage** is a measure of profitability. Generally 5% is the minimum desired number.

Operating margin consists of the dollars remaining after deducting direct and indirect expenses.

Revenue is the value of the services delivered by the laboratory.

Revenue deductions consist of the dollars that account for that portion of patient charges not collected, services determined not to be covered by insurers or Medicare, or discounts for prompt payment; also called "disallowances."

19

Evaluating: The Sixth Management Function

OBJECTIVES

Upon completion of this chapter, the reader should be able to:

- Describe principles of evaluation that would be applicable in assessing the performance of laboratory personnel.
- Identify appropriate measurement tools to evaluate knowledge, skills (practical or application), and behavior (affective) as compared with predetermined and described criteria for both competence assessment and performance appraisal programs.
- Develop a model performance appraisal program, including how a manager can ensure that inadequate or inappropriate components are overcome before completing the appraisal.
- Describe principles of evaluation that would be applicable in assessing laboratory-related activities.
- Discuss issues regarding productivity measures in a laboratory, including the consideration of when and how managers should intervene.
- Given a specific activity, such as an employee orientation program, an employee recognition event, or continuing education seminar, write three to five questions that could be used to evaluate it.
- Discuss the benefit(s) of using evaluation principles for strategies designed to measure selected laboratory-related (clinical) outcomes.

KEY WORDS

evaluation
measurement tools
competence assessment
performance appraisal
feedback
outcome measures

Introduction

Managers and supervisors assess achievement of work goals and objectives as their sixth management function. They analyze and validate whether or not what they planned was delivered, either as performance of personnel or activities (services and programs).

In the management cycle, the manager should identify first what needs to be done and formulate a plan for doing it; organize the process of doing it; direct, control, and coordinate the process of doing it; and, lastly, evaluate the results. If the results are acceptable and fulfill the goals, the work continues as before. If the results are off the mark, inadequate, or unacceptable, then the cycle begins again. It is important to correctly identify what is *needed,* not just what is *wanted.* Talented, successful company owners and managers strive to fulfill both goals. The terminology falsely simplifies the concept: Do or make something according to a plan, collect data about it, look it over, and judge the outcome. In reality, many obstacles can prevent successful outcomes. Occasionally, good fortune intervenes and the outcome is acceptable in spite of erroneous procedures. Sometimes the opposite can occur—procedures can be satisfactory but the outcomes are not. The evaluation process provides a retrospective view of how things happened as well as the status of the outcomes. Evaluation findings can assist in predicting future results, when all factors are controlled.

PROBLEM-SOLVING ASSESSMENT REQUIREMENT AS STATED BY CLIA '88[1]

Each individual performing high-complexity testing must be capable of identifying problems that may adversely affect test performance or reporting of test results and must either correct the problems or immediately notify the (laboratory) general supervisor, technical supervisor, clinical consultant, or director.

Regulatory and accreditation agencies specify requirements and standards for evaluating personnel, methods, instrumentation, processes, outcomes, and products for human consumption (in blood banks); see the problem-solving assessment requirement as stated by CLIA '88, and Appendix 19–A.[1] Manufacturers who produce supplies, materials, and reagents used in clinical laboratory methodologies and human-use products and those who produce clinical laboratory instruments are obliged to demonstrate fulfillment of rigorous standards before selling their products. Health care employers rely on human resource staff to prepare legitimate job descriptions and develop policies for employee performance evaluations. While certain legalities exist for conducting performance evaluations, no one specific design is mandatory or ideal. Specifications regarding assessment and documentation of employees' competence and performance have been published by these agencies.

Benefits of evaluation are closely linked to improving quality, maximizing productivity, achieving standards, developing expertise of the workforce, and ensuring outcomes (therapy and cure for diseases). In medicine, evaluation impacts on patient care. Dr. O'Leary, Joint Commission on Accreditation of Healthcare Organizations (JCAHO) President, wrote, "There is now a social mandate for performance measurement . . . reform proposals at federal and state levels include a requirement for measuring performance outcomes and

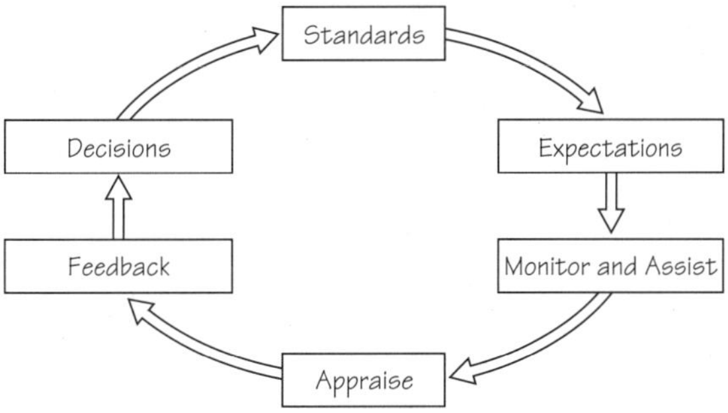

Figure 19–1 Evaluation cycle.

reporting performance information . . . people want to know what they're getting for their money, the value (to them)."[2]

In this chapter, the principles of evaluation are described, first to provide readers with an understanding of basic concepts. The processes of evaluation applied to two divergent subjects, people and activities, are presented next in general terms. Selected examples are explained for each subject. Readers should think of the similarities of these strategies in relation to evaluating laboratory methods and products for which they might become responsible.

Basic Principles of Evaluation

What should be evaluated? Nothing can escape being studied when the results are important or critical. Evaluation becomes pertinent to ensure that the correlation between *expected* outcomes and *obtained* outcomes remains high. Three basic goals support evaluation: (1) to provide adequate *feedback,* (2) to serve as a basis to *modify or change* a behavior or outcome, and (3) to provide information that will be used to *establish future* performance and activity criteria (Fig. 19–1). Evaluation becomes the process of documenting the fact that "something," when compared with expressed written criteria (standards), meets or exceeds the minimal levels of those criteria. When one knows the predetermined criteria, judgments can be made more accurately about the information obtained from measurement tools. The goal is to hit the bull's eye

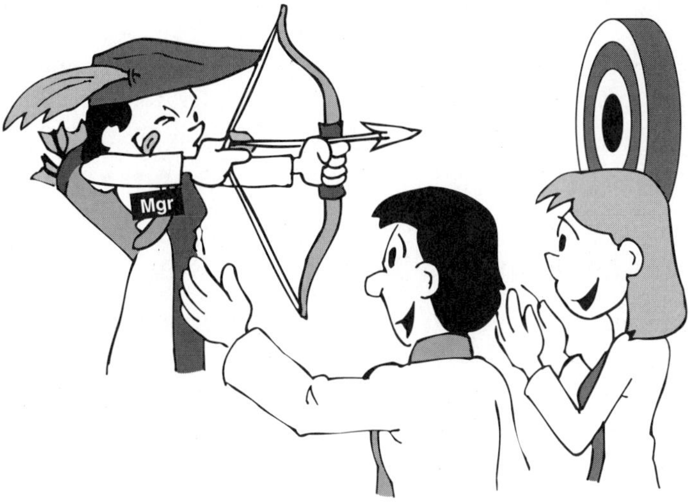

Table 19–1
STEPS OF MEASUREMENT

1. Identify and define *what,* i.e., quality or attribute, is to be measured.
2. Determine a "set of operations" to *demonstrate* the quality or attribute.
3. Establish a set of procedures or definitions to *quantify* the quality or attribute, preferably by units of degree or amounts.

Data from Thorndike RL, Hagan E. Measurement and Evaluation in Psychology and Education. 3rd ed. New York, John Wiley & Sons, 1967, pp 9–16.

every time one takes aim (action). This goal, like others, can be accomplished most often and most consistently with practice.

Traditional measurement implies assignment of an exact, quantitative number to an object and evaluation by placing a value on something on the basis of standards. Thorndike suggested that measurement in any field involves three common steps, as shown in Table 19–1.[3] Measurement procedures should be used only as tools with the results requiring *interpretation.* Thorndike also advised that attributes related to human behavior that are not subject to quantification can be documented as acceptable and consistent.

Certain assumptions modified from the field of education will enable readers to compare and contrast this model when applying it to a management model. In both models, the first assumption considers the goal of evaluation to improve (change) human behavior, knowledge, or skills. The desired improvements relate to objectives as learning or outcomes statements. Measurement tools display the degree to which the objectives have been achieved. Another assumption states that no single score should represent human behavior. The assessment of how a person *performs* his/her work is equal in importance to the *results* obtained. A person's whole actions should be considered rather than single isolated observations. Using a variety of measurement tools increases one's understanding of a person and enables one to help that person better understand him/herself. Once interpreted, the information enables employees to reinforce their strengths and identify those areas in which they might improve (their weaknesses). Measurement and evaluation should span the gamut of activities and behaviors executed by a person in his/her school or work setting. In the workplace, one more assumption promotes the concept that any evaluation program will be more successful if supervisors and employees are both involved with its development and implementation.

The concept of evaluation implies that managers first should plan the assessment to improve a person or activity. Secondly, they should use evaluation *with* rather than *of* an individual. Thirdly, they should evaluate an individual's progress based on his/her ability to perform.[4]

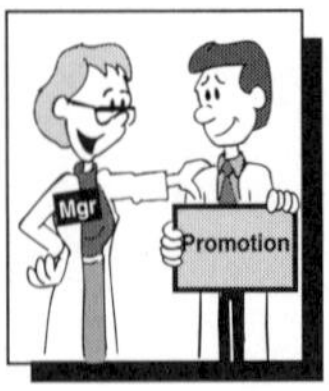

Activity 1A: Employee Behaviors for Evaluation

Each reader or group should describe one behavior expected of an employee that should be routinely evaluated. Briefly explain the benefits that improving this behavior would have for a patient, a physician, or the laboratory (workplace).

Activity 1B: Activity Outcomes for Evaluation

Each reader or group should describe one outcome expected of an activity, for example, laboratory service, product, or program, that should be routinely evaluated. Briefly explain the benefit that improving this outcome would have for a patient, a physician, or the laboratory environment (workplace). Record the employee behaviors, Activity 1A, and activity outcomes described for future activities.

Psychologically, effective personnel evaluation depends on the individual's acceptance that evaluation will help him/her personally. Individuals engage in those behaviors they consider successful or ones they like to do. They respond according to the maxim, "What gets rewarded, gets repeated." Likewise, negative behaviors, when inadvertently rewarded, will be repeated also. Habits, whether or not they are considered good or bad, are difficult to break—even improving "good" habits can be difficult. Individuals perform better, consistently and at a higher level, with constant or regular feedback rather than just a once-a-year perfunctory evaluation. When motivated, individuals perform at their peak level. Employees actively engaged in the evaluation process, for example, designing assessment tools and implementation, then "grading" their own exams, will subsequently change their behaviors to fulfill their own objectives.

Desired behaviors or outcomes should be formulated as objectives. Employees must have access to them and be able to understand them. Objectives can be best achieved by employees when they have complementary job descriptions, performance standards, dates for periodic review, and established instructions about how to proceed in doing their work. Similar success can be obtained when using objectives in activity processes.

Assessing without personal bias, called "being objective," becomes essential in the evaluation process. Evaluators must set aside preconceived ideas of what should happen, how it should be done or how someone should be doing it, and likes or dislikes of what or who is being evaluated. Results are all-important to some people. Managers too often focus on the "bottom line." Other managers and employees recognize the importance of the means by which the end was achieved. They strive for consistent performance in order to produce the same acceptable results, time after time, or better results the next time.

Evaluation of Personnel

Employees make up the major share of resources in an organization. One goal addresses maximizing their contributions. Managers and employees must agree on definitions of qualities and behaviors, which rarely comes easily. No single measurement tool suffices to provide comprehensive descriptions.[5] Attributes to be considered for evaluation reflect what individuals know, their physical abilities, their attitudes toward the situation, and their productivity—in summary, their performance.

Several decisions should precede implementing an employee evaluation process. First, identify which employee behaviors to measure; refer to Tables

Table 19–2
AREAS FOR PERFORMANCE EVALUATION

Old Paradigms	New Paradigms
Can state principle and steps of procedure	Conceptual: applies principle of old method to new instruments
Knows when to repeat procedure; verifies quality control	Integration: identifies and resolves problems, makes decisions; knows when to change process
Pays dues to professional society; recognizes roles of physicians, nurses, and other health care givers	Professional: demeanor and attitude beyond laboratory science, develops team building skills
Compliance to policy most of the time	Ethical: consistent in honesty, integrity, questions outmoded policies of potential harm in workplace
Can report results accurately; takes messages correctly	Communication: sends appropriate verbal and written information; actively listens to others
Promotes tradition; accepts progress at moderate pace; plans that research will become clinical applications in 10–15 years	Adaptive: learns new work; develops coping skills to handle stress, welcomes change; anticipates new technology from research in 2–5 years; computer literate
Promoted based on seniority	Contextual: plans career growth and scholarship activity, comprehends socioeconomics and government

Adapted from Mountain P. Automation solutions: What to look for and what to avoid. Clinical Laboratory Management Review 1996; 10(6): 637–644.

19–1 and 19–2. Many qualities or attributes that were previously held valuable under the *old paradigm* targeted punctuality, attendance, dress, and expected conformance in behaviors, often to the same laboratory method ± 2 Standard Deviation quality control (QC) rule. The *new paradigm* promotes different core skills and abilities, especially for technical personnel performing automated systems work, which is less easily defined or measured.[6] Roles for laboratorians are rapidly developing away from the traditional laboratory (hospital) workstation. The presence of employees at work when needed; compliance with rules, policies, and procedures; and conduct becoming a professional health care giver remain essential attributes. These might be considered even more important than before in the face of changing work modalities, customer service demands, and competition among organizations.

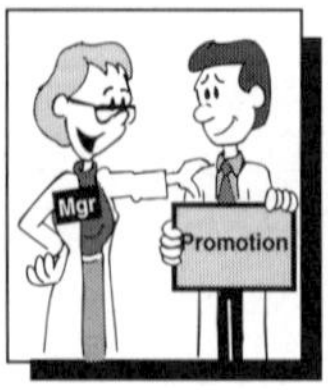

Activity 2: Personnel Attributes in New Paradigms

Each reader or group should select one attribute from the list of *New Paradigms* in Table 19–2 and write a description of it. Discuss how this attribute might be "measured" in a laboratory setting. Record the attributes and descriptions for future use.

Once the attributes have been chosen, confirming the appropriate domain they represent facilitates "demonstration." Attributes reflect knowledge (the Cognitive Domain), skill (the Psychomotor Domain), or attitudes (the Affective Domain). The level to be demonstrated must be considered also. *Recall* represents the basic level of learning in which an individual can demonstrate comprehension of facts, procedures, and affective phenomena and extend them to determine their implications in various situations. *Interpretation* or *application* represents the integration, execution, and employment of principles, values, and procedures in particular and concrete situations. *Problem solving* represents the analysis of information or situations in order to develop adaptations or courses of action and to make judgments about the impact or value of each. In clinical laboratories, regulatory requirements include assessing employees' problem-solving abilities.[1]

Readers can review Chapter 4 in the Education section for additional explanations of domains and taxonomy levels.

Measurement tools should be selected according to intended use. More than one tool might be advantageous (Table 19–3). Developing or adapting measurement tools for the situations in which they will be used can be challenging even for experienced evaluators.[7, 8]

After the evaluator has collected data or observed and documented behaviors, the evaluation process continues. The information and reports should be analyzed and interpreted. Decisions must be made regarding the course of action. Remember that the purpose of evaluation is to improve the situation. Occasionally, it supports the status quo as the best course. This also applies to human behavior and performance appraisals.

Difficulties with personnel evaluations and performance management arise when finances and the "bottom line" are deemed top priority. Lack of giving authority and support to middle managers and first-line supervisors from top-level administrators to formally recognize employee accomplishments (which is thought to be costly) or criticize performance (which is thought to be harsh) feeds the problem. The socialization and culture of the workplace endorse that everyone should be nice and mind his/her own business, which also stymies managers from effective personnel evaluations.[9, 10] Eccles advocates that businesses should change their philosophies to revolutionize the performance measurement process.[9] Measuring other aspects of business, for example, quality, customer satisfaction, and employees' performance, will affect decisions only when the status of these aspects is equal to or greater than that of financial ones.

Table 19–3
MEASUREMENT TOOLS ASSIGNED TO DOMAINS

Knowledge	Skills	Attitudes
(Cognitive)	***(Psychomotor)***	***(Affective)***
Written exams (1–3)	Checklists (1)	Rating scales (1,2)
Practical exams (2,3)	Practical exams (2,3)	Interviews (1–3)
Projects (3)	Observation reports (1)	Questionnaires (1,2)
Case studies (3)	Simulations (3)	Simulations (role-play) (2,3)
Oral questioning (1–3)	Demonstrations (1,2)	Rankings (1)
Simulations (2,3)	Critical incident reports (3)	Self-assessments (1–3)
Critical incident reports (3)		Critical incident reports (3)
		Anecdotal records (1–3)

Domains: (1) direct observation of routine test performance on patient sample(s), including patient preparation, if applicable, specimen handling, processing, steps of procedure, and results calculation and report; (2) assessment of test performance using previously analyzed specimens, duplicates, internal blind testing samples, and external proficiency testing samples; and (3) assessment of problem-solving skills.

PERFORMANCE STANDARDS

Criteria that state clearly and succinctly the expected performance of employees in the work environment become the performance standards. Reflecting the *essential* tasks or major job duties and responsibilities (MJRs), performance standards may be assigned *weights* based on time, importance, quality, output (productivity), or span of control. Like objectives, performance standards reflect the several components: specific, measurable, attainable, agreed to, realistic, and timebound (review SMAART in Chapter 12).

Both the employee and his/her supervisor can utilize performance standards in gauging how well the job is performed. Certain behavioral qualities are not easily quantified, such as innovation, the manner in which a task was performed, and degree of professionalism. Expectations should be discussed by employee and supervisor to ensure understanding of expectations and abilities *before* the employee is evaluated. When supervisors and employees compare their lists of expectations, differences should be discussed. Agreement, compromise, or improvement in the work environment might result in a change in the performance standards before (performance) problems develop.[11]

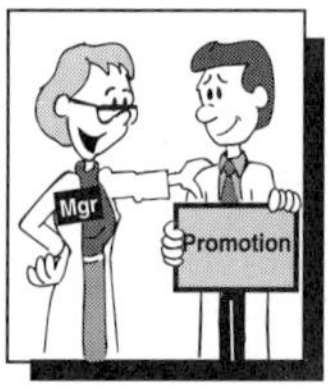

Activity 3: Writing Performance Standards and Weights[12]

Review the *major job duties and responsibilities* (MJRs) for laboratory medical technologists/clinical laboratory scientists. Write one performance standard (PS) for each; assign a weight (numerical value) for each MJR.

MJR #1 Performs complex clinical laboratory tests and procedures safely, with accuracy and precision, following accepted standards of practice; demonstrates ability to relate theory to test procedures and to make appropriate clinical interpretations.

MJR #2 Reviews test results for accuracy and reasonableness; verifies accuracy of results as reported either manually or via computer.

MJR #3 Performs quality control testing and evaluation on equipment and reagents, according to standards of practice.

MJR #4 Operates, maintains, and troubleshoots laboratory equipment and instrumentation according to standards of practice and protocol, regardless of sophistication or complexity.

MJR #5 Demonstrates effective interpersonal skills to work with others within the laboratory section, between laboratory sections, and throughout the hospital.

MJR #6 Manages time effectively, completes assigned daily tasks within a reasonable time frame; overtime, when used, is justified and assigned work that cannot be completed is reported to supervisor; upon early completion of assigned tasks, helps co-workers.

MJR #7 Instructs students, residents, and new employees according to established policies and programs.

MJR #8 Readily assumes additional duties and professional responsibilities.

See Activity Discussion 1 at the end of this chapter.

Many authors advocate that employees can do better when managers set their expectations higher, engage active participation from employees (involve them in determining how well the job should be done and how to do it), and encourage improvements (in work operations) without increasing resources or spending.[13, 14] (This phenomenon has been documented in classrooms when teachers who do not know the limitations of students apply the same standards regardless of abilities and the students achieve those standards.)

COMPETENCE ASSESSMENT

Competence is defined by Poe as the "possession of the critically required abilities, knowledge, judgment, skills, attitudes, and values, and (their) proficient use."[15] Behaviors should be classified as effective or ineffective, not good or bad. The ability to learn the mathematical concepts that underlie balancing a checkbook does not ensure that a person really can perform this task. On the contrary, a person may be able to balance a checkbook but not possess math knowledge beyond addition and subtraction.

In determining competence of employees, managers should consider intervening variables. A competency, such as motivation to learn and do well, might be responsible for successful demonstration of other competencies. Variables such as motivation have little predictive value. For example, studying the dictionary may enable a person to score higher on verbal achievement tests, but possessing an extensive vocabulary doesn't make the person a good writer or conversationalist. Competence assessment in the workplace serves a role similar to formative evaluation in teaching. Both measurements—competence assessment and formative evaluation—occur *during* a period or event rather than at its end. Both measurements identify the knowledge, skills, and behaviors that are still to be developed or improved. Both processes consider an individual's ability to perform.

CRITERIA TO SELECT LABORATORY TESTS FOR COMPETENCE ASSESSMENT

1. Risk
2. Frequency
3. Difficulty
4. Cost
5. Subject to error
6. Result-reporting intricacy
7. Mandatory

Competence assessments in health care have developed into serious activities. Competence assessment is viewed as the means to *ensure* accuracy, compliance, and functionability of employees to supervisors, owners, inspectors, and customers. Specifically for laboratory testing, anyone who performs laboratory tests must participate. For example, nurses, cardiac catheterization technicians, and respiratory therapists must adhere to these requirements and demonstrate their competence in performing the tests they are assigned to do. Laboratory supervisors often manage point-of-care testing (POCT) or ancillary site testing (AST) operations, including training, competence assessment (CA), quality control (QC), and quality assurance (QA) (Table 19–4). This challenge

Table 19–4
COMPETENCE ASSESSMENT POLICIES FOR NONLABORATORY PERSONNEL PERFORMING WAIVED/DESIGNATED LABORATORY TESTS

CA examinations will include specimen handling, results-entry into computer, and safety warnings.
CA will include review of QC log sheets, which include Quick Reference on corrective action/troubleshooting/reagent storage instructions at regular intervals.
CA will not include *any* test procedure's stepwise instructions.
Individuals producing unacceptable CA results on first attempt will be allowed a second attempt. If second CA results are unacceptable, then review with an on-site instructor or evaluator will be conducted. Another attempt with different materials will follow. Failure to produce acceptable CA results on the third attempt will require retraining.
CA results will be documented in Monthly QA reports.

comes from a question in the CLIA '88 requirements, "Can you show a list of technical personnel competent to run instruments and perform procedures?"[1]

Since competence for any endeavor or work has to be viewed as multidimensional, involving Cognitive, Psychomotor and Affective Domains, it is important to incorporate the best assessment tool(s) for the task (Fig. 19–2). Competencies being assessed should be linked to job performance. Assessment tools should be validated for accuracy in measuring what has been selected to be measured, determining the "passing" score, and discriminating between effective and ineffective behaviors (refer to tests in the Education section of this book). These tools should be reliable in that once used, they will produce the same results when used the next time. Activities or procedures used to assess employees' competence should be identified and the assessment protocol described in the laboratory's policy manual.

All laboratory testing procedures are subject to assessment but are selected based on specific criteria (see Criteria to select laboratory tests for competence assessment). Procedures should be selected if there is high risk while performing the procedure, such as the use of radioisotopes. Procedures that are rarely done in the laboratory (but cannot be done by an outside laboratory owing to need for fast turnaround time) or by the same employees should be included. Also, consider procedures that are difficult to perform because of complex steps, sophistication of instruments, or handling of reagents. High costs to perform procedures puts them on the assessment list. Procedures that are subject to error, such as nonautomated endocrine, toxicology, and molecular tests, should be included. Those tests in which reporting the results is a special, intricate process would be assessed. Lastly, those procedures that are mandatory are assessed. All phases of the testing process are subject to assessment: preanalytical, analytical, and postanalytical. Preanalytical assessments might include specimen acceptability, accuracy of patient identification, and thoroughness of test request. Postanalytical assessments might include QC validation, acceptance of results, reporting of results, confirming that the results intended for a patient actually appear on that patient's records, and billing accuracy. Employees should be assessed only on those activities that they are responsible for performing. A grid of task assignments for a microbiology laboratory is displayed in Table 19–5. A cross section of domains should be assessed: knowledge and recall through the judgment/problem-solving level; technical skills, critical thinking, and decision making; and communication. Managers should first review job descriptions for critical

Problem Solving Skills Competence Assessment Documentation Form

Skill in solving problems associated with: ______________________________

Those employees for whom problem solving **IS** within their scope of practice will complete this CA. Method(s) utilized for assessing and documenting PROBLEM SOLVING SKILLS and comments, especially for notable activities or to recommend additional training/review, will be identified by the Evaluator.

EMPLOYEE NAME ______________________________ ID# ______________

LAB SECTION ______________________________ DATE ______________

I have assessed this employee's problem solving skills using:

_____ Case study, external program

_____ Group discussion

_____ Individual discussion with Evaluator

_____ Case study, internal source

_____ Critical incident observation

_____ "Bugged" instrument or procedure

_____ Other: ______________________________

Evaluator's Comments:

_____ Employee demonstrated adequate problem solving skills.

_____ Employee requires additional training/review or independent study.

Employee's Comments:

DATE: _____ Evaluator ______________________ Employee ______________

. . . .

Additional training/review/independent study done: ______________________

DATE: _____ Evaluator ______________________ Employee ______________

Figure 19–2 Problem-solving skills competence assessment documentation form.

dimensions and requirements of critical characteristics. They should review employee reports regarding procedures and circumstances that are particularly effective and those that (occasionally) produce outcomes different from what is expected.

Certain benefits can be gained from competence assessment that QC and QA programs do not produce. In observing several employees performing the same procedure, a supervisor might note that a particular step is done differently by each person. The supervisor would then rewrite the step to ensure conformity. Errors and inconsistencies might be detected in procedure and policy manuals that would otherwise go undetected. Also, a supervisor observing employee performances might notice that a particularly efficient manual motion (dexterity) demonstrated by one employee can be taught to the others. During practical exams or simulations, supervisors might note that certain employees take significantly less time. Similar efficiencies in workflow could be established for other employees. Negative characteristics, such as lack of motivation or the inability to manage stress, displayed by an employee

Table 19–5

MICROBIOLOGY LABORATORY EMPLOYEE REQUIREMENTS FOR COMPETENCE ASSESSMENT

Task Description	MT	MLT	LA
Ordering/Accessioning	X	X	X
Quality control	X	X	
Parasitology	X	Part	
Mycobacteriology	X	Part	
Biochemical tests–Mycobacteriology	X		
Anaerobes	X	Part	
Respiratory cultures	X	Part	
Antigen/Antibody detection test	X	Part	
Blood cultures	X	X	Part
Bacteria and yeasts–Biochemical tests, substrate utilization	X	Part	
Susceptibility testing–Bacteria	X	Part	

(Selected descriptors only included here.)

Legend: MT = medical technologist/clinical laboratory scientist; MLT = medical laboratory technician/clinical laboratory technician; LA = laboratory assistant; X = complete responsibility; Part = partial responsibility.

might be identified as influencing his/her competence. The supervisor can recommend continuing education that could then help the employee strengthen the specific characteristic.

Proficiency testing subscription programs from external sources are required by regulatory agencies for clinical laboratories. Proficiency testing differs from competence assessment programs in that materials are analyzed and results reported by one (or maybe two or three) technical personnel. All subscribing laboratories' results are statistically compared and analyses of each laboratory's performance returned several months later. The specific proficiency testing event could be counted for that laboratorian's competence assessment. Also, survey materials, when in sufficient amount, or slide transparencies can be incorporated into the laboratory's competence assessment program for future use.

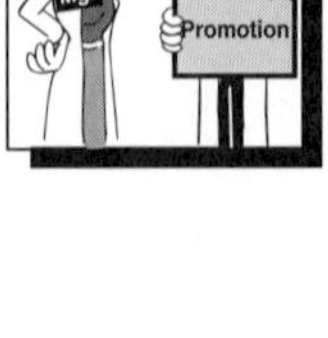

Activity 4: Measurement Tools for Competence Assessment

Discuss advantages and disadvantages of proficiency testing materials and direct observation as measurement tools for competence assessment.

See Activity Discussion 2 at the end of this chapter.

PERFORMANCE APPRAISALS

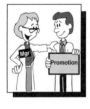

The process of appraising performance requires managers and supervisors to document behaviors and work accomplished by employees. The most signifi-

Table 19–6
GENERAL BEHAVIORS AND TASKS FOR COMPETENCE ASSESSMENT/PERFORMANCE APPRAISAL

Behaviors	Tasks
Problem-solving skills	Safety
Decision-making skills	Confidentiality
Interpersonal skills	Computer operations
Conceptual thinking skills	Fire extinguisher use
Critical thinking skills	Blood-borne pathogens: general; TB; Universal standards
Communication skills: verbal—face-to-face, telephone; written	CPR, if required by Department
Interpersonal/interaction skills: bosses, co-workers, customers	
Team-building skills	

cant benefit gained from performance appraisals for the organization comes from enhancing its human resources. The following four strategies should be initiated with employees by managers: (1) identify new areas of knowledge and skills (desired by employee and needed by employer); (2) implement structured training of employees including practice in order for them to develop their expertise; (3) document and promote (Jacobs says, "store") expertise for use when needed or to replace if lost; and (4) recognize expertise when it is used (Table 19–6).[16]

The performance of employees is most often documented and discussed once a year, usually their employment anniversaries, by their supervisors or managers. Only when a troublesome situation occurs or the circumstances change does performance warrant discussion and documentation at other times. Evaluations should be positive, although criticism might be the real reason for the interview. Even in the most negative evaluation, some comment should be made on any effective behavior demonstrated by the individual. Although honesty in the evaluation process as well as the report is crucial, criticism should be done with temperance and consideration for other people's feelings.

EMPLOYEE DEVELOPMENT THROUGH PERFORMANCE APPRAISALS

- Identify new knowledge and skills
- Develop expertise
- Record expertise
- Recognize expertise

These strategies apply to all employees regardless of their education, training, experience, or position, particularly when the "promote from within" philosophy is advocated in a corporate culture. For employees, favorable performance appraisals of their previous year's endeavors often mean eligibility for promotion or transfer, career development opportunities, or just job security in their current positions. In some situations, merit salary increases, commissions, or bonuses are allocated depending on performance appraisals rated superior, excellent, or outstanding. (Salary programs identified as merit or commissioned are usually linked to attainment of specific objectives for designated times, often based on numerical calculations of revenue generated or costs saved, under employment contracts that detail objectives as well as proposed payments and can vary from one period to the next, depending on the owners' and stockholders' arrangements.) For employers, unfavorable performance appraisal of an employee's endeavors, including documentation that training, retraining, and counseling have produced little or no improvement or change, may support demotion or firing of that employee.

Managers and supervisors rarely enjoy the task of doing performance appraisals. If their expertise lies in science, medicine, finance, engineering, or technical fields, they may lack training in the (human) appraisal process. Keep in mind that owners and administrators have similar feelings about appraising the performance of managers and supervisors. Frequently, greater importance is placed on doing managerial appraisals because producing external reports, fulfilling organizational goals and objectives, and achieving self-planned objectives carry a heavier weight at this level of responsibility. Still, no one likes the tedium and legalities of performance documentation, especially if the behaviors are negative or require correction.

The performance appraisal process consists of two points: how did the employee perform his/her work in the past (year), and how will that employee do his/her work in the future?[17, 18] Unfortunately, the emphasis, even on the form itself, can fall on past performance rather than correction of deficiencies or determination of objectives during the next period. Managers should commit to dividing the emphasis on unacceptable as well as future performance *with* employees. An optimal performance appraisal sequence consists of planning, managing, evaluating, and developing the performance of employees (Fig. 19–3). Components of planning performance were presented in earlier sections of this chapter.

Managing performance consists of collecting data representative of the

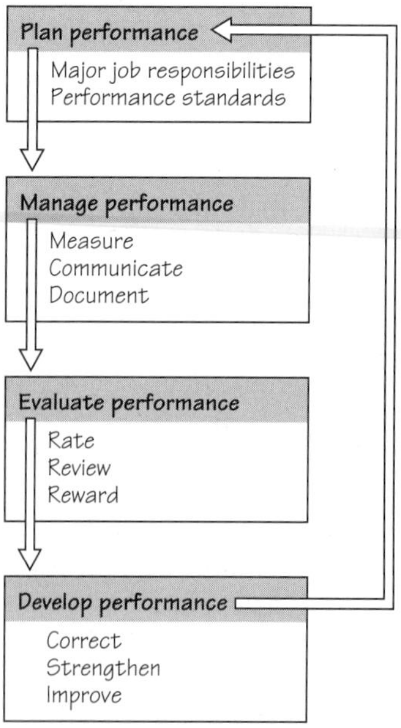

Figure 19–3 Performance appraisal sequence.

employee's work such as critical incidents (for correction). Information might come from comments, both complimentary and critical, from customers, other departmental personnel, and co-workers. For specific concerns, communication in the form of feedback is necessary. Appropriate feedback is addressed in the next section of this chapter. All data and comments should be dated and filed in order to track the employee's subsequent actions.

The evaluating performance step incorporates rating, reviewing, and rewarding. Using data and documentation, managers can more easily select the score for each major job responsibility and provide examples that rationalize the scores. Most performance appraisal forms contain both a rating scale and space for comments for each major job responsibility.

Activity 5: Rating Scales for Performance Evaluation

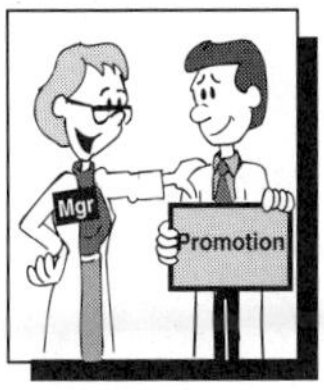

Refer to the major job responsibilities (MJRs) in Activity 3 and the performance standards developed by the readers/group/class (see Activity Discussion 19–1). Discuss each rating scale in Table 19–7. Select one or create your own for the MJRs.

In *participative* performance appraisals, employees complete self-assessments. During the interview, discussions would compare theirs with the supervisors' appraisals of them plus the explanations of why certain criteria were met (or not met), including examples.

Coaching relates to performance appraisal but should be kept separate. Some employees need coaching to realize the course they should be taking and get on it. This provides an employee developmental opportunity for the manager. The formal performance appraisal process documents when a behavior problem produces ineffective performance that has not been corrected.

PERFORMANCE INTERVIEW

The purpose of appraisal interviews is to provide an opportunity for discussion of an employee's performance at a designated time and place. The infor-

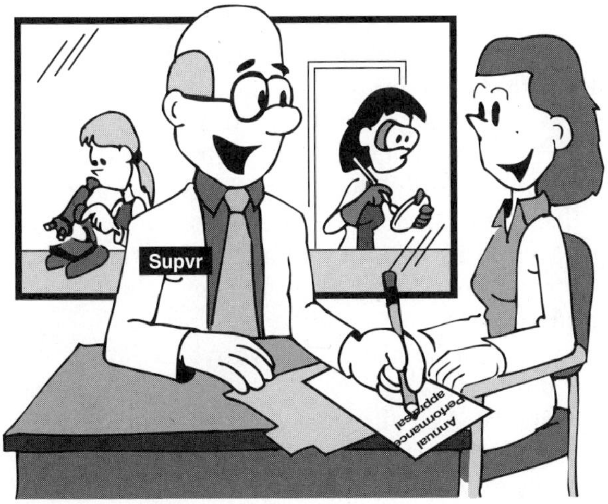

Table 19–7
RATING SCALE EXAMPLES

I. Graphic Rating Scale Directions: Check the Appropriate Box for Each Major Job Responsibility				
Unsatisfactory	***Fair***	***Good***	***Superior***	***Exceptional***
a. Fails to meet standards most of the time b. Employee requires retraining c. Reason to release/ dismiss	a. Minimal; does not meet standards some of the time b. Employee requires observation	a. Meets minimal standards most of the time b. Suggest areas for improvement	a. Exceeds minimal standards some of the time b. Demonstrates ability to maintain this level	a. Exceeds minimal standards most of the time b. Distinctly and consistently outstanding c. Model employee

II. Behaviorally Anchored Rating Scale (Numerical) Directions: Select the point value which corresponds to the level of performance	
A. Three-point scale:	1 point = fails to meet standards 3 points = meets standards 5 points = exceeds standards
B. Four-point scale:	0 = unacceptable 1 = below average 2 = average 3 = above average 4 = excellent
C. Five-point scale:	1 point = seldom meets standards 2 points = occasionally, but not consistently, meets standards 3 points = consistently meets standards 4 points = consistently meets and frequently exceeds standards 5 points = consistently exceeds standards

mation to be exchanged focuses on the past from the perspective of both the employee and the supervisor and the future as agreed to by both persons. Supervisors should plan and control the arrangements for interviews. They should concentrate on the employee and attend to details, that is, schedule the interview at a time convenient and less stressful for the employee, forward telephone calls, use a room with a door that can be shut to ensure privacy, hang a "Do not disturb" sign on the door, reduce physical barriers by sitting at a small table with the employee rather than behind a desk, make eye contact even when giving negative information, and maintain a cordial and friendly demeanor as in the ongoing work relationship. Likewise, employees should prepare for their interviews. Employees' preparation should include review of their past performance, perhaps as part of filling out the same performance appraisal form, and they should note examples to support acceptable or above-average behaviors. Both persons should start the interview calmly and at ease.

Both individuals should engage in two-way communication techniques. Goodale advises the supervisor to give feedback and recognition of the employee's performance "as often as is necessary for the benefit of both parties."[19] An example of *performance and results* that are related to the job are behavioral observations during the course of the year both to commend for recognition and to recommend for improvement. At the beginning or end of the interview, questions or comments might be included regarding the employee's family, personal interests, or professional desires that would indicate the supervisor's interest in the employee as a person. The "meat" of the interview focuses on the work environment and the employee's performance there. When supervisors ask employees direct questions about what they do well on the job and what they want to do, the employees will do their own assessment. During the interview, supervisors should remember to state the positives first and the negatives last. According to Goodale, "probe first, prescribe later."[18] The individual's future performance should be mutually agreed to at the conclusion of the interview. Astute supervisors will also ask employees' opinions about the way the work environment could be manipulated to improve their performance.

The personal relationship between the supervisor and the employee is crucial and ongoing. It is not just important at performance appraisal time. Months of poor supervision cannot be wiped out with one good interview.

Feedback

Three types of feedback occur within the workplace.[11] *Informative* feedback portrayed by numbers reflects quantities without interpretation: number of fasting blood sugars performed daily, number of "couldn't get" blood specimens by each phlebotomist, average number of service calls on an instrument per month for a year, or a score on a test. Without comparison to standards, these numbers lack meaning. Even if plotted graphically, day after day or month after month (Appendix 15–A), one can only state, "This is what was done," *not* "The performance is 90% under the goal," or "We've achieved the standard!" Informative feedback is valuable and must be collected accurately. It must be handled appropriately, with certain elements requiring coding for anonymity to ensure confidentiality.

Reinforcement or *rewarding* feedback focuses on positives: verbal compliments, written letters of commendation, special privileges such as attending a national professional meeting, salary increases, or promotions. Through some mechanism of interpretation or comparison to standards, the behavior is considered acceptable or effective. Rewards given for effective behavior should be designed to stimulate continuation of that behavior. Attentive managers adjust the way they deliver rewarding feedback by considering the needs of the individual employee. Most employees accept (some bask in) public appreciation with feedback displayed before their colleagues, friends, even family. Others prefer a quiet verbal thank you or note or an office meeting with the door closed. *All* people like to know when they've done a "good" job. Thoughtful managers consider others' personal likes and select "rewards" accordingly.[20]

Corrective feedback informs an individual that a change (in behavior) is necessary. It indicates that behaviors less than satisfactory should be improved, changed, or stopped. In addition, people deserve explanations and reasons why change is necessary, what the change should be (specific actions or behaviors), and what effect the change will bring (restate the desired expectations, goals, and objectives). Managers must avoid the pitfall of comparing one employee with another. This critical step always ensures comparison of the person's behavior to an objective or standard. Another trap managers fall into occurs when negative behavior is rewarded. This can easily happen as most people dislike giving reprimands or dealing with confrontation. Managers may not recognize that when they don't say anything, they inadvertently reinforce the negative behavior! Without feedback, employees often assume that what they're doing is acceptable. Some people will continue negative actions just to challenge their superiors or co-workers, even when they know they may violate a rule or policy. Corrective feedback not only identifies the negative behavior but describes the expected behavior. For critical incidents, there may be no tolerance for anything other than immediate and complete change: that is, now, not by the end of the month, or stop the behavior completely rather than progressively change.

Motto for effective feedback: Go *public* with *positive*. Go confidential with *corrective*.

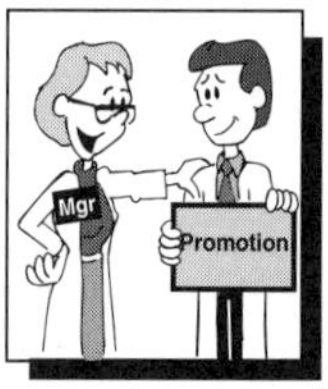

Activity 6: Turning Criticism Into Corrective Feedback

A manager criticizes a phlebotomist, "You had four 'couldn't gets' this morning. I thought you were trying to do better but I don't think you care." Readers or groups should write a dialogue between these two people as *corrective* feedback.

Feedback is preferred over criticism to let employees know what is thought of their work, not their personal worth or personality. Worthwhile and significant or critical behaviors should be targeted. Feedback, appropriately staged, encourages employees to offer opinions and reasons for their behaviors. To initiate the employee's performance plan, restate the behaviors that could be strengthened, improved, or corrected. The employee should be closely involved in developing this plan and the target date when it should be accomplished.

HANDLING FEEDBACK: PRAISE OR CRITICISM

Many employees need to change the way they think about and handle feedback. Bias and egotistical mannerisms of all persons involved have to be

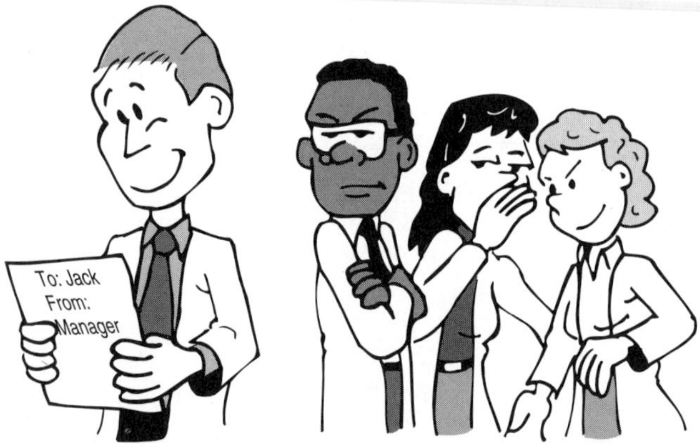

eliminated from the feedback process. Praise can be just as difficult to give and accept as criticism. The giver must be sincere. The praise must be justified. The praise must go to the right person(s). Even if a supervisor influenced the employee's effective behavior, sharing the credit just isn't appropriate. Occasionally, employees will not trust that the praise of their performance is legitimate; they may have experienced so much criticism or sarcasm in spite of their hard work that this is what they've come to expect. Supervisors can help employees overcome this by citing the reason for the praise directly to the person. They can also adapt the praise to the form the employee feels most comfortable receiving—private or public. Praise should be noted in employees' files when given throughout the year to be included in their annual performance appraisal. Individuals sometimes are embarrassed by praise, especially if they think that the work they do isn't important or that they were just doing what they were supposed to do. They should be encouraged to just say "Thank you," and not negate the praise with statements such as, "It was easy; anyone could have done it." Praise is rewarding feedback, a strong motivator, and a nice way of showing appreciation for efforts or contributions in the workplace.

Contrary to effective performance warranting praise are those inadequate or problematic behaviors that warrant correction. Managers can alter confrontational meetings. Control of hostility and anger is important in order for criticism to be accepted as corrective feedback. Both parties should project negotiating and accepting attitudes instead of defending and rejecting attitudes. People who become defensive are less likely to hear or consider what the other person is saying. The manager should communicate the impact of the ineffective behaviors on the organization and services. Feedback itself is effective if "incorporated into one's behavior repertoire"[21] instead of simply being ignored. The object is to have the person think about the feedback and not react emotionally.

If the information is valid, then agreement should be offered by the employee. If the information is invalid, but not from the superior, then the comment should be acknowledged without agreeing or arguing. When the superior states an invalid criticism, the employee should ask for examples. If the examples are vague or erroneous, then the comment should simply be acknowledged, again without agreeing or arguing. When valid information is given, agreement should be followed by a decision whether or not to change the behavior, and if change is feasible.[22, 23] Most importantly, how an employee behaves must remain separate from his/her value as a person.

Other Evaluations

Other methods of personnel evaluation play a role in the workplace. Performance evaluations can be prospective and conducted before an individual is hired. Evaluation based on group endeavors can confound the assessment of each member's contribution unless clear and specific criteria are delineated before the group begins its functions. "Upward" evaluations can contribute to the improvement or change of performance of supervisors, managers, or administrators.

PREPLACEMENT ASSESSMENT

Determining the knowledge, skill, and behavior of a prospective employee happens before the individual is placed in a new organization, department, laboratory section, or job. Preplacement assessments, validated and in written policy, have become extremely helpful in determining the abilities and potential *before* investing in hiring and training employees.[24]

Assessment protocols may be professionally developed or self-developed for one's own organization. Certain assessments require administration and interpretation by trained counselors, for example, the Myers-Briggs Type Indicator (MBTI).[25] Any assessment requires validation for accuracy and reliability. The written policy must state to all candidates the type of assessment that will be given.

EVALUATION OF TEAM PERFORMANCE

The new paradigms developing in laboratories are driving the formation of teams. Now managers are forced to think about the evaluation process differently. Will it be the same for all? How can it be different if all members do the same thing? Traditional individual rewards and promotions do not match up with team efforts. All members should feel they can influence overall group performance without compromising the recognition of individual excellence. Often a dual reward system is developed: one for individuals and one for the team. Any reward system can be utilized more readily when performance standards and the design mechanism determine the contributions each person makes to the team effort.[26, 27]

EVALUATION OF MANAGERS, SUPERVISORS, AND OTHERS

Administrators, managers, and supervisors should ask employees why one activity was done very well and why another one was not. Interested administrators do ask. In addition to the outcome, they want to know how *their* behaviors influence the employees' behaviors. A turnabout strategy, called the *360-degree feedback method,* can be done as a group performance appraisal from employees, customers, and other department personnel who use services or interact with the top echelon of managers.[28] This method, considered a diagnostic and assessment tool, keeps administrators informed of the status and process from the very people who are doing the work and from those who are receiving the service (or product).[29, 30]

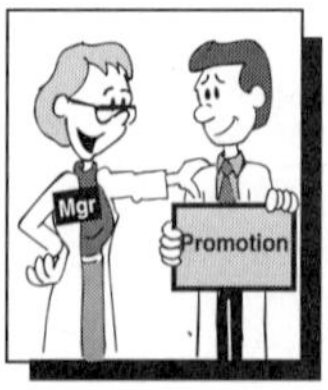

Activity 7: Rate the Boss

Each reader or group should develop a questionnaire for "upward" evaluation of laboratory supervisors by employees. For each of the following traits, write one (or more) question. Compare all questions, selecting one to three questions per trait. Develop a rating scale (Table 19–7).

1. Leadership
2. Communication
3. Teamwork
4. Role model for quality
5. Planning

If other traits are presented in class, write questions for each one also.

Policies

Employee rights are supported by three policies usually developed by organization and human resource administrators. One policy provides recourse for employees who think they have been wronged or treated unfairly. Known as a *grievance* or *appeals procedure,* it should be written and made available to all employees. Managers and supervisors should be trained in the use of this procedure, particularly because of documentation that would be required from them, when an employee who reports to them initiates this procedure.

Another policy explains *disciplinary* or *corrective action* that can be given. Specific penalties are explained according to the misconduct, infraction, or violation. In most instances, the policy is designed to be progressive, with employees offered additional opportunities to change or improve their behaviors or to comply with procedures, rules, and policies. In severe circumstances, especially if the violation is proven to be a violation of a law, such as theft, immediate dismissal is the disciplinary action. This policy must also be written and made available. Managers and supervisors must be informed about the use and process of this policy.

The third policy involves *confidentiality.* In Chapter 14, communication channels were described. The "grapevine" can be a very active source of misinformation, especially when an employee is observed being called into the supervisor's office. At all times, managers and supervisors should maintain policies regarding confidentiality related to employee information. Casual discussions regarding a specific employee's performance or discipline should not be condoned. Before any information is shared about an employee's unacceptable behavior and subsequent action or discipline, this action should be carefully considered. Breach of confidentiality warrants discipline also. (Clinical program officials frequently include employee and colleague confidentiality along with patient confidentiality as a part of laboratory science students' performance appraisals in their laboratory courses.)

Evaluation of Activities

Evaluation procedures in the laboratory can be conducted on many activities. Internal evaluations enable managers to select methods and procedures, instruments and equipment, and one test instead of another. External evaluations are conducted to determine the status of services and operations using customer surveys, financial reports, and accreditation inspections. Acceptance of and perception of the value of services (products) determine the choices that customers will make in purchasing those services. Health care and laboratory testing are not exempted from unrealistic expectations and misperceptions by customers. One purpose of evaluation is to enable administrators to ascertain whether they should offer services that do not, in fact, fulfill customers' needs or meet their expectations but are nonetheless requested.

Laboratories may evaluate test kits prior to mass production, an instrument before it is purchased, and test procedures before those currently in

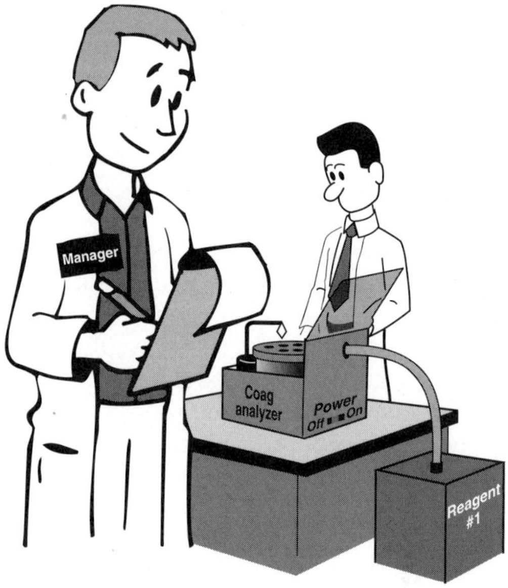

use are discontinued. Method evaluations designed for laboratory tests and instruments focus on accuracy and precision.[31] Other studies consider costs, personnel, efficiency, quality control, and interpretation of results.

Services can be evaluated as the "product" offered by laboratories. Services vary from organization to organization on the basis of customer population and their needs, cost of performing tests, and competition. Evaluations enable managers to determine such services as the variety of tests performed: glucose but not lactose or the scheduled availability of tests: (1) hepatitis analysis offered Mondays, Wednesdays, and Fridays 0700 to 1500 hours, with specimens received at other times being processed and frozen; (2) 24-hour availability for STAT tests: blood gases; or (3) the efficiency of reporting test results: STAT glucose results in 45 minutes or urine protein electrophoresis within 72 hours (3 days).

Programs, events, or a series of activities can be evaluated either during their progression or at completion. Applications in pathology and laboratory science include such activities as:

- A one-hour lecture on one issue: specificity and sensitivity, tumor markers;
- a one-day seminar on one topic: "DNA Technology in the Clinical Laboratory;"
- a training program for a new employee in one laboratory section of several weeks' duration: microbiology (see tasks listed in Table 19–5);
- an educational training program of several months' or years' duration: MT/CLS, MLT/CLT, phlebotomy, point-of-care testing, pathology residency

Voluntary professional evaluations for accreditation provide opportunities for organizations to be compared with predetermined criteria developed by their peers. "Essentials" or requirements and "guidelines" or recommendations form the criteria. Although successful accreditation is the goal, even the seeking of voluntary accreditation represents an effective attitude in itself. Licensure mandates compliance with standards in order to exist and/or function at all; it is not a voluntary process. Documentation is required as well as on-site inspections. License approval and renewal depend on achieving the designated level of the standards.

Comments solicited in external evaluations represent feedback. This feedback reinforces the activity or indicates that change is needed and in which areas. Selected comments can appear in brochures as benefits that participants might receive when they seek services or attend future activities at that organization.

LABORATORY PRODUCTIVITY MEASURES

Productivity in the workplace represents the output as compared with the input.[32] This ratio can be calculated in different ways. Certain measurements are task defined and quantifiable, making the ratios fairly easy to calculate. Others are more difficult to calculate, especially if they relate to creativity and quality. These results rarely produce numbers. The overriding concern regarding productivity relates to finance, considering factors such as best test ordered (utilization), test volume, and labor and materials costs. Each factor generates its own productivity information. This information shows how well things get done.

National productivity ratios, calculated from income data obtained from the U.S. Commerce Department, are influenced by "investment, the organization of production, managerial skill, and workforce characteristics."[33] This statement should trigger the realization that productivity, whether high or low, does not fall solely on the shoulders of workers/employees.

The productivity ratios of greatest concern to laboratory managers are shown in Table 19–8. Through comparisons with other laboratories,[34, 35] managers can assess the efficiency of personnel, procedures, and instrumentation (ratios of billable tests per paid hours and ratio of technical personnel to total number of employees), and policies from the organization, department, and

Table 19–8
PRODUCTIVITY RATIOS FOR LABORATORIES PER MONTH

	Laboratory A	Laboratory B	Laboratory C
a. $\frac{\text{billable tests}}{\text{FTE}}$			
b. $\frac{\text{billable tests}}{\text{technical FTE}}$			
c. $\frac{\text{technical FTEs}}{\text{total FTEs}}$			
d. $\frac{\text{worked hours}}{\text{paid hours}}$			
e. $\frac{\text{billable tests}}{\text{paid hour}}$			

Legend: FTE = full-time equivalent; a person who is full-time and works a 40-hour workweek is counted as 1 FTE; a person who is part-time and works 24 hours per workweek is counted as 0.6 FTE. Billable tests are those that are ordered, usually tabulated by an organization's finance systems.

laboratory section (ratio of work hours to paid hours). (Note: In this chapter, financial information as related to productivity has been excluded.)

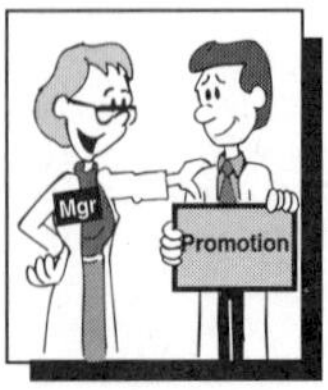

Activity 8: Laboratory Productivity Ratios

Given the following information for three laboratories, calculate the ratios using Table 19–8. Discuss which laboratory appears to be the most efficient, the most profitable, and delivers the highest quality test results. Discuss data for each laboratory that most likely indicate a need for change or improvement (action by managers). Discuss what additional information would be necessary to make these decisions.

	Laboratory A	Laboratory B	Laboratory C
Billable tests per month	85,000	122,550	52,078
FTEs	95	107.5	85
Technical FTEs	60	65	55
Worked hours	124,800	18,633	14,733
Paid hours	141,820	20,476	16,190

See Activity Discussion 3 at the end of this chapter.

Activity 9: Other Laboratory Productivity Ratios

Each reader or group should brainstorm and write a list of other productivity ratios that they, as employees and managers, would want to consider. From the list, they should discuss what changes they might have to consider.

See Activity Discussion 4 at the end of this chapter.

Activity 10: Value of Productivity Measurements

Discuss at least five managerial changes or improvements that might be considered on the basis of information obtained from productivity measurements.

See Activity Discussion 5 at the end of this chapter.

> Motto for productivity: Efficiency is doing this right; effectiveness is doing the right things.

Obligations for fiscal responsibility to customers (patients and physicians) override all other concerns for managers, supervisors, directors, and owners facing the task of making it possible for employees to accomplish more, and making employees want to accomplish more.

Factors, categorized as either "extrinsic" or "intrinsic," can prevent personnel from achieving their maximum level of productivity. Extrinsic factors represent those associated with the work environment. Intrinsic factors relate to or come from individuals themselves.

Activity 11: Barriers to Top Productivity

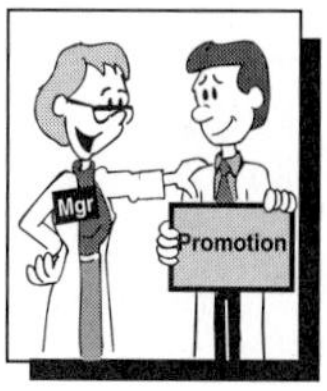

Describe three to six factors considered "extrinsic" and three to six factors considered "intrinsic" that reduce productivity levels. Discussion should address how managers can intervene to reduce these barriers.

See Activity Discussion 6 at the end of this chapter.

OUTCOME MEASURES

Selection of appropriate measures for outcomes evaluation can be as difficult as identifying those for personnel. In this case, what gets attention, gets measured! Issues that trigger negative customer reactions, influence patient care, justify resources, or dominate financial statements demand attention. These concerns become key indicators to measure those aspects of performance that are important and *meaningful to laboratory customers.*[36]

Several authors describe strategies that they would challenge laboratorians to consider in order for laboratory services to be improved or enhanced: improve turnaround time (TAT), reduce laboratory errors, deliver information efficiently and correctly to physicians and designated health care givers, eliminate inappropriate testing, control system failures, minimize unnecessary variations in patient care practices, and increase quality of testing methods.[37–42] Not much different from other evaluation processes, this one presents unusual circumstances to overcome. Identifying the appropriate measurement tools and putting them into place and securing (access) and collecting data have been major constraints in successful outcomes evaluations. Statistical analysis slightly confounds the process. Interpretation and implementation of improvements compound and propel the process throughout laboratories and health care organizations. Truly, no one system suffices when laboratory managers and others tackle these issues.

Outcome management has been defined by Spath as the "analysis, evaluation, and dissemination of the results of medical processes or procedures to improve health-care outcomes."[43] Four elements of the evaluation process require explanation: (1) *specification,* which defines the expected outcomes and measures to assess outcomes achievement; (2) *measurement,* which is the design and confirmation of valid and reliable assessment tools; (3) *information systems,* consisting of computer hardware and software for data collection, input, retrieval, and analysis; and (4) *process improvement,* which includes the design and implementation of quality improvement techniques.[43]

Dr. O'Leary described outcomes as descriptions of the past to provide standards that are designed to predict the future. He advises collecting data that would link performance to outcomes and, subsequently, to improvement. Health care givers and laboratorians should think of data as a "red flag" to point out why something "bad" happened and then determine ways to fix it.[2] Recent health care reform issues focused on cost and access (to medical care) issues. A movement has begun for equal time to the issue of *quality*. Improvement of quality can be accomplished with models for clinical pathways, test utilization protocols, and case management guidelines.[44]

Problems Associated with Evaluation

Problems, when not identified or resolved, can interfere with evaluation processes and outcomes. Circumstances and people do not differ in this regard—sometimes problems are obvious and at other times covert. When accounting for known factors, one may overlook, unintentionally, the subtle human elements.

PROBLEMS INVOLVING PEOPLE

The Pareto principle applies here also: 20% of the people produce 80% of the problems. Several primary factors create employer-employee problems. One significant cause relates to perceptions of job responsibilities that do not match with what the organization puts forth. Another major cause is associated with miscommunication. A third serious cause correlates to inadequate or inappropriate coping skills; this is especially noticeable in health care environments in which stress is high and its occurrence often unpredictable. Do-gooders and saboteurs alike interfere with endeavors, making them ineffective. Their intentions, based on their personalities, reactions, or lack of objectivity, cause havoc in the workplace.

Several authors describe "difficult" people, who may be the bosses as well as the employees. They recommend strategies for handling these people and avoiding becoming a "difficult" person in response.[45–49] Common occurrences and viable solutions appear daily in newspapers, magazines, professional journals, and seminars.[50–53]

EVALUATORS

Problems arise when evaluators are uncertain about the standards or expectations. The standards may not be appropriate or clearly written. The actual rating scale descriptors may not be well defined—for example, "What is meant by 'good' or '3'?" Without clear information, evaluators must rely on their own interpretations, which can be subjective or prejudiced. They associate the descriptors with their own experiences. These problems apply to both employee evaluations and activity evaluations. Additional problems are described related to evaluation of personnel, but likewise can occur during evaluation of activities.

The *halo effect* describes the influence of one rating on another. Supervisors who have not had close contact with the employees or think of them as unfriendly may rate them lower on items such as "demonstrates effective interpersonal skills to work with others" (see Activity 3 MJR #5). The supervisors may be influenced to rate other responsibilities lower also, such as "readily assumes additional duties" (see Activity 3 MJR #8). For activities, the expectation is that a group known for giving valuable seminars with useful handouts will give future seminars of equal or greater value. One would feel uneasy giving a low rating if this turned out not to be true.

Evaluators who feel uncomfortable with giving high and low ratings often select middle scores or "average." This *central tendency* effect hampers effective (top) performers from being recognized and rewards ineffective (poor) performers. It also narrows the distinction between those who might be qualified for promotion and those who would not be qualified. Other supervisors demonstrate tendencies toward either *leniency*, and rate (almost all) employees high average or high, or *strictness*, and rate (almost all) employees low average or low. This likewise inhibits the discrimination between acceptable and unacceptable behaviors among employees.

Another problematic phenomenon can occur when the employee realizes his/her performance appraisal is coming up in a month or so. Called *recency*, this represents the situation when a mediocre performing employee becomes an exceptional hard working one for the month. Without on-going documentation of performance, an unsuspecting supervisor can be impressed and can rate the employee on the basis of the most recent observations.

One more problem can exist, and that is *bias*. Laws support employees' rights against certain prejudices entering into the appraisal process. Poor ratings based on characteristics such as age, race, religion, and gender have been documented as illegal in lawsuits.[54] Other, more subtle discriminations occasionally prevent accurate performance appraisals by an inexperienced supervisor: for example, poor performance in one position or workplace will be expected to continue in another; people who don't have money won't be courteous; a person in a wheelchair can't learn a complicated procedure; or a person who rides the bus to work won't be punctual. These *perceived* inadequacies often require that employees expend extra effort to convince supervisors of their potential and abilities.

Activity 12: Biases to Avoid in Evaluations

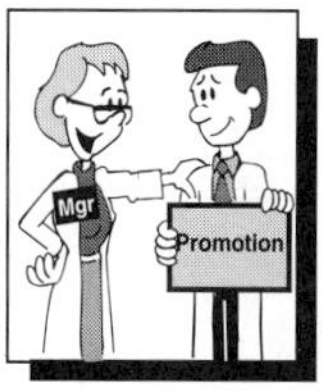

Develop a list of biases that can present problems in evaluation. Examples can be taken from readings, knowledge of experiences others have had, and personal (school or work) experiences. Descriptions of the biases might include appearance, physical or other disabilities, names or other identification, economics, social aspects, and education.

Managers can assist supervisors in developing their evaluating skills through coaching. Knowledgeable supervisors can share their experiences

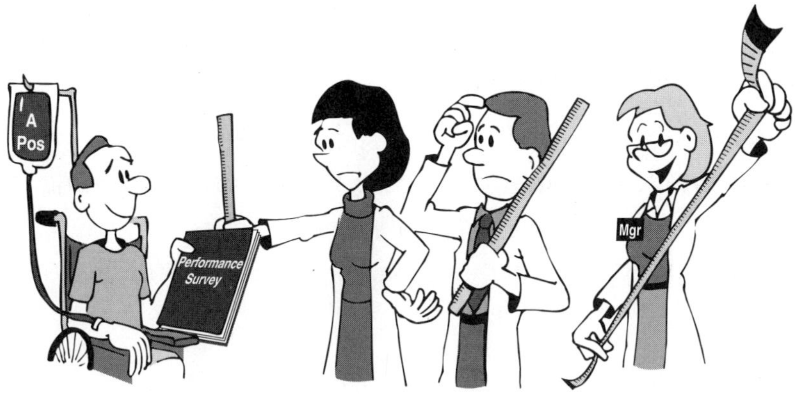

Table 19–9
EVALUATION SYSTEM CHECKLIST

1. Why was the evaluation done?
2. How do you know that what was measured was what was wanted? How do you know that the results are valid? How do you know that the results are accurate? How can you determine that the results are relevant?
3. How do you know that what was measured was reliable? Are the findings precise, dependable, and consistent?
4. Was the measurement tool used objective?
5. Was the evaluator objective both in collecting the data and in interpreting it?
6. Are the conclusions similar to others? If not, is there a reasonable explanation? What will be done about the situation?
7. Is the evaluation system practical? Can it be done in an appropriate length of time? Is it readable and clear? Is it easy to administer? What is the cost?
8. Is it legal? Does it apply to all persons in the same environment? Does it discriminate but is not discriminatory?

regarding both employee and activity evaluations. Names of employees should not be included. New supervisors can study professional materials and literature for guidance and examples of cases.

In all of these situations, subscribing to fair practices is the legal obligation of employers and supervisors. Managers who fail to adequately inform or train the supervisors can be held accountable for the (inappropriate or illegal) actions of the supervisors.

Process

Obviously, any evaluation system produces results that can drastically affect the employees or activities. For employees, this can mean more money, increased benefits, recognition, and even being promoted or being fired. In the case of activities, such as a test, a method, or a seminar, this can determine whether or not they are continued or dropped. Results of evaluation of instruments determine which, if any, will be purchased and which will not.

Beyond the human factors identified previously, several process problems can interfere with or prevent the production of accurate results. A review of evaluation systems should be conducted, even if only briefly (Table 19–9).

Acceptance and perception of value of product determines choices customers will make in purchasing products. Health care and laboratory testing are not exempt from these considerations. The point of evaluation verifies that what you said you would do, you are, in fact, doing. This applies to hiring and retaining individuals expected to behave or perform in a prescribed manner and whether or not they do.

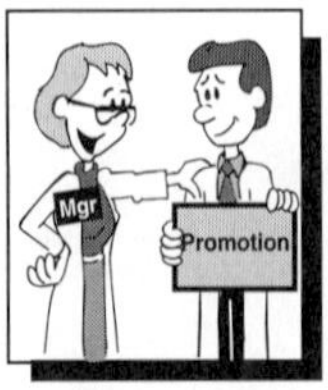

Activity 13: Evaluation Process Problems, Symptoms, and Possible Solutions

For each of the four areas and corresponding questions listed, identify one to three *symptoms* that indicate a problem exists. Describe *possible solutions* for each symptom.

1. *Measurement problem*: What should be evaluated?

2. *Decision problem*: How can behavior and performance, or activity be evaluated?
3. *Policy problem*: What should be done with the results?
4. *Organization problem*: What is the organization culture? How do managers and supervisors work?

See Activity Discussion 7 at the end of this chapter.

Summary

Evaluations take much time, require concentration, have legal ramifications if handled incorrectly, can cause anxieties among employees, and rarely produce immediate effective responses. Managers often ask, "Why should I bother?" Mandatory reasons come from regulatory agencies. More importantly, human resources still make up the biggest component of the management pie (see Fig. 11–2). Although advancing technologies may replace personnel performing routine tasks in the laboratory, knowledgeable, caring personnel provide the applications and resolutions to problems. Jacobs touts managers who identify "emerging management expectations to help employees develop job knowledge and skills."[16]

> What gets measured, gets done.—Mason Haire

Evaluation is an appropriate method to determine how and what a person or activity does in comparison to predetermined standards. Analysis and interpretation of data ascertain whether or not the behavior of a person, the activity itself, or the results of services meet or exceed the minimal level of the standards. Evaluation concludes the process after objectives and expected outcomes to be achieved are set. The process encompasses utilization of task analysis, job descriptions, performance standards, and dates for periodic or annual review. Developing and selecting appropriate tools for the designated type of evaluation are part of the duties of the evaluator. Functions of evaluation include *feedback, modification or change,* and *establishing future* activities and criteria. Assessments must be conducted objectively in order to eliminate bias and produce constructive conclusions. The role the evaluator plays is significant to the success of the total process. Feedback can be praise or criticism but always should include positive comments. Manager and employee should agree on the steps leading to effective behavior. All employees' performance appraisals deserve to be reviewed by laboratory administrators because this provides a real benefit to overall improvement of the operation.

Health care reforms dictate new paradigms for managers. They must meet many challenges. First is identifying new performances and expectations in terms of knowledge, skills, abilities, and attributes (KSAAs). Next is creating new definitions in standard and measurable formats. Managers may have to quickly recast these definitions when they become inadequate. Managers will have to consider how to recognize and reward. Another challenge is determining how employees' beliefs and value systems will motivate them in the new and changing workplace. Last is figuring out when this has been achieved.

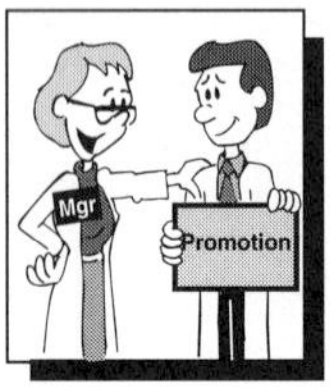

Activity Discussion 1: Performance Standards (PS) and Weights (WT) for Major Job Responsibilities (MJR) (Refer to Activity 3 for MJR statements.)

***MJR #1* WT = 20**

PS 1. Produces accurate results with three or fewer errors per year.

PS 2. Comprehends and performs duties independently with little or no direct supervision.

PS 3. Demonstrates ability to act and/or follows through (when appropriate) in situations not covered by written or verbal instructions.

***MJR #2* WT = 15**

PS 1. Verifies questionable/abnormal/flagged results by repeat testing according to standards of practice (SOP) and written policies of the laboratory. Makes no more than six errors per year.

PS 2. Relates critical (panic) laboratory reportable results to appropriate nurse/physician, documenting these communications every time.

PS 3. Notifies team leader, supervisor, and/or pathologist/director of exceptional or abnormal results according to established criteria. Secures additional patient information when necessary.

***MJR #3* WT = 15**

PS 1. Prepares and determines validity of solutions, reagents, and stains; notifies team leader or supervisor when supplies and materials are low. When authorized, can order inventory items in appropriate quantity and quality.

PS 2. Makes sound judgments and interpretations based on test results. Recognizes discrepancies. Attempts to resolve discrepancies according to training and SOP.

PS 3. Performs required QC procedures on equipment and reagents according to SOP; accepts any discrepancies into use only when appropriate criteria are met.

PS 4. Notifies team leader and/or supervisor of discrepant results, problems with QC, or malfunctioning equipment. Completes Corrective Action forms as necessary with no more than three instances of omission per year.

***MJR #4* WT = 15**

PS 1. Performs daily and preventive maintenance on instruments according to schedule; documents findings with rare exceptions.

PS 2. Troubleshoots whenever possible; calls service when necessary.

***MJR #5* WT = 10**

PS 1. Demonstrates effective communication skills by conveying information accurately, being polite, using appropriate language, and applying active listening skills to interpret communication correctly.

PS 2. Promotes hospitality by acting in a friendly, courteous, and professional manner with all hospital personnel, patients, and visitors.

PS 3. Responds to new ideas and changing environment.

***MJR #6* WT = 10**

PS 1. Habitually completes testing within the established turnaround times.

PS 2. Utilizes free time to the advantage of the laboratory section and department. Consults team leader and/or supervisor for additional assignments.

PS 3. Able to perform several tasks simultaneously during peak workload situations.

PS 4. Able to prioritize and reorganize workload in response to STAT requests according to SOP.

***MJR #7* WT = 5**

PS 1. Trains new employees, students, residents and/or peers. Uses appropriate educational practices for training and evaluating behavior and performance.

***MJR #8* WT = 10**

PS 1. Assumes responsibility for own competency assessment and continuing medical laboratory education (CMLE) by attaining required yearly contact hours and keeping records up to date. Participates in laboratory section, department, and hospital assigned competency assessment and continuing education activities.

PS 2. Accepts and completes other tasks and special projects as assigned. Reports to team leader and/or supervisor regularly of ongoing project status.

Activity Discussion 2: Advantages and Disadvantages of Two Measurement Tools for Competence Assessment

1. Repeat testing of proficiency testing materials; equivalent to unknown or real activity.

Advantages:	Can compare with survey results
	Explanations provided
	If unacceptable, can review with supervisor
Disadvantages:	Specimen may be insufficient for more than one person to analyze
	Lack of immediate answers, that is, survey reports

2. Direct observation of technical personnel performing ____________ test.

Advantages:	Explanations provided immediately after performance
	If error, can review with supervisor
	Verified protocol followed
	Can assess compliance with changed protocol
	Can validate consistency among personnel in performing procedure
	Evaluators can be persons other than supervisor who are trained
Disadvantages:	Time consuming
	Requires high-level objectivity by evaluator

Activity Discussion 3: Answers to Table 19–8

	Laboratory A	Laboratory B	Laboratory C
a. billable tests / FTE	*894*	*645*	*612*
b. billable tests / technical FTE	*1417*	*1140*	*947*
c. technical FTEs / total FTEs	*0.60*	*0.57*	*0.65*
d. worked hours / paid hours	*0.88*	*0.91*	*0.91*
e. billable tests / paid hour	*4.05*	*3.86*	*2.89*

Activity Discussion 4: Other Laboratory Productivity Ratios

1. Ratio of tests per FTE per shift
2. Workload versus staffing for each laboratory section
3. Turnaround time (TAT)
4. Number of assays a technologist/technician can do in 30 minutes, 60 minutes, 2 hours, 4 hours

Activity Discussion 5: Value of Productivity Measurements

Managerial changes or improvements that might be considered based on productivity measurements:

1. Change total number of FTEs and/or number of technical FTEs.
2. Schedule personnel—start times, shifts worked, flexible hours.
3. Compare ratios between laboratory sections; look at processes used in the most productive laboratory sections.
4. Change test methodologies.

5. Determine instrument needs.
6. Monitor employee performance.

Activity Discussion 6: Barriers to Top Productivity

EXTRINSIC BARRIERS

1. Physical layout
2. Equipment
3. Supplies
4. Information system (computer—LIS)
5. Interdepartmental rapport
6. Environmental control
7. Parking
8. Staffing and schedules
9. Policies
10. Interruptions
11. Workload

INTRINSIC BARRIERS

1. Lack of motivation
2. Norm of convergence and conformity (individuals work at lowest average level of group; peer pressure to work at same level of productivity)
3. Lack of empowerment (authority)
4. Emphasis on output standards and bottom line rather than process
5. Lack of ownership in activity
6. Self-esteem of individuals
7. Responsibility not assigned to/taken by employees
8. Competence to perform procedures

Activity Discussion 7: Evaluation Process Problems, Symptoms, and Possible Solutions *(continued on next page)*

Measurement Problem: What should be evaluated?	**Decision Problem:** Appraising behavior and performance, or activity	**Policy Problem:** What should be done with the results?	**Organization Problem:** What is the organization culture? How do managers and supervisors work?
Symptoms: Uncertainty about roles and responsibilities of each job. Work behavior and job performance are difficult to quantify. Lack of clear statements of objectives for organization and departments. Data consist only of numbers; no documentation or descriptions.	**Symptoms:** Lack of written standards: competencies and criteria. Lack of agreement on ratings or scores. Manager or director changes data: ratings or scores. Evidence of bias, discrimination. Lack of fair appeals and grievance process.	**Symptoms:** Managers and supervisors who conduct and analyze evaluations thoroughly and appropriately are treated the same as those who do not. Employees, regardless of evaluation, stay on their jobs, receive raises, and some are even promoted. Activities producing less than desired outcomes continue with no change.	**Symptoms:** Evaluation forms and reports are not completed or lack documentation. Time not allocated for managers and supervisors to perform evaluations. Employees perceive evaluation of their work and environment as something managers do to keep busy. Required without value addressed. New process every year.

Possible Solutions:	Possible Solutions:	Possible Solutions:	Possible Solutions:
Managers and employees together: write objectives for organization and department and promote them. Develop job descriptions with major job responsibilities and duties. Written outcomes identified for each (work) activity. Train managers to document assessments without bias.	Managers and employees together: write performance standards with observable, behaviorally based criteria. Performance documented and outcome data collected over time. Communicate clearly performance and outcomes expectations. Train evaluators and include practice.	Management institutes internal and external evaluation: customer satisfaction surveys; self-assessments; employees of bosses. Regular and consistent application of evaluation policies. Institute performance-contingent reward system.	Impose requirements with time allocation of evaluation activities of all managers. Promote collaborative efforts between managers and employees. Communicate value and changes based on evaluations. Improve, not change, evaluation process as needed.

Review Questions

1. One of the primary reasons to evaluate employees is to
   a. Reduce salaries.
   b. Improve their performance.
   c. Reassign tasks.
   d. Determine who needs retraining.
   e. Fulfill management obligation.
2. Describe the relationship between job descriptions, major job responsibilities, and performance standards. Explain how each would be best used for personnel employed in a clinical laboratory.
3. For each of the following measurement tools, identify the corresponding domain and taxonomy level
   a. Written exam.
   b. Case studies.
   c. Interviews.
   d. Demonstrations.
   e. Checklists.
4. In Table 19–6, general behaviors and tasks for competence assessment and performance appraisal are listed. Select two items: one general *behavior,* and one *laboratory task.* For each item, write a brief statement or question that could be used to determine competence.
5. Using the questions and rating scale developed in Activity 19–7, Rate the Boss, interview three people: a senior in college/university who has (any) supervisory experience, one of the clinical instructors in a laboratory science program, and someone who has been a supervisor, manager, administrator, professor, or company owner for at least five years. Tabulate the ratings for each group of people. Review their comments. Are there any significant differences in the ratings between the groups? Are there any similarities between the groups regarding their comments?

See p. 412 for answers.

References

1. Health and Human Services. Clinical Laboratory Improvement Amendments of 1988, Federal Register, 42 CFR, February 28, 1992. Part II, 493–1495, p 7183.
2. O'Leary DS. The measurement mandate: Report card day is coming. Clinical Laboratory Management Review 1994; 8(1): 84, 74–81.
3. Thorndike RL, Hagan E. Measurement and Evaluation in Psychology and Education. 3rd ed. New York, John Wiley & Sons, 1967, pp 9–16.
4. Troyer ME. Accuracy and Validity in Evaluation Are Not Enough. The J.R. Street Lecture for 1947. Syracuse, Syracuse University Press, 1947.
5. Downie NM. Fundamentals of Measurement: Techniques and Practices. 2nd ed. New York, Oxford University Press, 1967, pp 4–14.
6. Mountain P. Automation solutions: What to look for and what to avoid. Clinical Laboratory Management Review 1996; 10(6): 637–644.
7. NCCLS Training Verification for Laboratory Personnel; Approved Guideline GP21-A, NCCLS, December 1995; 15: 9–10, 38–39.
8. Nevalainen DE, Berte LM. Training, Verification and Assessment: Keys to Quality Management. Malvern, Penn, Clinical Laboratory Management Association, 1993.
9. Eccles RG. The performance measurement manifesto. Harvard Business Review 1991; 69(1): 131–137.
10. Nolan RL, Hammer M, Paul N, et al. Letters re The performance measurement manifesto. Harvard Business Review 1991; 69(2): 194–204.
11. Haynes ME. A system for managing performance: Improve both the performance and the productivity of your staff. Clinical Laboratory Management Review 1987; 1(3): 125–132.
12. Procopio N, Ramirez NF, Mattson JC. Major job duties and responsibilities, performance standards, and weights for medical technologists performance appraisals in the Hematology laboratory section, Department of Clinical Pathology. William Beaumont Hospital, Royal Oak, Mich, 1996.
13. Schaffer RH. Demand better results—and get them. Harvard Business Review 1991; 69(2): 142–149.
14. Umiker WO. Performance standards make evaluations almost easy. Medical Laboratory Observer 1979; 11(8): 63–74.
15. Poe G. Quote in Educational Technology 1975; 15(1): 19–25.
16. Jacobs RL. Improving performance through an organization culture of employee expertise. Clinical Laboratory Management Review 1996; 10(6): 307–617.
17. Dessler G. Personnel Management. 3rd ed. Reston, Vir, Reston Publishing Co., Inc., 1984, pp 461–470.
18. Kuzmits FE, Herden RP, Sussman L. Effective Performance Evaluations. Homewood, Ill, Dow Jones-Irwin, 1984, pp 7–25.
19. Goodale JG. Six steps to improve discussions of employee performance. Clinical Laboratory Management Review 1995; 9(1): 7–14.
20. Pacetta F with Gittines R. Don't Fire Them, Fire Them Up. New York, Simon & Schuster, 1994, pp 112–113.
21. Bushardt SC, Jenkins JM, Cumbest PB. Less odious performance appraisals. *In* Petrini C, ed. Training 101. Training and Development Journal 1993; 47(10): 29–33.
22. Harmon S. Receiving criticism with confidence. Handling criticism: Part II. Medical Laboratory Observer 1991; 23(4): 56–59.
23. Rider EA, Longmaid HE. Feedback in clinical medical education: Guidelines for learners on receiving feedback. Journal of the American Medical Association 1995; 274(12): 20.
24. Pawlak J. Get ready for a pop quiz before you take the job. Detroit Free Press, 1995; November 20: 9F.
25. Myers IB, McCaulley MH. A Guide to the Development and Use of the Myers-Briggs Type Indicator. Palo Alto, Calif, Consulting Psychologists Press Inc., 1995.
26. Harrington-Mackin D. The Team Building Tool Kit. New York, AMACOM, 1994, pp 120–126.
27. Jackman M with Waggoner S. Star Teams, Key Players. New York, Fawcett Crest, 1991, pp 59–60.
28. Hoffman R. Ten reasons you should be using 360-degree feedback. Human Resource Magazine 1995; 40(4): 82–85.
29. Weisinger HD. Productive criticism Part 2: A new environment for criticism. Clinical Laboratory Management Review 1996; 10(1): 27–34.
30. Martin BG, Morris MW. Measuring performance and promotability of middle managers. Medical Laboratory Observer 1991; 23(9): 38–41.
31. Rosales JL. How to design method evaluations for laboratory tests and instruments. Tech Sample®. Management and Education MGM-2. Chicago, ASCP, 1996.
32. Smith EA. The Productivity Manual. Houston, Gulf Publishing Co., 1990.
33. Despeignes P. Productivity up 2.2% in 4th QTR, but long-term trend still weak. Investor's Business Daily February 12, 1997, p B1.
34. Sodeman TM. Your lab's productivity. CAP Today. 1993; 7(6): 24–36.
35. Castañeda-Méndez K. Statistician suggests LMIP improvements. Advance/Laboratory 1996; 8(17): 4.
36. Zinn J, Getzen T. Developing key laboratory performance indicators: A feasibility study. Clinical Laboratory Management Review 1995; 9(3): 178–197.

37. Wong ET. Improving laboratory testing: Can we get physicians to focus on outcome? Clinical Chemistry 1995; 41(8B): 1241–1247.
38. Jones H. A method for developing outcome measures in the clinical laboratory. Clinical Laboratory Management Review 1996; 10(2): 115–119.
39. Hammond HC. Applying the value-of-information paradigm to laboratory management. Clinical Laboratory Management Review 1996; 10(2): 95–106.
40. Winkelman JW, Mennemeyer ST. Using patient outcomes to screen for clinical laboratory errors. Clinical Laboratory Management Review 1996; 10(2): 134–142.
41. Mittman BS, Hilborne LH. Applying practice guidelines, outcomes, research, and research recommendations. Check Sample®. Laboratory Practice Management No. LMP 95-4. Chicago, ASCP, 1995.
42. Jackson JA. Extending the concept of outcome-based medicine. An overview of the 14th International Conference on Human Functioning. American Laboratory 1995; 14(10): 6.
43. Spath PL, ed. Clinical Paths: Tools for Outcome Management. Chicago, American Hospital Publishing, 1995, pp 31–45.
44. Bissell MG. Defining laboratory-related outcomes measures—establishing a link to patient-focused care. Editorial. Clinical Laboratory Management Review 1996; 10(2): 95–97.
45. Cousteau V. Translated by Johns RJ. How to swim with sharks: A primer. Perspectives in Biology and Medicine 1973; Summer: 525–528.
46. Umiker WO. Coping with Difficult People in the Health Care Setting. Chicago, ASCP Press, 1994.
47. Lussier RN. Increasing performance through counseling and discipline: Models for dealing with problem employees. Clinical Laboratory Management Review 1993; 7(2): 112–118.
48. Kuzmits FE, Herden RP, Sussman L. Improving Supervisor Productivity through Managing the Unsatisfactory Employee. Homewood, Ill, Dow Jones-Irwin, 1984.
49. Gill SL. How to cope with difficult people. Clinical Laboratory Management Review 1988; 3(4): 208–212.
50. Fred Pryor Seminars. "How to handle difficult people." Shawnee Mission, Kan, Pryor Resources Inc., 1995.
51. Scheele A. Why it doesn't matter if your boss doesn't like you. Working Woman. 1992; 18(10): 34–37.
52. Palmer C. Little things in the workplace can trigger office rage. The Detroit News, July 20, 1996, p 1C.
53. Klosinski DD. Positive interaction with problem people. In Common Sense Supervision workshop. ASCP Workshop Week, Boston, 1990.
54. Synder JR. Assessing the legality of performance appraisals. Clinical Laboratory Management Review 1991; 5(6): 483–489.
55. Klosinski DD, Collins SL. We do good work, don't we? Document it! Competence assessment workshop. American Association for Clinical Chemistry Annual Meeting, Chicago, 1996.

Suggested Reading

1. Berte LM. Developing Performance Standards for Hospital Personnel. Chicago, ASCP Press, 1989.
2. Livingston JS. Pygmalion in Management. A manager's expectations are the key to subordinates' performance and development. Harvard Business Review 1988; 66(5): 121–129.
3. Praestgaard A, Rankenburg J. Laboratory management index program. Advance/Laboratory 1996; 8(14): 10–13.

Competence Assessment

4. Baer DM, Ellinger P. Q&A: Should competency tests be used punitively? Laboratory Medicine 1996; 27(6): 370.
5. Ehrmeyer SS, Laessig RH. Bedside: Teaching competency at the point of care. Advance/Laboratory 1996; 5(2): 16–21.
6. Jobe M. Competency testing as a management tool in today's lab. Laboratory Medicine 1991; 22(8): 523–524.
7. Martin S, McClure K. Competency testing in the hematology laboratory. ASCP Teleconference. November 21, 1996.
8. McCaskey L, LaRocco M. Competency testing in clinical microbiology. Laboratory Medicine 1995; 26(5): 343–349.

Performance Appraisals

9. Henerson ME, Morris LL, Fitz-Gibbons CT. How to Measure Attitudes. Newbury Park, Calif, Sage, 1987.
10. Martin BG. The continuing search for solutions: Maximizing human resources. Clinical Laboratory Management Review 1991; 5(6): 507–509.
11. Performance Appraisals: The Latest Legal Nightmare. Alexander Hamilton Institute, Inc. (Modern Business Reports, 197 W. Spring Valley Ave., Maywood, NH 07607), 1990.

Outcomes Measures

12. Bernstein LH. Outcomes management: A key factor that can "make or break" a lab. Advance/Laboratory Professionals 1996; 8(23): 18–20.

13. Kaul K, Cohen R, Dranove D, et al. Direct sputum analysis for tuberculosis by polymerase chain reaction vs conventional techniques in a public hospital. In Assessing Clinical Outcomes. AACC/Leadership Series, 1995, pp 3–6.
14. Salmon BC. Is your hospital over-ordering STAT lab tests? A utilization review might work wonders. Advance/Laboratory Professionals 1995; 7(18): 22–23.

Regulatory Agencies

15. Food and Drug Administration (FDA), Docket No. 91N-0450. Quality assurance in blood establishments. U.S. Govt. Printing Office, Washington, DC, pp 9–12.
16. American Association of Blood Banks (AABB), Accreditation Requirements Manual (ARM), 4th ed. Fall, Bethesda, 1993. 2.000 Quality assurance and quality control. pp 10–11.

APPENDIX 19–A

Regulatory Agencies' Evaluation and Competence Assessment Requirements
(Selected portions only)

I. State Operations Manual (SOM), Survey Procedures and Interpretative Guidelines for Laboratories and Laboratories Services, *Appendix C*, Revision 256.

493.1451 Standards: Technical Supervisor responsibilities.

D6120 (8) Evaluating the competency of all testing personnel and ensuring that the staff maintain their competency to perform test procedures and report test results promptly, accurately, and proficiently.

D6121 The procedure for evaluation of the competency of the staff must include:

(i) Direct observation of routine patient test performance, including patient preparation, if applicable, specimen handling, processing, and testing;

D6125 (v) Assessment of test performance through testing previously analyzed specimens, internal blind testing samples of external proficiency testing samples; and

D6126 (vi) Assessment of problem-solving skills; and

D6127 (9) Evaluating and documenting the performance of individuals responsible for high-complexity testing at least semiannually during the first year the individual tests patient specimens.

D6128 Thereafter, evaluation must be performed at least annually.

D6129 Unless test methodology or instrumentation changes, in which case, prior to reporting patient test results, the individual's performance must be reevaluated to include the use of the new test methodology or instrumentation.

II. Accreditation Manual for Pathology and Clinical Laboratory Services (AMPCLS), JCAHO, Oakbrook Terrace, IL, 1996.

PA.1.4.1 Qualifications include current competence in the technical skills and knowledge required for the position;

Intent Evidence that such staff are qualified must emphasize demonstration of current competence which will be assessed by a surveyor at the time of survey. The following are evaluated when assessing current competence for this standard:

Documentation of performance evaluations;

PA.1.4.4 Initial and continuing competence of staff is assessed and maintained:

PA.1.4.4.3 performance reviews for staff . . .

Intent Staff are evaluated for competency in performing required laboratory tasks, as well as for other parameters specified in job descriptions; technical staff will be evaluated by an individual qualified to provide technical judgments regarding their performance. In addition, other staff, including supervisory staff, are evaluated for performance of their job responsibilities, as defined in their job descriptions.

5. Test performance assessment as defined by laboratory policy. Examples of ways to evaluate include testing previously analyzed specimens, internal blind testing samples, or external proficiency-testing samples, and
6. Assessment of problem-solving skills, as appropriate to the job being performed.

III. Commission on Laboratory Accreditation Inspection Checklists. College of American Pathologists (CAP). Northfield, IL, 1995.

Hematology Section II. Phase I, Question # 02.1135: Does the hematology laboratory have a defined, documented system to ensure consistency of morphologic observations among all personnel performing blood cell microscopy? Phase I, Question # 02.1450: Does the hematology laboratory have a defined, documented system to ensure consistency of morphologic observations among all personnel performing body fluid cell differentials? Transfusion Medicine Section V. Phase I, Question # 05.0320: Is there a mechanism for monitoring adherence to policies and procedures in the laboratory and throughout the transfusion process and are the results reviewed by the medical director?

20

Management Synopsis and Synergy

OBJECTIVES

Upon completion of this chapter, the reader should be able to:

- Summarize management in terms of its roots and rationale as a process.
- Identify potential new roles and new work for laboratorians associated with the six functions of management.
- Describe the effects of change on laboratory management and explain at least two strategies associated with change.
- Compare and contrast knowledge, skills, and behaviors previously needed by leaders and managers in laboratories and health care organizations to those projected to be needed in the 21st century.

KEY WORDS

management synopsis
management synergy
future roles
new work
benchmarking
empowerment

Introduction

In the previous nine chapters, readers were introduced to basic management concepts and information. Opportunities for practice (labeled "Activity") representing a variety of managerial skills were also included. Development of appropriate attitudes (by readers of this text as well as people in the laboratory workforce, regardless of their roles) ranks as the authors' greatest concern of the three domains (Knowledge/Cognitive, Psychomotor/Skill, and Affective/Behavior). We ask, "Have you, as one of our readers, become convinced that accomplishing management functions requires more than knowledge and skill? Are you interested in developing effective managerial values and attributes for yourself and in helping others do the same?"

In this chapter, a *synopsis* written as brief summaries is presented. Readers will be encouraged to identify and relate to the forces coming together in *synergy* as they decide whether supervision and management should become the goal of their career path.

A Synopsis of Management

Management should be considered an *improvement process*, a process by which improvement of one's self and work occurs through skill development, knowledge acquisition, and growth in awareness, appreciation, and valuing of people, surroundings, and environments. This process of development, when it takes place in thriving operation environments, almost always guarantees improved products, activities, and outcomes.

A retrospective look at the emergence of management will enable readers to better understand what might be expected of them as future managers and supervisors. The maxim is, "History repeats itself." Management as it is known today was created by a British statesman, Sir Stafford Cripps. He conceived it as a "force" to restore Britain's economy and help in solving his nation's tremendous problems after World War II. He believed that the concerns to be dealt with involved (1) organization of work for mass production, (2) leadership of workers toward productivity and achievement, (3) responsibility for the social impact of management, and (4) obligation for producing results.

Similar issues exist today in health care management for owners and employees, leaders of the country, and customers. These issues focus specifically on rising costs of health care, national health insurance, National Labor Relations Board (NLRB) decisions regarding the workforce (especially concerning union membership), Health Maintenance Organizations (HMO) and Managed Care Organizations (MCO), third party payers, privatization (for profit) and consolidation of hospitals and health care entities, Occupational Health and Safety Act (OHSA) and other regulations, and liability. No one person can master the responses these challenges mandate. Only with people working in teams—delegating and sharing authority and responsibility, communicating, and evaluating—will effective resolutions be found and implemented.

Management Functions

New roles and new work for managers and employees continue to develop throughout the health care field. Work and tasks are assigned differently as

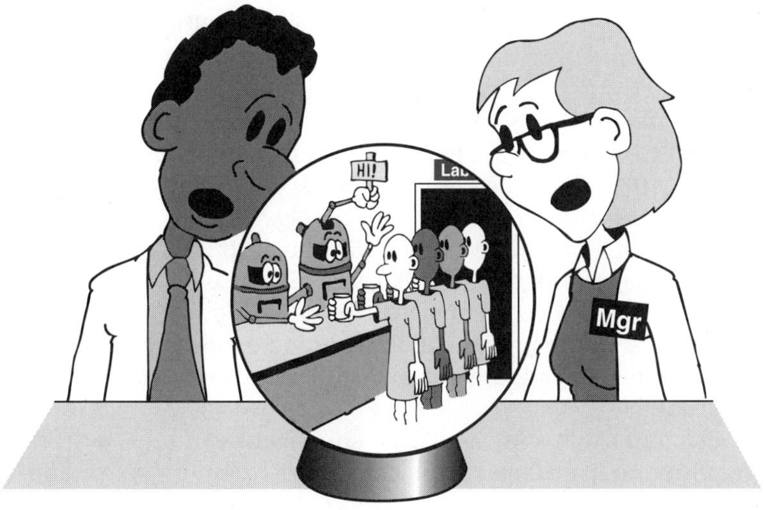

education and training needs of employees are reassessed with system changes due to automation, robotics, and reengineering. Academic and clinical training programs struggle to determine and implement courses to fulfill these changing needs. Together, educators and managers quickly assemble their ideas and schemes in order for graduates and new employees to be prepared for revamped laboratory settings.

Activity 1: New Roles and New Work for Laboratory Managers

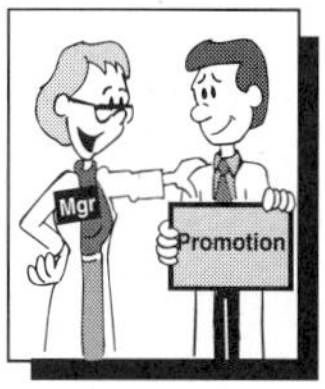

In Table 20–1, management topics from several sources are listed.[1–3] Describe each topic according to how you perceive its application and importance. Discuss how each topic might be incorporated into a structure curriculum or outlined as a self-study program.

EMPOWERMENT

The concept of empowering employees received rave reviews at the onset of this management strategy. More responsibility and freedom were delegated

Table 20–1
MANAGEMENT TOPICS* FOR LABORATORIANS

Knowledge of mission, vision, and goal statements
Professional commitment
Communication
Information management
Improvement management: people, activities, processes, resources
Quality assurance and regulatory compliance
Evaluation: people, activities, processes, resources
Finance: revenue and expenses
Interdisciplinary team participation
Education and training
Marketing

*Listed in random order.

downward to employees for making decisions, handling difficult situations and customers, and solving problems. This released managers from "micromanaging" and supported their time and energies for creativity and attending to economic needs.

Somehow this management tool seems to have missed its intended target. Kennedy reported conflicts between the work ethics and expectations of the "baby-boomer generation" managers and the "generation X" workers.[4] A few reasons for the failure of empowerment that she described fit into the dilemma of laboratory managers. One reason is that workloads had increased by 25% since 1989; another is that training had been overlooked, with the mandate issued but no rationale or guides included; and a third reason is that while the work structure changed, the associated performance appraisal and reward systems had not.

Kennedy[4] and Atchison[5] advocate empowerment in health care. They offer suggestions that managers can apply: use common sense and not just rules; teach and train in separate "focus" groups each composed only of workers with similar attitudes: the naysayers, the maybes, and the "I am empowered!" people; and address rewards and recognition and performance appraisal systems. Another suggestion is to listen carefully and supportively to employees.

MANAGING CHANGE

Do new paradigms displace old paradigms or do patterns just recycle? Doing the same or new work is no longer sufficient for business to survive and succeed. The theme has become one that promotes doing the work better at less cost. Employees ask managers, "What do you mean when you say 'better'?" To answer this question requires setting objectives with specific criteria or standards, then comparing the results to the standards. Improving care has become the major theme in medicine. Much activity and many meetings occur in efforts to resolve this ongoing dilemma.

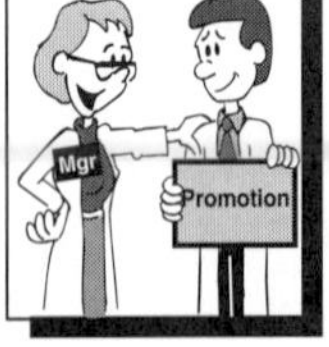

Activity 2: The Dilemma of Resolving Health Care Issues in the 21st Century

From the following list of topics (or any of interest to you), select one and research two to four articles about it for class or session discussion. Focus discussions on the roles laboratorians will be asked to play or should proactively pursue in improving the quality of care these patients will need. Create a list of skills for managing and training future laboratorians to fulfill these roles.

1. Medical care of the elderly[6, 7]
2. Infectious disease: tuberculosis, hepatitis, AIDS, cytomegalovirus (CMV)[7, 8]
3. Genetic disease: cystic fibrosis, sickle cell anemia, muscular dystrophy
4. Chronic disease: diabetes, depression, heart disease, arthritis
5. Drugs: for therapy, of abuse[9]

Trends and Innovations

New technology? New tests? New diseases or conditions? New resources? New reimbursement rules? Trends build and mold business and jobs. Uncertainty about future needs and services is a crucial issue in all medical disciplines. Expectations remain that *more* is not necessarily better but *new* and improved is essential. Like the education process, management cannot determine where it should go unless it determines where it is.

Several strategies enable managers to determine the factors impacting on organizational operations. Benchmarking and needs assessment (discussed under Marketing Services) provide information to guide decisions about which services to offer. Marketing "sells" those services to customers.

BENCHMARKING

BENCHMARKING
Benchmarking is defined as the measurement of one's own product or services against specific standards for comparison and improvement.

By its definition, benchmarking fits a niche that laboratory managers and technical people find comfortable in which to work. Most uses have involved internal comparison between laboratory sections for staffing, cost savings, and reducing errors. Occasionally, internal comparisons have been made between the laboratory and other departments in the same organization. Hilborne cites a benchmarking example of blood (ordered and) transfused into patients in orthopedics if their hematocrit results fell to 27% and obstetrics patients, who did not receive blood until their hematocrits were less than 25%.[10] Closely studying this example generates questions regarding what is the acceptable standard, what justifies maintaining different criteria (levels), and how can costs be reduced and quality be improved without making changes in policies (including criteria and standards). More aggressive studies are being conducted within organizations to establish standards that deliver consistent quality patient care with savings of time, supplies, and money across several departments.[11]

External benchmarking, well established in business since 1979, addresses comparisons with either companies of similar interests or competitors.[12] Studying work processes and products of highly successful companies can be helpful to improve similar activities in health care organizations because business acumen and savvy are also necessary in the health care field.

Several benchmarking processes exist. The most successful reported have been from Xerox and Motorola. Using a similar approach, the College of American Pathologists developed the Q-Probes program.[13] Benchmarking closely resembles basic evaluation processes.

Accepting the value of benchmarking to compare and improve is one method of reevaluating and reestablishing standards. Proponents of personal goal setting don't rely on the standards of others to determine their goals—they want to be *number one* and will work with, coach, push, pull, drag, and carry anyone who wants to be *number one* with them.[14–16] They want you to do what you think is right for you and do it rather than questioning what is happening down the street and then doing what others are doing. This puts you behind before you've started. Authors Hilborne[10] and Schifman[11] list excellent references for further study of benchmarking.

OUTCOMES MANAGEMENT

Readers should apply the knowledge they've learned in previous chapters in creating their own titles (terms) for and descriptions of quality improvement processes. Personalization fosters ownership in a concept or activity. Think about continuous improvement processes or total quality management as a "persistent improvement penta-points system" (PIPPS); see Figure 20–1.[17]

Some methods are complex, such as clinical pathways and continuous quality improvement (CQI) teams, which review major activities and resources, especially if high costs are involved. Others can be relatively easy and within the purview of laboratory management to investigate. Examples are redesigning of laboratory test order forms or (computer) menus; restructuring or eliminating panels of tests, such as an electrolyte panel changed to a cardiology panel; and developing algorithms or reflexive testing, which assist physicians in selecting the next test(s) to order.[1]

Clinical pathways have been created to improve patient care. They are a set of sequenced required interventions to support a positive outcome.[17, 18]

Clinical pathways should be monitored continuously for:

- effectiveness–whether a particular job is done or objective is achieved.
- efficiency–incorporates process, personnel, and cost required to accomplish the task.[17]

MARKETING SERVICES

The positive meaning of marketing infers promotion of one's best assets, including value to customers. Planning this new activity is sometimes difficult for laboratorians. They must step away from their testing workstations and tasks and think about "selling" themselves and their work. Fortunately, those who tackle this assignment find their analytical skills valuable.

Marketing begins with an assessment of the customers' needs. Needs assessment questionnaires or surveys can be basic if they are straightforward, thorough, and clearly stated. Once the needs assessment information has been collected, it should be categorized and analyzed. This means matching current

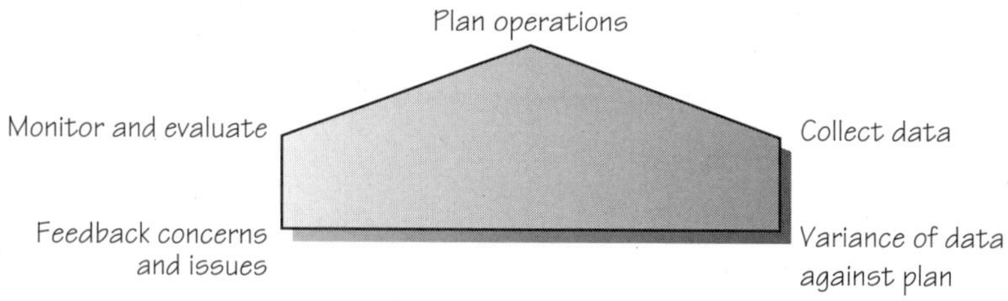

Figure 20–1 Persistent improvement penta-point system (PIPPS). (Data from Cordell JL: Laboratory cost management and clinical pathway development. Workshop at the ASCLS Annual Meeting, Anaheim, Calif, 1995.)

Table 20–2
FIVE COMPLAINTS AND PROBLEMS FROM PHYSICIANS

Lack of timely information and results.
Absence of coordinated and completed follow-through.
Results are not accessible by the right physician at the right place.
Results are not specific or suitable for purpose.
Report is not comprehensible.

Adapted from Riggs L, Winsten D. How to improve your image with physicians. Clinical Laboratory Management Review 1996; 10(1): 35–39.

services to those needs. Next comes promoting what those services are to be for customers. Managers can secure information from customer feedback about the services, many times by how much the services are used as well as compliments and complaints.[19–21]

COMPLAINTS AND CUSTOMER RELATIONS

Several authors advocate that profitability and survival of laboratories will be based on how well they determine the benefits of their services.[9]

Activity 3: Handling Complaints for Customer Satisfaction

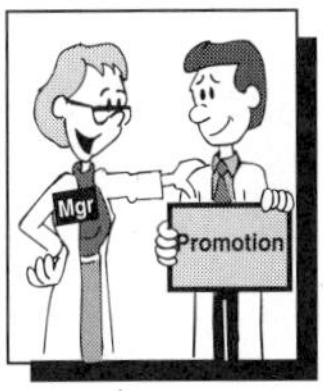

From complaints from physicians listed in Table 20–2,[22] each reader or group should select one and write two descriptions: how the complaint should be handled: the process, by whom, and possible solutions; and how customer satisfaction will be attained. During group discussion, procedures derived by consensus should be developed regarding:

1. how complaints should be handled
2. who the best person(s) is/are to handle the complaint
3. which solutions (at least three) are the most likely to be effective
4. implementation plan(s) and time
5. measurement tools and evaluation methods to determine level of customer satisfaction

See Activity Discussion 1 at the end of this chapter.

Who the Leaders, Managers, and Educators Will Be

"If you are in the business of health care, you have become a change-master, an expert at adapting, reshaping, resizing and repositioning yourself and your organization. You have to be in the right place at the right time with the right services, and now at the right cost." This statement was made by Maggie Morehouse, President of the Michigan Organization of Nurse Executives and

Director of Nursing, Chelsea Community Hospitals, Michigan, in response to the need for programs on patient-focused care.

Review the list of topics in Table 20–1 and the information developed in Activity 1. Complete the following activity.

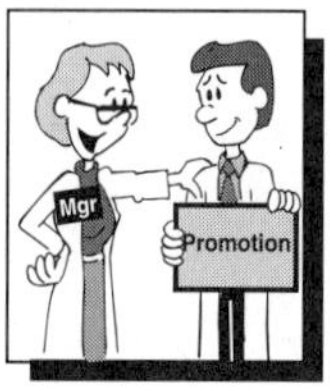

Activity 4: Performance Standards (PS) for Supervisor's Major Job Responsibilities (MJR)

Eight major job responsibilities (MJR) for laboratory supervisors were presented in Appendix 11–A. For each MJR, write one to three (or more) performance standards (PS). Describe each PS as it applies now and discuss how it might be changed as new roles are assigned to laboratory supervisors. See Appendix 11–B.

As you complete the readings and activities presented in these 20 chapters, you should begin to realize that similarities parallel each other for educators and managers. In the disciplines of education and management, leaders are essential but they may not always be in administrative or supervisor roles. In Figure 20–2, a model of the structure and concepts of the knowledge, skills, and attributes for education and management is presented. Very different forces sway a technically and/or scientifically competent laboratorian to become a teacher or a manager.

Summary

The selected topics and explanations presented in this chapter represent only a small part of the subjects, writings, and presentations available in laboratory science literature and resources. Readers are encouraged to continue learning and seeking opportunities to study and contribute their ideas to promote the improvement of laboratories and their management.

The forces in laboratories and health care will come together in *synergy* with effective management and leadership. If you, as a laboratory professional, select supervision and management as the goal of your career path, you will find challenges and opportunities each day.

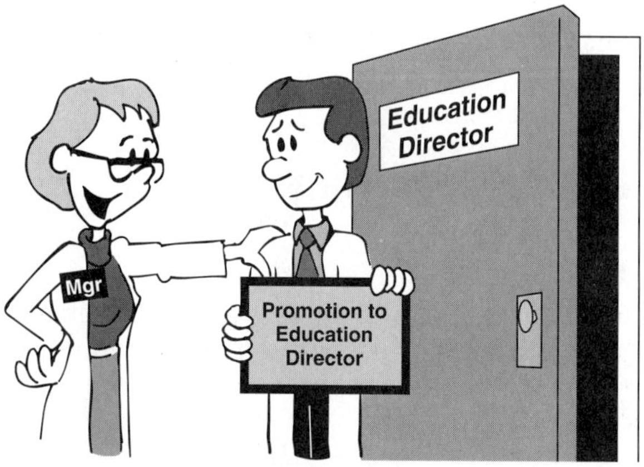

EDUCATION	CONCEPTS	MANAGEMENT
TEACHING		SUPERVISING
	Functions	
Planning		Planning
Organizing		Organizing
Instructing		Directing
Active teaching (Controlling and Coordinating)		Controlling
Testing		Coordinating
Evaluating		Evaluating
	Skills	
Communicating		Communicating
Motivating		Motivating
Selecting, retraining, dismissing		Hiring, firing
	Attributes	
Common sense		Common sense
Analytical thinking		Analytical thinking
Interpersonal skills		Interpersonal skills
• students		employees •
• other teachers		other managers •
• administrators		bosses •
Handling difficult students		Handling difficult employees
Conflict supervision		Conflict management
	Topics of concern	
Policies, regulations	Legal	Regulations
Program, operations	Accreditation	Activities, operations
Students and faculty	Confidentiality	Patients and employees
	Ethics	
	Finance	
	Outcome assessment	
Program, graduates		Services, employees
	Professional	
Students, graduates		Managers, employees

Figure 20–2 Model comparing education and management topics.

Activity 5

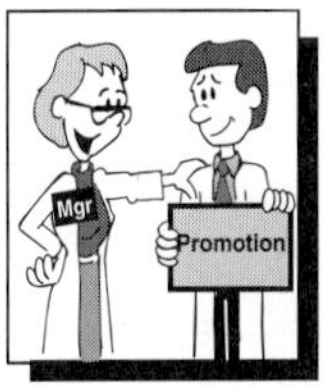

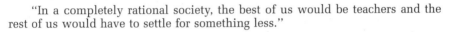

The following quotes are provided to be transcribed and posted periodically to inspire you and your colleagues as you pursue your dreams and ambitions. (NOTE: Please remember to acknowledge the source of any quotes posted.)

"In a completely rational society, the best of us would be teachers and the rest of us would have to settle for something less."

—Lee Iacocca, Chairman and CEO, Chrysler Corporation, 1993

"Superb execution and performance naturally come to visionary companies not so much as an end goal, but as the residual result of a never-ending cycle of self-stimulated improvement and investment for the future."

—James C. Collins and Jerry I. Porras. Built to Last: Successful Habits of Visionary Companies. New York, Harper Business, 1994

"The phantasmagoria of health care: Can you reform an oxymoron?"

—Frederick I. Scott, Jr., Editor's page, American Laboratory 1993; May:6.

"Scientific leadership requires both financial resources and the personal confidence to lead." (paraphrased)

—Robert L. Stevenson, Technology and trade: The Japanese way. American Laboratory 1996; December:4.

"Great management is about character, not technique."

"Managing is not a series of mechanical tasks but a set of human interactions."

"Integrity in management means being responsible, communicating clearly, keeping promises, knowing oneself."

"Great managers serve two masters: one organizational, one moral."

—Thomas Teal, The human side of management. Harvard Business Review 1996; 74(6):35–44.

Activity Discussion 1: Handling Complaints for Customer Satisfaction

Only brief suggestions are provided here.

Timely information and results: Make every attempt to adhere to established turnaround times designated as appropriate for tests that are offered on a STAT, Urgent, and Routine basis.

Coordinated and complete with continuity: Development of electronic data handling systems, such as Community Health Information Networks (CHIN), to provide sequential, combined, and correlated patient laboratory data throughout patients' medical care regardless of site of care. Provide safeguarded access and confidentiality.

Accessible by the right physician at the right place at the right time: Previously, results were usually sent to the location from which the orders were placed; now the patient or physician or assigned health care giver may no longer be at this site. With HMOs and MCOs, the family practice physician initiating laboratory test orders may have referred the patient to a specialist who is the one who needs the results when seeing the patient, now at a new location. Providing assistance and training to physicians in obtaining information from information systems has become a new responsibility for laboratorians. Another factor to consider may come from the physicians themselves; it is related to how they will indicate where and when (and to whom) a patient's results should be sent.

Specific or suitable for purpose: Information may be used in different ways by different physicians, i.e., to surgeon from internist. Flexible information formats or the ability to modify presentation of information may be highly desired by physician groups as customers of the laboratory.

Comprehensive: Lengthy, detailed, irrelevant information often accompanies laboratory test results. Reports can be designed that contain succinct, essential, and most recent information first, and supportive, explanatory, and additional information if needed. Physicians develop preferences, analytical and critical thinking processes, and applications based on the type of patient (their customers who are also the laboratory's) in their care.

Review Questions

1. Five complaints have been identified that concern physicians and their opinions of laboratory services. Of the following, which one would be the easiest for a laboratory manager to resolve?
   a. Use of laboratory language instead of medical terminology.
   b. Test results sent to the primary care physician's office rather than the necessary site.
   c. Test results not produced within specific time limits.
   d. Purpose of orders not met.
   e. Test information not understandable.
2. The management boom in Britain was created to
   a. end World War II.
   b. increase the number of employees who wanted to become managers.
   c. make citizens aware of safety hazards in the workplace.
   d. develop effective methods for mass production.
   e. assign the responsibility for results to employees.
3. Describe the impact and influence that the following issues are expected to have on managerial roles and responsibilities in the future.
   a. Reimbursement
   b. Reengineering
   c. Regulations
   d. New technology related to tests
   e. New technology related to procedures (automation)
   f. New (generation of) employees
4. Define the following terms/acronym.
   a. Synergy
   b. Empowerment
   c. CHIN
   d. Benchmarking
   e. Marketing

See p. 412 for answers.

References

1. Pomerantz P, LoSciuto L. Results of Clinical Laboratory Management Association's industry trends survey. Clinical Laboratory Management Review 1996; 10(6): 597–605.
2. Health care is changing: are you? ASCP Course presented November 1–3, 1996, Rosemont, Ill.
3. McDonald JM, Smith JA. Value-added laboratory medicine in an era of managed care. Clinical Chemistry 1995; 41(8B): 1256–1262.
4. Kennedy MM. Empowered or overpowered? Clinical Laboratory Management Review 1995; 9(2): 152, 149–151.
5. Atchison TA. Turning Health Care Leadership Around. San Francisco, Calif, Jossey-Bass Publishers, 1991, pp 130–135.
6. Klosinski DD. Collecting specimens from the elderly patient. Laboratory Medicine 1997; 28(8): 518–522.
7. Hook WC. Gastrointestinal bacteria. Advance for Administrators of the Laboratory 1995; 4(8): 43–49.
8. Guisti D. Emerging infectious diseases. Advance for Administrators of the Laboratory 1996; 5(7): 80–83.
9. Brzezicki LA. Drug abuse on the rise. Advance for Administrators of the Laboratory 1996; 5(7): 49–57.
10. Hilborne LH. Benchmarking. Check Sample®. Laboratory Practice and Management No. LPM 96–1. Chicago, ASCP, 1996.
11. Schifman RB. Utilization of external databases for benchmarking and quality management in medical microbiology. ASCP Teleconference. November 12, 1996.
12. Kelly LA, Street BS. Seeking improvements through laboratory benchmarking. Clinical Laboratory Management Review 1996; 10(3): 244–251.

13. Q-Probes program. College of American Pathologists, Northfield, Ill, 1995.
14. Pacetta F, with Gittines R. Don't fire them, fire them up. New York, Simon & Schuster, 1994, pp 21–37.
15. Cook J. From lab administrator to health care administrator. Advance for Administrators of the Laboratory 1995; 4(8): 67–72.
16. Senge PM. The Fifth Discipline: The Art and Practice of The Learning Organization. New York, Currency Doubleday, 1990.
17. Cordell JL: Laboratory cost management and clinical pathway development. Workshop at the ASCLS Annual Meeting, Anaheim, Calif, 1995.
18. Nolin CE, McCormack KE. En route to critical paths. Advance for Administrators of the Laboratory 1995; 4(8): 73–76.
19. Ash KO, Weiss RL. Laboratory Management self-study course. Washington, DC: AACC, 1996: 113–129.
20. Varnadoe LA. Medical Laboratory Management and Supervision. Philadelphia, F. A. Davis, 1996, pp 276–285.
21. Brzezicki LA. Microscopes to marketing. Advance for Administrators of the Laboratory 1996; 5(7): 77–79.
22. Riggs L, Winsten D. How to improve your image with physicians. Clinical Laboratory Management Review 1996; 10(1): 35–39.

Suggested Reading

1. Bass BM. Leadership and Performance Beyond Expectations. New York, The Free Press, 1985.
2. Burtis CA. Converging technologies and their impact on the clinical laboratory. Clinical Chemistry 1996; 42(11): 1735–1749.
3. Diplomate in Laboratory Management (DLM) Certification Examination Content Outline. Board of Registry, American Society of Clinical Pathologists, 2100 West Harrison Street, Chicago, Ill 60612–6798 (312) 738–1336, 1995.
4. Evans D, Frantz DK, Ng VL, et al. Cost Containment in the Clinical Laboratory. Denver, A Berkeley Scientific Publication, 1995.
5. Examination Content Outlines for CLS, CLT, and Phlebotomy. National Certification Agency for Medical Laboratory Personnel, Inc. P.O. Box 15945–289 Lenexa, KA, 66285. (913) 438–5110, 1996.
6. Freedman DH. Is management still a science? Harvard Business Review 1992; 70(6): 26–38.
7. Kost GJ. Bedside know-how. Advance for Administrators of the Laboratory 1996; 5(7): 63–68.
8. Kricka LJ. Please do not be alarmed—we are experiencing a paradigm shift. Clinical Laboratory News 1995; 21(7): 26–36.
9. Mintzberg H. The manager's job: folklore and fact. Harvard Business Review 1990; 68(2): 163–176.
10. Reddick WT. Simulation: A complementary method for teaching health services strategic management. Proceedings, SCAMC, Inc. Philadelphia, Hanley and Belfus, 1990: 308, 312.
11. Umiker WO. The Customer-Oriented Laboratory. Chicago, ASCP, 1991.
12. Umiker WO. The Empowered Laboratory Team. Chicago, ASCP, 1996.
13. Waldroop J, Butler T. The executive as coach. Harvard Business Review 1996; 74(6): 111–117.
14. Wilde M. Lab management skills put to the test by Generation Xers. Advance for Medical Laboratory Professionals 1996; 8(21): 10–11, 18.
15. Wingenfeld JR. Developing professional skills for the future of health care. Laboratory Medicine 1995; 26(12): 810–813.

Information Systems

Forrey AW, McDonald CJ, DeMoor G, et al. Logical observation identifier names and codes (LOINC) database: a public use set of codes and names for electronic reporting of clinical laboratory test results. Clinical Chemistry 1996; 42(1): 81–90.

Skjei E. Parsing the puzzle of patient ID. CAP Today 1996; 10(3): 62–64.

Managing Change

Castañeda-Méndez K. Time to change. Advance for Administrators of the Laboratory 1995; 4(8): 20–27.

Harmon S. Strategies for handling imposed changes. Medical Laboratory Observer 1993; 25(9): 60–64.

ANSWERS

Chapter 1

1. The educational process consists of the following steps:
   a. Statement of objectives
   b. Instruction
   c. Testing
   d. Evaluation (Recycle if necessary)

2. Competency-based education (all CLS courses) should reflect this process.

3. An *effective teacher* is one who can inspire learning.

Chapter 2

1. Instructors' responsibility toward students in their classes is to teach the material they will need to function in the workplace. This includes understanding the body of knowledge and acquiring the skills that represent *entrance level* to the clinical site. To achieve this, the instructor must be available to students, and offer opportunities to achieve this goal.

2. The three categories that encompass essential attributes of an instructor are: (1) technical skills (2) teaching (instructional) skills, and (3) personal attributes (qualities).

3. Answers may vary regarding what students think about the instructional preparation of instructor. Most are surprised that instructors/professors do not have to acquire a teaching certificate to teach in a university.

Chapter 3

1. True

2. Activity, conditions, criteria

3. The covert verb *understand* is not observable. Add to the statement, "by drawing a series of illustrations. . . ."

4. (ASCLS-Producing accurate results). After completion of instruction, students will perform automated blood counts with 100% accuracy.

5. (NAACLS-confirming abnormal results). After performing red counts of unknown specimens and calculating one to be abnormal, students will repeat the count and reproduce the result within a 0.5% deviation.

Chapter 4

1. f. Evaluation

2. b. Comprehension

3. a. Knowledge

4. c. Application

5. e. Synthesis

6. b. Comprehension

Chapter 5

1. Demonstration

2. Role play

3. Lecture, CAI

4. Problem-based, instruction, CAI

5. Small group learning

6. Problem-based learning

7. Role play

8. Distance learning

Chapter 6

1. Reliability

2. True

3. 1. d
   2. a
   3. f
   4. e
   5. b

4. Comprehension

5. (Various answers.) Preparing a Review Session should include (1) studying the course syllabus and noting how much time the instructor dedicated to various topics. This relates to the emphasis placed on the subject. (2) Reviewing your hand-out notes and additional notes you took during the lecture together with specific readings designated to be studied from the accompanying text. (3) Plan a test grid and list the topics to be studied on the y axis (vertical) against the Cognitive Level of the subject matter on the x axis (horizontal). Students often ask the instructor for study questions that would assist them in planning a test grid.

Chapter 7

1. d

2. Grades are meant to reflect *academic* achievement (ability), whereas *evaluations* reflect behavior (attitudes).

3. Transcripts of students who have attended some community colleges have been identified as containing "inflated grades." This could result from the student having been taught less difficult material; thus the student has achieved a high grade. At the university level, the difficulty of material increases and the transferred student does not perform as well. In the case of this student, a prior grade of an A (Community College) relates to a B or C from the university. This causes conflict affecting both the student and the program that has admitted the student with high community college grades.

4. Statistical central measures that are easily calculated and can generate basic information regarding students/testing include the *median* (listing high to low scores and determining the central grade), the *mode* (the most often repeated grade), and the *mean* (listing all grades from an exam and dividing the sum by the number of students having taken the exam).

5. When dividing a grading system for your course, (1) establish criteria of performance, achievement that represents all levels of ability (outstanding, below average, average, borderline and failure) and relate these levels to the objectives you have presented in your course syllabus. Consider your objectives as either major (must be achieved) and minor (would like them to be achieved but not mandatory). (2) in your syllabus, establish how the final grade is achieved—how much quizzes and exams are weighed (all adding up to 100), so students know exactly what contributes to their grade. (3) usually the clinical or the academic program has determined the inclusive numbers that represent an A (90 to 100, or 94 to 100).

Chapter 8

1. True

2. Among the responsibilities of students listed in the Undergraduate Bulletin are these three: (1) must fulfill conscientiously all assignments and requirement of their courses, (2) maintain a scholarly, courteous demeanor in class, and (3) adhere to the instructors' and general university policies (attendance, withdrawal).

3. These all reflect the *Affective* Domain.

4. Examples of *diversity* not listed in the Box include homeless, alien, eccentric, hyperactive, part-time student, motherless/fatherless.

5. McKenzie discussed these general points regarding learning: (1) See relationship of general science to a specific science. Recall the meaning and application of subject matter, words. (2) Understand the meaning of what you are learning.

Chapter 9

1. Recourse available to students who believe that the grades they received were not fair includes (1) discussion with the specific instructor regarding the derivation of the grade, (2) appeal to the chairperson of that department, and (3) appeal to the dean of the college.

2. (From the Undergraduate Bulletin of Wayne State University, Detroit, Michigan)

   College/School Grade Appeal Procedures: Each college and school has established grade appeal procedures. These procedures are available from the Dean's Office of the College or School. Once these have been exhausted, the student may request the Provost to review the decision on the record. Following established protocol, the Provost will inform the student and the Dean of his/her decision within three school days after receiving the request.

3. Reasonable accommodations for handicapped students within a college building would include (1) installation of "push buttons" to open doors, (2) an area of stalls enlarged in rest rooms to accommodate a wheelchair, (3) the lowering of drinking fountains, and (4) areas in lecture rooms and laboratories that can accommodate a wheelchair.

4. Four resources the university provides students with regarding legal matters are (1) the appeal process, (2) hearing panel, (3) the ombudsman, and (4) federal and state laws.

5. Three laws affecting admission standards are (1) No individual may be denied admission on the basis of race, or (2) handicap and (3) admission policies can be based on an individual assessment of an applicant's credentials and potential for achievement.

Chapter 10

1. c

2. ASCP, NCA or both

3. False

4. True

Chapter 11

1. c
2. d
3. d
4. b
5. b
6. c

Chapter 12

1. c
2. d
3. b
4. Given the five characteristics—*SMAART*—of good objectives, define each and cite an example of each characteristic.

   *S*pecific–limited to one idea; focused on a single target.

   *M*easurable–quantitative or qualitative as compared to some predetermined criteria or existing standard.

   *A*chievable–has been done in a similar manner; resources, talent, finances are available; assumptions, obstacles, and contingencies have been addressed and tested.

   *A*greed upon–objectives have been approved in writing among the group members or those who will evaluate your achievements.

   *R*ealistic–of worth to the individuals, the organization, or customers; makes sense; has practical value.

   *T*ime-bound–predetermined date of completion.

   Examples for each characteristic can be discussed with the instructor.

5. Given a list of activities, describe how you would go about prioritizing according to importance:

   - *High* priority–critical, goal-related, must be done today or is urgent.
   - *Medium* priority–important, goal-related, must be done soon or can be delegated.
   - *Low* priority–would be nice to get done, may or may not be goal-related, can wait, has no significant time pressure.

Chapter 13

1. a
2. c
3. c
4. d

Chapter 14

1. Directing is considered the most important step in the management process because it consists of essential skills: communicating, motivating, delegating, and coaching. All of these skills require effective interpersonal aptitudes and abilities.
2. d
3. c
4. Examples of using "silence" in conversations are:
   - encourage other people to talk or continue to say more.
   - give oneself time to think about response.
   - indicate attention on speaker.
   - allow message to sink in.
   - provide opportunity to shift from one theme to another theme.
   - break emotional tensions.
5. Compare descriptions written by readers with those authors provided in section on Motivation Theory.

Chapter 15

1. e
2. b, c, d
3. Examples of desired outcomes when monitoring TAT of glucose on IIT patients consist of:
   - provide consistency in care for all patients.
   - improve delivery of patient care.
   - improve laboratory service when standards are met or raised.
4. c

Chapter 16

1. c

2. b

3. What is your certification number? What is your age? Will you provide me with a photograph of yourself? Who should be contacted in case of emergency? What is your marital status? What is your ethnicity? (Ask if required by Human Resources or an external agency.) Are you unable to work certain days of the week or holidays based on your religious practices? What are specifics of your medical history that warrant any special accommodations? Will you agree to the following tests: (1) drug testing (system must follow confidentiality protocols with testing performed by an external, unaffiliated laboratory.) (2) Color-blindness test (this may be required in order to adjust test analysis procedures.) What special accommodations might you need in order to perform work? (ADA requirements.)

4. Meeting checklist:

   BEFORE: (1) Determine plans regarding attendees, date, time, place, equipment or materials and supplies, set-up, refreshments, guests and others who have an interest in attending. (2) Define purpose (and goals). (3) Set and prepare agenda (consult others as appropriate). (4) Notify attendees (members and guests) and distribute agenda. (5) Collect resource materials.

   DURING: (1) Conduct meeting according to plan: roles of attendees; assign items: "discussion only" first, most difficult at mid-meeting, decisions at end. (2) Secretary or appointee records minutes. (3) Motivate participants. (4) Effective communication. (5) Summarize/adjourn.

   AFTER: (1) Make a list of unfinished business (if there is any). (2) Evaluate the meeting—was the purpose fulfilled? Was the agenda completed? (3) Follow-up with unfinished business. (4) Discharge decisions. (5) Distribute minutes. Ask if there will be another meeting.

Chapter 17

1. b

2. Various answers could be considered: responses should be reviewed by the course instructor or a laboratory supervisor.

3. c, d, e

4. c

Chapter 18

1. a

2. e

3. d

4. b

5. See Activity Discussion 7.

Chapter 19

1. b

2. See Activity 3 and Activity Discussion 1.

3. Domain and taxonomy level:
   a. Written exam: Cognitive—1, 2, and 3
   b. Case studies: Cognitive—usually 3
   c. Interviews: Affective—1,2, and 3
   d. Demonstrations: Psychomotor—1, 2, occasionally 3
   e. Checklists: Psychomotor—1, 2, occasionally 3

4. Refer to Table 19–3 for examples of tools.

5. Various answers

Chapter 20

1. c

2. d

3. and 4. Answers can be found in Chapters 11–20.

Index

Page numbers in *italics* refer to illustrations; page numbers followed by t refer to tables.